I MAKE A DIFFERENCE:

Making the Transition from Clinician to Educator!

Larry Hudson, *Editor*
Nancy Raynor, *Associate Editor*
Phyllis Olmstead, *Assistant Editor*
with 44 contributors

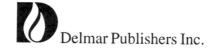
Delmar Publishers Inc.

Notice to the Reader

Publisher does not warrant or guarantee any of the products described herein or perform any independent analysis in connection with any of the product information contained herein. Publisher does not assume, and expressly disclaims, any obligation to obtain and include information other than that provided to it by the manufacturer.

The reader is expressly warned to consider and adopt all safety precautions that might be indicated by the activities described herein and to avoid all potential hazards. By following the instructions contained herein, the reader willingly assumes all risks in connection with such instructions.

The publisher makes no representations or warranties of any kind, including but not limited to, the warranties of fitness for particular purpose or merchantability, nor are any such representations implied with respect to the material set forth herein, and the publisher takes no responsibility with respect to such material. The publisher shall not be liable for any special, consequential, or exemplary damages resulting, in whole or in part, from the reader's use of, or reliance upon, this material.

Delmar Staff
    Executive Editor: David Gordon
    Administrative Editor: Marion Waldman
    Project Editor: Carol Micheli
    Senior Production Supervisor: Karen Seebald
    Production Coordinator: Barbara A. Bullock
    Art Coordinator: Judi Orozco
    Design Coordinator: Karen Kemp

For information, address Delmar Publishers Inc.
Three Columbia Circle, Box 15–015
Albany, New York 12212

All rights reserved. No part of this work covered by the copyright hereon may be reproduced or used in any form or by any means—graphic, electronic, or mechanical, including photocopying, recording, taping, or information storage and retrieval systems—without written permission of the publisher.

Printed in the United States of America
Published simultaneously in Canada
by Nelson Canada,
A division of The Thomson Corporation

10 9 8 7 6 5 4 3 2 1 XXX 99 98 97 96 95 94 93

Library of Congress Cataloging-in-Publication Data

I make a difference : making the transition from clinician to educator
        / [edited by] Larry Hudson.
    p. cm.
    Includes bibliographical references and index.
    ISBN 0-8273-4990-4 (textbook)
    1. Medicine—Vocational guidance—Study and teaching. 2. Allied
health personnel—Vocational guidance—Study and teaching.
    [DNLM: 1. Health Occupations. 2. Teaching—methods.
3. Vocational Educational—methods. 4. Vocational Guidance—
methods. W 18 I11]
R690.I18   1993
610.69—dc20
DNLM/DLC
For Library of Congress   92-10180
                                               CIP

TABLE OF CONTENTS

Table of Contents	*iii*
Dedication	*vii*
List of Figures	*viii*
Preface Larry Hudson	*ix*
Acknowledgments	*xi*

1 The Transition: From Clinician to Educator! — 1
- Using your prior experience as a clinician — Larry Hudson
- Changing "hats" from clinician to teacher of clinicians — Larry Hudson
- Defining your new role as a teacher in vocational health occupations — Holly Bennett
- Surviving the first day — Rebecca Osterhout
- Talking "Educationese" as a new language — Michael McCumber

2 Classroom Instruction: Becoming a Teacher — 13
- Motivating students — Jane Rocque
- Selecting teaching techniques — Holly Bennett
- Receiving feedback from students — Roberta Driscol
- Assessment — Jack Powers
- Test construction — Holly Bennett

3 Laboratory Management: Practicing the Job — 29
- Maintaining student safety — Shirley Baker
- Following infection control procedures — Maxine Hudson
- Planning simulations — Shirley Baker
- Assessing student performance — Shirley Baker
- Ordering supplies — Shannon Manuel
- Acquiring equipment and tools — Shirley Baker

4 Clinical Instruction: Teaching the Job — 51
- Planning clinical experiences — Janice Sandiford
- Clinical supervision of students — Janice Sandiford
- Making clinical practice relevant — Janice Sandiford
- Answering the assertion: Hey, that's not the way we learned it! — Holly Bennett
- Evaluating student performance — Janice Sandiford
- Developing affiliation agreements — Jacquelyn King, Janice Sandiford

- Recruiting and orienting clinical faculty   Rita Richardson
- Placing students in their first job   Rita Richardson

5 The Learners: Knowing the Students   65
- Characterizing middle school students   Larry Holt
- Describing high school students   Brenda Benda
  Lou Ebrite
- Assisting special needs students   Lou Ebrite
- Describing adult students   Larry Hudson

6 Student Relations: Charting Unknown Territory   79
- Conferencing and advisement   Jacquelyn Page
- Adapting to the changing work force   Steven Sorg
  Carol Darling

7 Program Survival: Marketing the Program   95
- Recruiting students   Rita Richardson
- Marketing the program   Judith Mabrey
- Using advisory committees   Rita Richardson
- Developing partnerships with the health care industry   Judi Hansen
  Chandra Bandhu
  Karen Shores
  Sharon Thomas
  Beverly Campbell
- Ensuring program accreditation compliance through quality audit mechanisms   Tom Edwards

8 Curriculum Development: What the Instructor Will Teach   127
- Identifying the curriculum   Nancy Raynor
- Steps for identifying curriculum   Nancy Raynor

9 Performance Objectives: What the Students Must Learn   135
- Performance objectives   Beverly Richards
- Performance assessment   Beverly Richards

10	**Competency-Based Education: Did They Get It?**	**145**
	○ Design	Nancy Raynor
	○ Implementation CBE in a VHO program	Judy Sheehan
		Barbara Matthews

11	**Legal Issues: What You Don't Know Can Hurt You**	**167**
	○ Due process and its application to VHO	Elaine Mohn
	○ Reducing tort liability	Elaine Mohn
	○ Failing an unsatisfactory student	Elaine Mohn
	○ Handling student grievances	Elaine Mohn

12	**The VHO Teacher's Role in HOSA: Advising in a Hands-Off Format**	**183**
	○ Becoming a chapter adviser	Joan Mucciarone
	○ Using the handbook	Joan Mucciarone
	○ Organizing a chapter	Joan Mucciarone
	○ Integrating HOSA into the classroom	Joan Mucciarone
	○ Local officers' perspectives	Judith Mabrey & Students
	• Secondary school students' perspectives	Judith Mabrey & Students

13	**Health Occupations Students of America: Our Vocational Student Organization**	**197**
	○ Understanding VSOs in general	Joan Mucciarone
	○ Revisiting the development of HOSA	Ruth Ellen Ostler

14	**Vocational Education: Our Umbrella**	**211**
	○ History of vocational education	Cynthia Woodley
	○ Federal vocational education legislation	Cynthia Woodley

15	**Health Occupations Education: Our Focal Area**	**223**
	○ Reviewing HOE in general	Elizabeth Kerr
	○ Describing HOE as a Division of AVA	Nancy Raynor

16	**Perspectives of VHO Professionals: From the School to the Federal Level**	**239**
	○ Middle school teacher	Phyllis Olmstead
	○ High school teacher	Brenda Benda
		Lou Ebrite

- Adult vocational center teacher — John Gentry / Carla Maloy
- Community college instructor — Lisa Long / Karen Allen
- Department chairperson — Elaine Mohn
- School district supervisor — O. J. Drumheller
- State department personnel — Nancy Raynor
- Teacher educator — Larry Hudson
- U.S. Department of Education personnel — Nancy Raynor

17 Uses of Current Technology: What's Available Now?   271
- Audiovisual equipment — Richard Cornell / Lois Drumheller
- Using computers — Janice Sandiford
- Incorporating the telephone — Phyllis Olmstead
- Combining the telephone and the computer — Phyllis Olmstead / Richard Merriam
- Television — Larry Hudson

18 Uses of Future Technology: What's Next?   301
- Applying interactive video — Anne Barron
- Promising virtual reality — Richard Dietzel

19 Making a Difference as a VHO Teacher: What It's All About   323
- Welcome to a new beginning — Arnie Warren

Appendixes   327
A. Recommended References
B. List of Final Authors

Index   337

DEDICATION

It is for our teacher colleagues that this Handbook is dedicated. We know how difficult the transition is and we know how rewarding teaching is so this Handbook really is for YOU.

The preparation of health care workers is very important and when you are a Vocational Health Occupations (VHO) teacher you can say "I Make A Difference" and know that it is true!

FIGURES INCLUDED IN TEXT

Chapter 2	Figure 2-1	Microteach
Chapter 3	Figure 3-1	Performance checklist, phone messages
	Figure 3-2	Descriptive rating scale, dental assisting
	Figure 3-3	Numerical rating scale, oral examination
	Figure 3-4	Product checklist, recording patient data
	Figure 3-5	Product rating sheet, illustrating anatomy
Chapter 8	Figure 8-1	VHO programming format
	Figure 8-2	Implementation plan
Chapter 9	Figure 9-1	Checklist, mitt restraints
	Figure 9-2	Checklist, radial pulse
	Figure 9-3	Rating scale, selection/use/care of equipment
	Figure 9-4	Rating scale, radial pulse
	Figure 9-5	Rating scale for testing instruments, (Mitstifer, 1983)
Chapter 10	Figure 10-1	Assignment Sheet
	Figure 10-2	'The Wheel'
Chapter 11	Figure 11-1	Student progression plan
Chapter 13	Figure 13-1	National VSO programs, (By Vaughn, Vaughn, & Vaughn, 1990)
	Figure 13-2	VSO Teacher's Creed, (By Vaughn, Vaughn, & Vaughn, 1990)
	Figure 13-3	HOSA Creed, from National HOSA
	Figure 13-4	HOSA Competitive Events, from National HOSA
Chapter 16	Figure 16-1	Educational organization chart
	Figure 16-2	One middle school vocational model
	Figure 16-3	Model of state division of vocational and technical education
	Figure 16-4	USDOE organizational chart
Chapter 17	Figure 17-1	Facsimile methods
Chapter 18	Figure 18-1	Features of CLV and ALV formats
	Figure 18-2	Sample barcodes
	Figure 18-3	Level III configuration

PREFACE

This *Handbook* began as an idea to give back to teachers and students something that has been given to us who work in vocational health occupations (VHO). That something is that they "made a difference" to us—thanks!

The creation, development, writing, and editing of this book have been a labor of love. All of the royalties generated by the *Handbook* will be distributed, equally, to two different organizations. That describes the sincerity of the authors involved in trying to provide a resource for teachers. One half of the royalties will be distributed to Health Occupations Students of America in order to provide scholarships for students to further their education in health related programs. The other half of the royalties will be distributed to the Health Occupations Education Division of the American Vocational Association so it may provide scholarships or stipends for teachers to attend their first American Vocational Association Annual Conference. We hope a million copies of the *Handbook* sell and that members of these two organizations benefit greatly.

Ideas for topics in the book were requested at the 1989 National Leadership Conference for Health Occupations Students of America, in Orlando, followed by input from participants at the Health Occupations Education Division meetings during the 1989, 1990, and 1991 American Vocational Association Annual Conferences, held, respectively, in Orlando, Cincinnati, and Los Angeles. During these conferences many people demonstrated their support for such a work. Over 75 persons provided topics and/or ideas for the *Handbook*.

Who is the intended audience for this handbook? The *Handbook* is intended for the teacher during the transition from being a clinician to becoming a teacher. Such instructors can be found in middle schools, high schools, adult centers, vocational centers, technical centers, technical institutes, and community colleges. The authors provide relevant examples for the new teacher because we have been there. We understand the transition from clinician to teacher of clinicians; we were beginning teachers and we do remember.

The book is written in a conversational style instead of a more formal "researchy" style. The chapters have been sequenced by what we feel constitutes the most relevant content in your career progression as a teacher. In your job as a teacher this entire *Handbook* will be useful to you. We have also included ideas that are not yet being used in the classroom but will be in the near future.

Our sole interest in writing this book is to develop the beginning VHO teacher into a professional educator. As you teach people about careers in general or specifically, they will become more competent practitioners and, in turn, teachers of VHO.

On behalf of the editors and contributing authors, we very sincerely offer this *Handbook* to you, the VHO teacher—YOU DO MAKE A DIFFERENCE!!

Editors:
Larry Hudson
Nancy Raynor
Phyllis M. Olmstead

Contributing Authors:
Karen G. Allen
Shirley Baker
Chandra Bandhu
Anne Barron
Brenda Benda
Holly L. Bennett
Beverly Campbell
Richard Cornell
Carol Darling
Richard A. Dietzel
Roberta Driscol
O.J. Drumheller
Lois Drumheller
Lou Ebrite
Tom Edwards
John T. Gentry
Judi Hansen
Larry Holt
Maxine Hudson
Elizabeth Kerr
Jacquelyn King
Lisa Long
Judith Mabrey
Carla J. Maloy
Shannon Manuel
Barbara Matthews
Michael McCumber
Richard Merriam
Elaine L. Mohn
Joan Mucciarone
Rebecca Osterhout
Ruth Ellen Ostler
Jacquelyn T. Page
Jack A. Powers
Beverly Richards
Rita Richardson
Jane Rocque
Janice Sandiford
Judy Sheehan
Karen Shores
Steven Sorg
Sharon Thomas
Arnie Warren
Cynthia Woodley

Artist:
Barbara Matthews

ACKNOWLEDGMENTS

It is so difficult to even begin an acknowledgment section for a book that has multiple authors and so many people to thank. First and foremost, the authors extend sincerest appreciation to our families, significant others, and friends. Without your sacrifice in terms of both time without us and support, this *Handbook* would not have been completed. The editors want to say thanks especially to our families—Maxine and Benjamin, Jim, Jeff, Jill, Wayne, and Doc; we really do appreciate your support!

To all of the contributing authors, thanks very much for your commitment and follow-through above and beyond the call of duty for a cause you believe in—one great team. We would not have even attempted to write this book if we did not as a group believe in the need for such a resource. When so many authors write a book and donate all the royalties, a special commitment is demonstrated.

Our Delmar contacts have been outstanding: special thanks to Marion Waldman, who believed in the project from the outset and on a very modest proposal, we might add. What a great editor. Lisa Santy, Electronic Publishing Supervisor also worked closely with the editors; thanks so much for your perseverance. The staff at Delmar, Carol Micheli, Project Editor; Barbara Bullock, Production Coordinator; and Judi Orozco, Senior Design Coordinator including President Joe Reynolds, are most supportive and believers in vocational education. Thanks for being our partners in this project.

Sincerely,

Larry R. Hudson
On behalf of all the authors

1
The Transition: From Clinician to Educator!

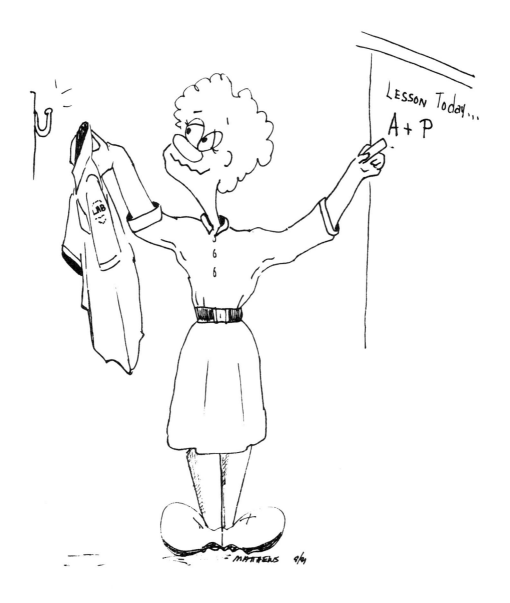

☞ USING YOUR PRIOR EXPERIENCE AS A CLINICIAN

Why were you hired as a health occupations instructor? Because of prior experience as a clinician, patient care person, or one who has expertise in a clinical setting are probably the foremost reasons people are hired as health occupations instructors. In many instances, prior experience as a clinician is *the* deciding factor for being hired as an instructor. In many educational institutions, prior clinical experience is a requirement to be a vocational health occupations (VHO) instructor. Such prior recent experience adds credibility to the classroom setting. Generally, a minimum of three years of prior recent experience as a clinician is required for employment or teacher certification in the public school sector. Your experience may be from three years to thirty years as a clinician prior to your considering the role of VHO educator. The program in which you will be teaching courses and the situations you will be teaching require that you have current relevant experience as a clinician for credibility and relevance in presenting the material. Your experiences are invaluable for students in that you can provide real-world and current examples from the clinical setting and experiences that they will be entering upon completion of the program.

The experience you have had as clinician will also count in your favor in another area — in some cases, as time toward an increase in the salary range as a new instructor. In some states, the number of years as a clinician count on the pay scale; even those without a bachelor's degree will qualify for the "equivalent-of-a-bachelor's-degree pay" in terms of the pay scale for instructors in the school system whether the school is a secondary school, postsecondary school, vocational center, adult center, or community college. In other words, you are recognized both in experience and in salary for prior clinical experience!

☞ CHANGING "HATS" FROM CLINICIAN TO TEACHER OF CLINICIANS

Role change can be rather traumatic both psychologically and emotionally. It is a challenging thing to make the transition from being a clinician — a person who gives a direct, hands-on clinical care (in whatever setting) — to being an instructor — a person who teaches clinical skills to other people. It is difficult for some to accept such new responsibility and the new role of being a teacher, an educator, and a professional person in a new area as opposed to being well respected and experienced as a clinician. Sometimes the transition may take years; for some, the transition is never quite complete. One of the first questions, of course, to ask is, "What am I?" If the answer "I am a clinician" rolls off your tongue right away and easily, then you have obviously *not* made the transition. However, if your answer is "I am a teacher," and it comes easily, you have in a sense accepted the transition and are willing to go forward from there.

Saying to yourself that you are a teacher of clinicians, an instructor, a VHO educator, a professional in education and saying that to yourself time and time again will help you to make that transition. This does not of course mean that you are giving up your clinical expertise, your clinical role, or your clinical "hat." For you can never give that hat up—you now wear two hats! The first is that of an expert clinician keeping current in your vocational health occupation, and the other is that of an educator staying current in the field of vocational education and in your particular health occupations field as an educator.

What were some of your old responsibilities? Maybe in some cases you were indeed teaching other staff, clients, or patients. You were responsible for patient-client care; you were the one with direct hands-on responsibility; you were the one who performed the tasks, and yet at times you were probably a teacher. Maybe you taught patients or clients self-care or you taught families how to assist with care. Maybe you conducted staff development training with new clinicians on the job and you demonstrated procedures or new products equipment to staff or students from other programs. Maybe you have carried out some of these teaching responsibilities in your career as a clinician, but they were only a small part of the overall responsibilities of the job. Do any of these teaching responsibilities ring a bell with you? Have you been a *teacher* and not realized it? Did anyone ever ask you, "Have you ever thought about being a teacher?" Has anyone ever said to you, "You would make a great teacher!" You said, "No, not me. I am not a teacher." But they said, "No, you really have the skill. You explained that procedure to me in a way no one else could have." Maybe you have thought about it. Some clinicians think they would like to be teachers but do not know of the possibility of teaching their occupation. It is quite a leap and it is intimidating to go from the secure role of clinician, especially if you feel pretty good about yourself and all of the people you are working with, to being the new kid in teaching. You have rapport and respect and now change career ladders altogether. It takes a lot of courage.

Let's look now at your new hat—that of being a teacher of clinicians—and preview just a few of the responsibilities in VHO education, your new profession. Some people perceive that a teacher's job is pretty easy: a few hours a day in the classroom, a day a week in a clinical setting, then having evenings and weekends free. Welcome to reality—this is not the case! Many a new teacher tries to make that transfer from clinician to teacher of clinicians only to comment, "You know, teaching is a lot more difficult than I thought." Teaching *is* a lot of work. You are always "on." You are really never off for the evening or a weekend as a teacher, but have you thought about that part of the job? As a clinician, you had a professional role; the same is true in teaching at whatever level — middle school, high school, vocational center, or community college. The professional role is assumed, with all of the responsibilities thereof. What are some of the new responsibilities as a teacher of clinicians, as a VHO instructor, a professional vocational educator, and an educator in general? It is more than being in the classroom, it is more than serving in the clinical setting, it is more than working in the laboratory, where students practice procedures.

☞ DEFINING YOUR NEW ROLE AS A TEACHER IN VOCATIONAL HEALTH OCCUPATIONS

Now that you have decided you would like to teach and have evaluated why you want to teach, it is time to do a self-assessment. As indicated earlier in this chapter, your clinical expertise makes a significant contribution to your teaching ability. How you translate your doable abilities and your hands-on skills to teaching those abilities and skills is important. You no longer are going *to do*, but you are going to aid the student in learning *how to do*. The art of teaching allows the student to do, to make mistakes and learn.

Your new role as a teacher is to convey information from you to your student. Easy . . . right? Think back for a moment. Do you remember a teacher who really taught you a lot? Take a moment to jot down what you remember about the teacher. What was it you learned? Did it take a long time? Was it a simple skill? Was it something that you still use today? Now think about a skill you learned. Did you learn it by repetition, that is, by making several attempts? Did you learn it with music, a catchy phrase, association, or mnemonics, or did you learn it by memorization or frequent writing? Evaluate each learning experience. Were they all different or did they duplicate certain methods?

As you have now identified, there are many ways we learn. In the last exercise, you probably came up with several instances of learning in which you learned in different ways to do something. These different modalities of learning are going to become the basic building blocks in your teaching repertoire.

As a new teacher, you will probably begin teaching using the modalities of learning that you learn best with and are most comfortable with and using the way you were taught, whether it is the most effective or not. Let's scrutinize the various ways of learning: auditory, visual, and kinesthetic. Your mission as a teacher is to identify and utilize all modalities of learning to the advantage of your students.

Another role of a new teacher is to establish classroom protocol. Before the first day of class, you will want to decide how to manage your class on a day-to-day basis. Something as simple as furniture arrangement is very important. If you want to begin with a standard classroom setup, with all the desks in line and in rows, then you will begin with a regimented classroom. Maybe you would like a more informal room, with long tables and chairs arranged in a U shape. Remember—it is rather easy to lose control of a classroom and much more difficult to regain it.

Secondary to your classroom protocol will be individual management. After you introduce yourself and tell a little about yourself and your background, you can have the members of the class identify themselves. Then you will want to describe to them how you will manage the class.

Punctuality: What time does class start? Must students be in the classroom or in their seats quiet and ready to go? Do you have a five-minute lag time, say, officially 8:00 but class starts 8:05? Must the students raise their hand with questions or may they just speak out? Must they listen to whoever is speaking in class or only when the teacher is speaking? It is fair to establish classroom expectation. It is also a basic right of courtesy to listen attentively when someone else is talking, but your students may not have that skill.

Classroom attire: What do you expect? Are you dressing your students for their profession, or do you believe in a casual environment? Both have positive implications. Can't decide? Leave Friday for casual day, or have Monday be "dress for success" day.

What about written assignments, tests, quizzes, and homework? What do you demand? One, two, three hours of homework a night? Is there a term paper due? Will students have to read news and magazine articles and write reports or give a five-minute oral report? Before your class begins, you will want to sit down with a calendar and assign each day with a lesson plan. Write what you will cover and what you expect students to read in advance for that day; indicate homework, quizzes, and tests. Also, very important to a new teacher, if you give a quiz, how will you grade it? Will you return it graded the next day? Will it be corrected and discussed in class with the test to follow later on the same material? Students need to know in a timely manner what questions they missed.

Finally, you need to decide about student participation. What is required? Must students contribute to class discussions? Does each student have to give an oral presentation? How about a demonstration? Again, in teaching strategies, we will discuss how to involve students, utilizing all their skills and abilities to achieve success.

As you can see, establishing some guidelines with short- and long-term goals before the first day of class is going to help you become organized.

One element not addressed is how you come across to your students. Remember—you are a role model. When you speak, meaning your language and your grammar, you should always be correct, never using poor language. What you wear will be observed and copied. While you lecture, your students will evaluate what you are wearing and notice everything about you: your personal hygiene and the condition of your clothes and hair, if you wear lots of jewelry, if you have dirty nails or hose with runs, etc. Some have found the stern approach a way of keeping control. They let three weeks go by before they crack a smile. Others of us believe in the open, friendly classroom. Add humor. Humor can be an important asset, but it should be appropriate; avoid off-color jokes. A comfortable student will be more prone to learn. Can that comfortable student eat in the classroom? How about drink coffee, water, or soft drinks in class? Again, to troubleshoot these areas will help you regulate and maintain control. Remember—you can always relax your style, but to tighten up once you've lost control is difficult, although it can be done.

We have discussed what you remember from your own experiences regarding memorable teachers and what ways you remember learning best. We then introduced learning modalities—how individuals learn—and then talked about what you need to do to prepare for your new role as a teacher.

We talked about your classroom protocol and how to organize your expectations for the students in conjunction with your daily, weekly, and monthly lesson plans, ending with a discussion about the day-to-day interpersonal management of your students.

☞ SURVIVING THE FIRST DAY

Help me make it through the first day! How many times have you made that plea? No other experiences is like it, the first day of class. You tremble with anticipation. What will the students be like? Will you meet their expectations?

The day begins before you are as prepared as you want to be.

You think of one more thing, a better idea, a new method. The bell rings and your first class begins.

Keep the first session simple, because both you and the students will be anxious in much the same way and for many of the same reasons. Once this is accepted it is easy to keep it simple.

Prepare a welcome packet for each student, including items such as the student policy handbook, calendar of the school year, sample evaluation sheet, clinical dates, and, last but not least, motivational messages. Gather words of wisdom from newspaper articles, comic strips, and magazines, or make some up yourself. This sets the tone for the classroom. From Benjamin Franklin to Ann Landers, start and end your courses with motivational inspirations.

Also, inside each packet, insert a name tag and a brightly colored marking pen. When students arrive, ask them to write their first name and draw a picture of something that best describes their interests. This exercise generates conversation with neighbors and allows you the opportunity to get to know each person.

The first day is notorious for interruptions: telephone calls from the administrative office, messages from the bookstore, questions about fees and insurance, you name it. Such interruptions may represent a source of anxiety until you stop to realize that the students actually benefit from these temporary diversions. Interruptions are a time for the teacher to listen. They give you time to quietly work at your desk and encourage students to read the material you have placed in their packet. They give your students an opportunity to adjust to the new environment.

As a VHO teacher, emphasize teamwork from day one, and refer to students as "the team" or "your team." This reference lays a foundation for each student to become a member of the health care team. Finally, take some time during the first day to share your love and commitment as a health care worker and as an instructor of each student.

The end of your first day arrives. You heave a great sigh of relief and satisfaction as students leave, eager for a new day. You have work to do before tomorrow, maybe even learn a "foreign" language!

☞ TALKING "EDUCATIONESE" AS A NEW LANGUAGE

Another World

You decide to try something new and visit another country, somewhere out of the way, a faraway place with a strange-sounding name. You meticulously pack everything you might need for the adventure — warm clothing, a raincoat, personal hygiene products, travelers' checks, air sickness pills, your passport, and, just in case, a list of emergency phone numbers. Your airline ticket is confirmed and hotel reservations made. The Concorde takes off at 7:00 a.m., and by noon you arrive at your destination. You step off the plane, pick up your luggage, walk outside to hail a taxi and . . . *no one understands a word you are saying.* To complicate things even more, you do not understand a thing they are saying. You are hungry and try to order something to eat. Try again! What a dilemma. You can't get to where you want to go. You can't get anything to eat. You have paid thousands of dollars and traveled first class over thousands of miles only to find out that, from at least one perspective, you are in deep trouble. After all of the careful planning, you forgot one of the most important tools for success: Communication. Someone — a native who speaks English — notices your situation. Light at the end of what could have been a long tunnel. At last, there is someone whom you can talk to and who understands you. Suddenly you do not feel so all alone in that foreign environment. And no, this is not intended to be a tale of suspense and intrigue.

This actually happened to me, but not in a foreign land. The tale that I spin henceforth is derived from my true adventures the first time I entered into the wonderful and mysterious world of vocational education focusing on health occupations. To say that I felt lost upon entering this foreign milieu would be an understatement. To describe myself as overwhelmed would be a most appropriate description. Beginnings: Let me describe to the best of my recollection some of the feelings and apprehensions of a fledgling vocational educator the very first day that I walked into the classroom. The course was General Methods of Course Construction in Vocational Education. As the instructor began a diatribe on the proper preparation of lesson plans and performance objectives, language that is second nature to me now, I cringed. A feeling of impending doom was upon me. Was I having a stroke? Was the left side of my brain not processing information properly? What language was this? Oh no, it's Educationese! After all, I speak fluent English, am well versed in medical terminology, and know a smattering of Spanish. How difficult could this language of vocational education possibly be? I hear words like condition, performance, and criterion referencing all in one sentence. Please, I am trying to be as objective as humanly possible, but the minutes and hours drone on, and instead of beginning to grasp the subject matter, I feel I have fallen into a deep well. Where is that sympathetic, understanding rescuer? Will someone please help me? I am drowning in an ocean of alphabet soup containing words, phrases, and acronyms so foreign to me. What makes me think I want to be a teacher in the first place? What's that you say? Next week's assignment will cover Modules B-2 and B-4? One more time! We will be covering lesson plans and objectives, modules and products: alive-alive-o. The clock works in my favor. Three hours have passed. A reprieve? I have a whole week to get ready for the next class.

Next week comes all too soon. Using examples shown in the books, I have roughed out some crude (believe me) objectives and pasted them on an even cruder lesson plan. I am soon to discover what could only be interpreted as the coup de grace. Of the ten students in the class, one other person and I were not teaching. A wise man once said, "You can keep your mouth shut and make everyone wonder if you are ignorant, or you can open your mouth and remove all doubt." Initially I opted for the former course of action.

One of my more astute classmates is discussing the value of the student "cum folder" and something called anecdotal entries. Not wanting to appear uninterested, I venture into the realm of questions and answers; I raise my hand and ask what I think is a well-put question concerning the value of performance objectives. The instructor fires back a response. "Performance objectives outline under what condition something is to be done, what is to be done, and to what degree of proficiency it is to be done." I can understand that. Why didn't the instructor say so in the first place? The teacher continues, "These objectives and related task statements are correlated with the DACUM chart based on a carefully conducted needs assessment." A bridge too far! DACUM? Howcum? I return to the labyrinth. The Minotaur senses my nervousness. It becomes quite apparent that I have my own needs assessment to perform.

The semester grinds on, and slowly but surely I am beginning to assimilate the language. I have begun to blossom, or should I say bloom? Bloom? Yes, Bloom's Taxonomy. It certainly taxed me for all I was worth. Just when I thought I was about to make ends meet, somebody moves the ends. Cognitive, affective, psychomotor: application, evaluation, receive, respond, imitate, naturalize. Is there no end to this nightmare? If I learn Educationese, will I forget my native language? I imagine myself speaking in three distinct languages at the same time. I need more rest. Write objectives in all three domains, at least four or five levels. That assignment alone sent me near the edge. Can they make a silk purse out of this sow's ear? Where is my Pygmalion or my Henry Higgins? Oh no, I am beginning to sound like them! Has it happened? Am I . . . multilingual? Not unlike my acquisition of medical terminology, will my future utterances in this new and strange language alienate those around me — my wife, my children, my colleagues? This was put to the test sooner than I expected.

The Pepsi Generation. At last I think I have found something to hang on to. Tonight our learned professor of vocational education says, "I wish to address the effect of the (what sounds like) Pepsi Commission on the future of vocational education in the high schools." Finally, I can converse intelligently. After all, I have taken nine hours of psychology including six hours of developmental/educational psychology. In those classes we discussed the influence of many outside stimuli on the learning styles and abilities of high school students and those entering college for the first time. Why not the effect of the caffeine in Pepsi, or Coke, or Mountain Dew, which possesses twice as much caffeine as most other soft drinks? My exhilaration was short-lived. Once again I realize my lack of educational literacy as he writes on the chalkboard the following: Postsecondary Education Planning Commission, ergo PEPC. I am stunned! If I were an ostrich I would hide my head. My only saving grace is that I did not share this bit of astute ignorance with anyone up until this writing. I did, however, garner some knowledge in the arena of educational policies that night.

I Think I Can, I Think I Can: A long sequence of classes that takes place in what feels like a very short period of time lands me my bachelor's degree.

Graduate school. Never let it be said that I know when I have had enough. Graduate school, here I come. Classes come and classes go. My writings speak of CBE (competency-based education) and the land of USDOE (United States Department of Education). I am consumed with thoughts of advisory committees, regional coordinating councils, and—watch out, here comes a new word—algorithms. I fear the language not. After all, I belong to the AVA (American Vocational Association), FVA (Florida Vocational Association), AARC (American Association for Respiratory Care), NBRC (National Board for Respiratory Care), FSRC (Florida Society for Respiratory Care), HOEAF (Health Occupations Educators Association of Florida), and FACC (Florida Association of Community Colleges), and I am seriously considering joining AVERA (American Vocational Educational Research Association). Behind my name I can add enough alphabet soup to feed a small contingent of well-fed soldiers: M.Ed., B.A., A.A., A.S., RRT, CRTT, CPTT, and CPFT, and I went to school at UCF and DBCC. Whew! And if that's not enough, there is always one more encounter, which is designed specifically to test your mettle.

Chanting helps: Picture it, December 1989, Orlando, Florida, the American Vocational Association Annual Conference. I am asked to become involved as a member of the local planning committee and to present to the Health Occupations Division a brief account of my internship at the U.S. Department of Education in Washington, D.C. I have never been to a meeting of this magnitude, and I am quite impressed and a bit nervous. Just a few hours into the meat of this conference for health occupations educators, Educationese once again rears its fickle head. Within the USDOE, DVACE, OVAE, and HOE, there are some other organizations that exist and by which I am later asked to join at least two. The National Association of Health Occupations Teachers (NAHOT) and the National Association of State Administrators of Health Occupations Educators (NASAHOE) are but two of the acronyms that become daily commonplace utterances. As the time nears for my presentation (late Sunday afternoon), the butterflies begin. These butterflies have hiccups. Because a portion of my past included some musical involvement, I devise a clever way of remembering the names of the revered organizations, and so as not to offend, I practice a chant. I pronounce the abbreviations as though they were ordinary words.

Let's see—DOEs and HOEs and NASAHOEs and NAHOTs standing in a row. One more time: DOEs and HOEs and NASAHOEs and NAHOTs standing in a row. A paralyzing fear strikes at my very soul when I suddenly realize that these sound like names of Indian tribes. I fear that if I chant them aloud, there is a good possibility that it will rain. (My maternal grandmother once told me that I am part Indian; which part was never indicated.) Very discretely during my brief presentation, I make reference to the fact that these acronyms remind me of Indian tribes and to the fact that all tribes are actually part of one great nation (smiles, light applause, I have won at least some of them over). Have you ever said something and then wished that you had those words back in your mouth? Why-oh-why-oh-why, did I ever leave Ohio (that is where I was born)? I am once again a victim of Educationese. The rest of the day and the remainder of the AVA/HOE Conference went quite well. I was able to meet numerous individuals from all areas of the country and to increase my Educationese vocabulary significantly. I joined NAHOT and receive quarterly correspondence concerning meetings and other functions.

Epilogue. Now I am a doctoral student in education, and the echoes of the ghost of language-past are still heard on quiet, lonely nights. I have moved into new dimensions. Electronic messaging, computer teleconferencing. I have gone beyond the telephone and now I am empowered; at least that is what it says on a bumper sticker I was sent. On-line telephone-computer conversations with me and my modem, my PS-2, my FIRNMAIL, ADVOCNET, TELENET, and I can do it all thanks to PROCOMM II. Sometimes, late at night when there are no messages for me on the network, I reflect on the time when I knew not the language and when a NAHOT and a DACUM and CBE were as foreign and as distant as any words could be. Good luck to you — the novice, the new entrant into the vast and rewarding field of VHO education, the aspiring teacher — I leave you with some good advice. Study hard and wear galoshes when it rains. Master the language called educationese. There is no thesaurus, no pocket dictionary for this language. The reason no such reference exists is that the language of education is dynamic. It is pulsing and alive, ever growing. You must learn it on your own, but once mastered, it is, as they say on "Wheel of Fortune," yours to keep until the end of time.

One of the first challenges faced is the language. The language that you are used to speaking is connected with a particular health occupation; you know that language well and have spoken it for years. What you are going to face now is a new "foreign" language that you must learn to speak, to write, to read, and to use. However, in learning this new language, you must not forget that your students are learning clinician language as well, the language of health occupations in general, so you are going to have to maintain your linguistic skill in the clinical language and learn to speak, write, interpret, and read the new language of education and vocational education in particular.

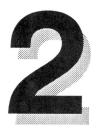

Classroom Instruction: Becoming a Teacher

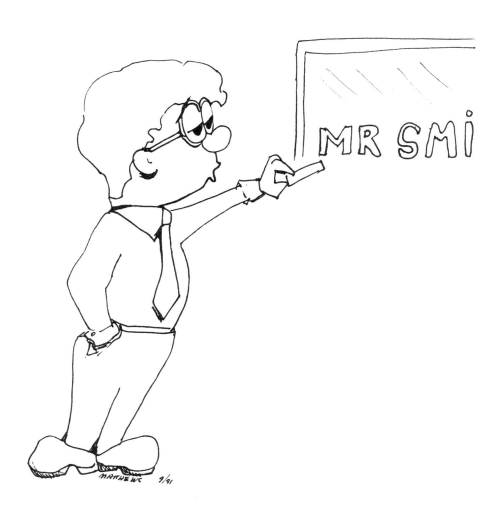

👉 MOTIVATING STUDENTS

Good Morning, Viet Nam

Now, everyone must have heard that line, right? The commercial success of this enthusiastic greeting to soldiers everywhere started the day off with a smile and a care. This is how you can make a difference. Start your classes with excitement and real enthusiasm! Take the opportunity to visualize a sunny day, class, and future. This is a new beginning. Your new beginning. Seize the day!

So you were hoping for a good class . . . you want your students to listen and be attentive . . . you have to transmit so much information . . . there is so little time . . . you are only one person . . . there are so many of them . . . .

You want them to be eager learners. You want them to be the best caregivers. You want them to respect you. You want to be the best teacher they have ever had. You must keep them awake. YOU MUST CREATE ENTHUSIASM!

Good morning, Viet Nam . . . .

Those of you who saw the movie *Good Morning, Viet Nam* know that Robin Williams' radio character brought excitement to the listeners. He knew what the soldiers needed and therefore created an enthusiastic audience. Part of that was due to the good ol' songs he played on the air, but also because the caregiver, Robin, enjoyed what he was doing and energetically spoke to those listeners.

You are one up on being a radio broadcaster. Your audience will see you every day. So, interject your lectures with some craziness, some fun, some good ol' songs. Wear wild clothing or accessories once in a while. Set the mood for creating energy in your student audience, with perhaps some controversy. You will inspire them!

Relate your own success stories to theirs. Make it a real part of you and them. They will listen. They will want to know more. You will know that they have listened and learned. They will come back for more.

But you must believe. Believe in yourself. Believe in them. Believe in the success of each student. Believe that you will play a role in that success. And guess what? You will.

Your enthusiasm must come from the heart. True caring will follow naturally. Your students will know. They will believe in you. What makes you enthusiastic about something? Is it the pleasure you receive? Is it the reward? Is it the fact that you feel appreciated? Or is it just knowing that what you have given your students is worthwhile? Any or all of this will initiate enthusiasm.

Well, students are human like you. One or more of your traits will surely be one or more of theirs. It can help to think about what you liked as a student. Naturalness is the best.

Act One . . .

The real scenario . . .

Monday morning, 8:00 class. First day . . . never had this teacher before . . . heard she (he) is new. Wonder if she'll (he'll) be hard . . . easy . . . good . . . bad.

You see, you have no reputation to uphold. You have a new beginning. You get to create a first impression. Wow, the responsibility . . . the pressure. But oh, the challenge and the fun. Scared? Yes! But everyone is the first day.

Think of your first time doing something you were afraid of, for example, riding a two-wheeled bike. There it stood, waiting for you to take a seat. You have seen your neighbors do it. Your brother did it before you. Why, even that younger child next door did it.

It can't be that hard, can it? Yes, that is why you have been putting it off. Well, today is the day and you have decided to seize the moment.

Handlebars in hand. Is this like a horse? Do you get on it standing on the left? Ah, this is your brother's bike. You somehow have to figure out how to get over the bar. Okay, you are partly on the seat, but your feet are still touching the ground — or your toes are, that is. Now, one foot on the pedal, two feet, push . . . crash. Again, pedal, push, wobble, very wobbly, crash. Stop. Rethink. Is anyone watching? Try again and again. And then, wow! You are riding. Oh, what a feeling — the air that surrounds you, the breeze — great, that is what it is. You thought you could and you did! So what if you fall again. That is what knee bandages are for — and scars.

Fear is real, mistakes will be made, sometimes you will fall, but never will you fail. Because, you see, you tried. You won't be perfect all the time. No one ever is. You will have good days and not-so-good days. But you will never have a bad day, unless you let that happen. You really are in control.

Remember — each student has his or her own specialty to bring to the class. It is fun to seek that out and share that uniqueness with others. Sometimes, students don't even know they have it. You could be the lucky one who spots it and makes it stay.

Good morning, Viet Nam . . . Yes, the role that Robin Williams portrayed was one of an unusual, very special person. But recognizing that fact does not take away from the enthusiasm you will display to your class in caring and sharing. Your days will surely be sunny, and your students will learn and be enthusiastic. You cannot lose this new beginning! *You will make a difference!*

☞ SELECTING TEACHING TECHNIQUES

This section will help evaluate the various modalities of learning so you can choose the methods that will get your message across.

You have been given a wealth of information up to this point, and now you need to evaluate the various methods so you may select the most appropriate ways to get the message across. Please note that the past sentence was written using plurals. There is *no one best way* to teach anything. What helped you to retain learning material? You have probably identified how you learn from lecture, videotapes, audiotapes, hands-on practice, return demonstration, reading, assignments, written papers, tests, and quizzes.

How you learn is completely different from the way that the next individual. Teachers cannot ignore this point. In order to be an effective teacher, you must be organized, knowledgeable, clear and succinct, patient, and personable.

How do you select teaching styles that allow you to emulate these five criteria? Organization is imperative. Your students must know what you expect of them, what they will be learning and when, how they will be graded, and what they must do to successfully complete and pass your course. You must have daily, weekly, monthly, and term lesson plans so that at a glance everyone knows what the class will be doing on a given day or week; what readings, assignments, and tests will be given; and all the due dates. It is okay to build in some downtime, because depending on the speed of the students, you may find that you need more time for an area of study. This should raise a red flag for you. Many otherwise well-organized classes have failed because there were no allowances for learning, assimilation, and processing. Each day should allow time for an evaluation of learning, assimilation, and processing. Each day should allow time for an evaluation and processing, as well as the same before a test or after a quiz.

Your teaching style should demonstrate that you are knowledgeable. This message needs to be conveyed as clearly and concisely as possible. Do not use fancy words or terminology unless you are making a point. KISS (Keep It Short and Simple) is imperative in teaching. If you use convoluted terminology, speak too quickly, lose your train of thought frequently, pepper your speech with umms, ahhs, ya knows, or profanity, you are going to lose your students. A teacher, whether first time, ten, or twenty years' experienced, benefits from practicing in front of a mirror and in front of a video camera. Tape yourself.

STOP – FIGURE 2-1 – MICRO TEACH – is an exercise to be completed. – STOP

Try this exercise. Pick a subject, any subject. How about how to take a pulse. Write an outline of the points you will cover. To the side of each point, jot down how you are going to get that point across. Ready?

Give your presentation in front of a video camera. Now take the video and give it to a family member or neighbor, someone who does not know how to take a pulse.

A. What happened?
B. Did your message get across?
C. Did you give that person an outline?
D. Was the outline necessary?
E. How did you teach taking a pulse?
F. Did you only lecture, and if so, was it effective? Retention from lecture alone is very small.
G. Did you demonstrate how to take a pulse?
H. Did you concentrate on only the radial pulse, or did you add in other arterial points as well?
I. Did you request a return demonstration?
J. Was the student competent?
K. Did you give specific criteria ahead of time so the student knew what was expected? If you did not, was that fair?
L. Finally, how much time was consumed in this one teaching session with one student?

Now you are ready to evaluate yourself. Bottom line – was the "student" successful? Hurray for you! If not, this was only a practice exercise, but valuable because you had the opportunity to see your teaching style. Was it good? Even if you didn't encompass all the above parameters, were you successful or partly successful? What did you do that you liked? Keep that. Now ask your student, "What did I do that you liked in the micro teach?" Keep that. If you were to offer this teaching session to another student, you might get the same feedback, or the student might identify another helpful area. Keep that. The result of this exercise is that you had the opportunity to select your teaching strategies. Again, notice the use of the plural of the term *strategies*.

In order to use successful learning modalities, review what happened or did not happen in your micro teach. Were your directions clear? If the student had a question, were there written instructions or criteria to refer to? Did you use visual as well as auditory reinforcement? Was the student expected to practice the procedure?

Active participation by doing often aids in both the learning process and retention. In order to pass, did the student have to verbally tell you how to take a pulse, write out an answer, or take your pulse? Again, you can use one or more of these ways to evaluate your student. Which way will best help your student to remember long term?

There is another aspect of teaching that must be considered in selecting effective teaching strategies. Know the audience that you are addressing. Just as we all learn in different ways, our expectations and how we learn are different. Some students simply start memorizing the lesson or trying task. Others want to watch and hear first. Everyone wants to succeed, but some students will not try unless they are assured of success immediately. Learning a skill takes lots of practice. Make sure students know this. Make sure that you have created a safe and comfortable environment to allow your students to make mistakes and learn. If you select a rigid style of teaching, your students will not want to attempt a skill unless they can succeed in pleasing you. This learning opportunity is not for you but is for the students.

In selecting teaching strategies that allow you to develop a teaching style, you need to consider the following: how you are going to make material appropriate, how you are going to relate it to previous knowledge, and how you will explain the importance to what students will be learning in the future. This is the answer to the why-do-I-need-to-learn-this question. Why is this important? Do I have to know this for the test? An answer might be that it is important because it constitutes a building block for the health care occupation.

Consider the micro teach on taking a pulse. Why is that important? It is a basic building block for assessing a patient's cardiovascular rate. It is also important because it could tip you off to an impending crisis. Or, on a very personal level, it can acquaint you with your own resting heart rate and your target heart rate for maximum exercise. Then you need to connect this skill to something students already know or are familiar with. If you can motivate students to think about how this skill can apply to them, they will better remember the skill because of its relevant and personal application.

The fifth factor in being effective includes what is termed *personality*. Motivating your students is imperative. Usually students themselves have chosen to be in your course, but not always. If you are enthusiastic, then they may be. How can you pique their curiosity? Relate lessons to their past experiences. Stress the importance of the lesson to clinical work. Clear documentation is imperative, because when a clinician defendant loses a license or money because of poor or unclear documentation, then the lesson has relevance. You have just taught the importance of rules.

Summary

This section has discussed how to select your own teaching strategies to develop a style. Initially you need to consider all methods available to you. These include oral presentations, videotapes and audiotapes, readings, written exercises, skill practice, and return demonstration. Concentrate on what you are trying to teach, and incorporate at least three different modalities to get your point across. Videotape yourself, critique your presentation, and have someone else try to learn from the video. The video will give you a basic platform from which to view the way you come across to the student and what modality is appropriate for the specific topic.

☞ RECEIVING FEEDBACK FROM STUDENTS

This section is designed to assist VHO teachers in understanding the role and appropriate usage of feedback. Receiving feedback from students can also bring emotions to the surface for teachers, especially if they are new to the field. Discussion surrounding solicitation of useful feedback and how to use feedback effectively will take place.

What Is Feedback?

Discussion of one's perceptions of and relationship with other persons present in the classroom environment almost always constitutes what has become known as feedback in the jargon of behavioral scientists. It refers to information that tells a system what the result of its behavior has been. Only by processing feedback can the system know what adjustments must be made in order to ensure reaching its goal. If, for example, a person has as her goal being perceived by others as a warm person, she never knows whether or not she is on target unless she receives feedback (in either verbal or nonverbal form) that she is indeed being perceived as a warm person. If she overhears two of her colleagues discussing how aloof she often is, then this piece of feedback can help her to analyze her behavior and see how she is failing to create the desired impression.

Most of the feedback we receive during our life occurs naturally — we overhear a remark, we perceive nonverbal cues such as a facial expression or a change in posture, we notice a shift in tone of voice — and we process these cues almost automatically, often unconsciously. However, because the feedback is often covert rather than explicit, we are in danger of interpreting it incorrectly. More explicit feedback — that is, having people tell us directly how they are reacting to our behavior — is sometimes useful.

What Are the Characteristics of Effective Teaching?

Many techniques have been used over the years to identify potentially useful items for inclusion in formal systems of rating teachers and their courses. One often used method requests the opinions of students.

Wotruba and Wright (1975) summarized twenty-one studies in which several groups had been asked to identify the qualities of effective teaching. The most frequently named characteristics were:

- Communication skills — clearly interprets abstract ideas and theories
- Favorable attitude toward students
- Knowledge of subject
- Good organization of subject matter and course
- Enthusiasm about subject
- Fairness in examinations and grading
- Willingness to experiment
- Encouragement of students to think for themselves
- Interesting lecturer — good speaking ability

Studies such as this help a teacher to gain a deeper understanding of perceived strengths and limitations. It is also possible to request, formally or informally, students' perceptions of any number of items, including personal mannerisms, techniques used, tests, tone or pitch of voice, and keeping students informed about class progress.

Most rating instruments encourage students to add comments about the course and the teacher. Open-ended questions, such as "How do you think the course can be improved?" or "What did you like least (and most) about the course?" can be used to elicit more detailed information and student reactions. Sometimes students may hear that their course grade will be affected if they write negative comments. Typing would ensure anonymity, but the cost and time involved may limit its use. Responses to open-ended question are also vulnerable to more subjective interpretation than are answers to single-response questions.

How Reliable Are Student Ratings?

An instrument of poor reliability would be one that gives different information each time it is used. Student ratings are not like this. Their reliability or consistency, as indicated by numerous studies, is very good, provided that enough students in a given class have made ratings. For best information, it is also important to base judgments on several courses taught by the same teacher. For instructional improvements, average ratings based on as few as eight or ten students could provide the teacher with useful information, but larger numbers of students are preferable. The proportion of a class that rates a teacher is as important as the number of raters. If, for example, only ten out of forty students in a class respond to a rating form, it is possible that they do not represent the reactions of the entire class.

Do Student Ratings Improve Instruction?

There is a good deal of skepticism regarding the effect of student ratings on changes or improvements in instruction—particularly when the results are seen only by the individual teacher. It is assumed that teachers value student opinion enough to alter their instructional practices when needed. But do they? Howser (1989) profiled reluctant teachers, defining them as "stagnant in their professional growth and resistant to change." She was particularly interested in why some teachers continued to grow, change, and learn through middle adulthood, while others do not. She contends that adult development stages, individual learner characteristics, and professional growth experiences influence teachers' receptivity to new knowledge or new skills.

Although the tools are available for teachers to gain valuable feedback from students, the information is helpful only if a teacher incorporates suggestions and makes changes to improve teaching methods.

How Do We Give and Receive Feedback?

Both giving feedback and receiving feedback can be highly threatening experiences, and it is important for teachers to work at developing a high level of trust in the classroom. Once the teacher and the students feel this level of trustworthiness, it is helpful to teach students the criteria for useful feedback. Some criteria include the following.

- The feedback is descriptive rather than evaluative. By describing one's own reaction, it leaves the individual free to use it or to use it as he or she sees fit. Avoiding evaluation language reduces the need for an individual to react defensively.
- It is specific rather than general. To be told that one is "dominating" will probably not be as useful as to be told, "Just now when we were deciding the issue, you did not listen to what others said, and I felt forced to accept your arguments or be attacked by you."

- It takes into account the needs of both the receiver and the giver of feedback. Feedback can be destructive when it serves only our own needs and fails to consider the needs of the person on the receiving end.
- It is directed toward behavior that the receiver can do something about. Frustration is only increased when one is reminded of some shortcoming over which one has no control.
- It is solicited, rather than imposed. Feedback is most useful when the receiver has personally formulated the kind of question that those doing the observing can answer.
- It is well timed. In general, feedback is most useful when offered at the earliest opportunity after the given behavior depending, of course, on the receiver's readiness to hear it and the support available from others.
- It is checked to ensure clear communication. One way of doing this is to have the receiver rephrase the feedback received to see if it matches what the sender had in mind.

Feedback then, is a way of giving help; it is a corrective mechanism for the individual who wants to learn how well a specific behavior matches the intentions.

ASSESSMENT

Assessment of learning is as important as development of a curriculum. Many times, teachers wonder what is so hard about teaching and assessing learning. They believe they know when the students know the material. There is a better way to assess students' learning.

You will be continually changing and modifying your curriculum and assessment instruments. If you have access to a computer with a word processor, you will find this process much easier and more enjoyable when you need to update. Computers allow you to be creative because they make it easy to add, delete, and correct a composition without having to retype everything over.

It is important to understand the relationship between curriculum and assessment of your students' learning. You should be asking yourself: What learning domain will the objective evaluate? How will I measure the objective? Is the objective measurable? As you develop your assessment instruments, you will be asking: Does this measure the objective? Is the assessment instrument valid and reliable?

Domains of Learning

Consider the three domains of learning:

COGNITIVE: Includes those behavioral objectives that emphasize intellectual outcomes, such as knowledge, understanding, and thinking skill.

PSYCHOMOTOR: Includes those behavioral objectives that emphasize motor skills and task performance.

AFFECTIVE: Includes those behavioral objectives that emphasize feeling and emotion, such as interest, attitudes, professionalism, and methods of adjustment.

Assessment of these three learning domains is conducted using several methods depending on which domain is being evaluated.

Cognitive: Can be evaluated through *instructor-made tests* such as written exams, essays, multiple-choice questions, and true and false questions. Standardized exams are valid and reliable tests that can be purchased from recognized state and national agencies, professional organizations, and reputable education companies. Surveys are another method of evaluating the cognitive domain. Employer surveys are administered to determine employer satisfaction with employees' knowledge in their specialty area. Graduate surveys are administered to determine graduates' satisfaction with their educational training.

Psychomotor: Instructor-made, competency-based evaluations, such as practical exams (laboratory setting), formative clinical evaluations, and summative clinical evaluations, as well as surveys can be administered both to patients being treated by students and to employers and graduates to measure satisfaction.

Formative evaluation refers to many types of research on programs that are conducted during the early, formative stages of the development of a program. The intent is to provide data on program operations so that systematic refinement may proceed.

Summative evaluation is research conducted on a refined program to determine its effectiveness in meeting its goals.

Affective: Instructor-made evaluation instruments such as formative and summative evaluations of students' professional behavior may be used. Surveys may be administered both to patients being treated by students and to employers to measure satisfaction with employees' professional behavior. Remember—your evaluation instrument should be timely, should measure what it was meant to measure, and should address one of the three domains of learning.

Evaluation may be defined as a systematic process of determining the extent to which the goals and standards are achieved. As we consider the evaluation process, the instructor must try to identify the purpose(s) of that process. Ask yourself, "What am I trying to find out?" This is related to the validity of the evaluation instrument.

Validity directly relates to the degree the instrument focuses on the language of the standard that is being investigated. For example, some VHO programs have adopted standards that begin with the phrase "Upon completion of the program." This particular phrase specifies the time the instrument would be applied to the student. Thus, a final exam for the first course in a VHO program would not be valid as the measurement of a graduate of the program "at the completion of the program," thus affecting the focus or validity of an instrument. A number of other adverse factors can influence the level of validity of an evaluation instrument.

Some of these factors are:

1. The evaluation tool itself (i.e., the instructions for completion do not clearly indicate how the user should respond).
2. The questions may be poorly constructed, ambiguous, or even unintelligible.
3. The test or survey may be inappropriate for the behavior to be measured (e.g., the instrument chosen cannot be used to measure the skills or behaviors).
4. The person or group responding to the survey tool may be unqualified to do so (e.g., the person responding to the survey may have never worked with the student or graduate).

Hence, the major aims in constructing and administering evaluation instruments are to control those factors that have an adverse effect on their validity and to interpret the results of the evaluations according to the degree to which adverse factors can be controlled.

Once you determine that your evaluation instrument is valid, you must then consider whether it is reliable.

Reliability represents the qualitative judgment about the consistency of test scores or other evaluation results from one measure to another. It is the extent to which a test is consistent in measuring what it is supposed to measure.

The concept of reliability relates to the consistency of an instructor's test items from one testing date to the next. The same students taking the same test on two different dates would, on a highly reliable test, have similar test scores. Item analysis is one method of assessing the effectiveness, reliability, and validity of a particular test item or test.

It has been reported that on a good classroom test, the reliability coefficient should be .70 or higher. Calculations for this coefficient are based on the assumption that each question is worth 1 point.

☞ TEST CONSTRUCTION

How do you accomplish this? First, examine your testing procedures. Let the students take the written test first. Each exam should be a collection of at least two of the following: fill in, mix and match, true and false, essay, and multiple choice. Multiple-choice questions should assess if students know the basic information and should give a problem in that instance.

EXAMPLE 1

Jimmy Brown, 3 years old, has a febrile, acute rhinitis with bilateral otorrhea. What would you expect the doctor to prescribe?

    a. aspirin
    b. acetaminophen
    c. an otoscope
    d. anhydrase

• • •

The question tests students' knowledge of medical terminology, disease process, and treatment. Not only must students correctly identify that this patient has a fever, a bad cold, and drainage from both ears, but the higher order of thinking expects them to also identify that the patient is a child and a possible Reye's syndrome candidate. Therefore aspirin could be a correct drug but would not be the drug of choice, whereas acetaminophen would be.

EXAMPLE 2

Jorene is applying to work as a lifeguard this summer. She has her basic lifesaving card and took lessons in cardiopulmonary resuscitation (CPR) last summer. She will need to take the following with her on her interview:

    a. lifeguard/CPR cards, résumé, application
    b. application, résumé, current lifeguard/CPR cards
    c. application and résumé only
    d. cards, application, résumé, letters of reference

• • •

Here the student should choose (b), knowing that a CPR card must be renewed every year. In addition, depending on the state, the lifeguard card may also need to be updated.

These examples demand a basic understanding from your students and then expect them to take that information and choose the best course of action.

An open letter to the reader:

In August of 1978 when I graduated from the Respiratory Therapy program at Kirkwood College in Cedar Rapids, Iowa, the last thing I thought I would ever be doing is teaching. As a graduate I was anxious to begin working in the hospital with patients. In the back of my mind I had goals of becoming a supervisor or department head. Well, things worked out pretty much as planned. I did get a job working with patients and I did get into management. What I didn't plan on was the gradual attraction toward teaching.

One of my job titles was Educational Coordinator. I was doing staff development and inservice for the respiratory therapy department and for other departments within the hospital. The more I taught the more I liked it. This position gave me the opportunity to work with and teach the respiratory students who were rotating through our hospital. It was then I realized I wanted to be a teacher.

I applied for and was hired as the Program Director of the Respiratory Technician Program that had been affiliated with the hospital I was working in. This enjoyment was not without many sleepless nights and days of frustration. However, it was all worth it when I graduated my first class. There is no way to describe the feeling as you watch your students receive their certificate with family and friends watching.

This scenario is probably similar to your own story on "How I Got Into Teaching." I would like to point out that Larry Hudson, the person responsible for this book, was my respiratory therapy instructor at Kirkwood Community College, and I would like to thank him for allowing me the opportunity to contribute my thoughts. THANKS!

Jack A. Powers, RRT

References

Centra, J. A. (1979). *Determining Faculty Effectiveness.* San Francisco: Jossey-Bass.

Des Jardines, T., and H. Douce (1991). "Program Assessment and Its Relationship to Validity, Reliability and Cut Scores." *JRCRTE Newsletter.*

Gronlund, N. E. (1971). *Measurement and Evaluation in Teaching* (2nd ed.). New York: Macmillan.

Howser, M. A. (1989). "Reluctant Teachers: Why Some Middle-Aged Teachers Fail to Learn and Grow." *OSSC Bulletin* v33, n3. Oregon School Study Council, University of Oregon.

Joint Review Committee for Respiratory Therapy Education: Description of Current Standards for Essential VI Program Evaluation. *JRCRTE.* Euless, Tex.: Author.

Lewis, R., and J. Lucas (1988). *ExamSystem Software* Computer program. National Computer Systems, Inc; Economics Research, Inc.

Nedelsky, L. (1965). *Science Teaching and Testing.* New York: Harcourt, Brace, Jovanovich.

O'Reilly, R., and P. von der Heydt (1988). *A Handbook on Evaluation for the Allied Health Program.* Euless, Tex.: Joint Review Committee Services Corporation (full list of bibliographies on the topic found on pp. 100–104).

Stanford, G., and A. E. Roark (1974). *Human Interaction in Education.* Boston: Allyn and Bacon.

Wotruba, T. R., and P. L. Wright (1975). "How to Develop a Teacher Rating Instrument: A Research Approach." *Journal of Higher Education* 46(6), 653–63.

3
Laboratory Management: Practicing the Job

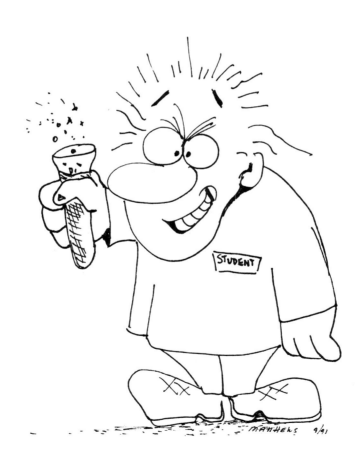

☞ MAINTAINING STUDENT SAFETY

Safety should be taught and emphasized from the first time your students step foot into your classroom until they complete the last day of your program. Losing one or both eyes, causing a disfiguring injury, or being responsible for a permanent injury due to carelessness and lack of safety's being taught is a very difficult way of learning your lesson.

When students enter the lab work area, they should be wearing eye protection, a lab coat or jacket, and gloves. You must not forget that *you* set the example for your students. When you put on your eye protection, lab jacket, and gloves, they automatically know that to participate they must do the same. In the lab area, do not allow students without protection while procedures are being performed.

The easiest way to prepare students for lab work is:

1. Read about the procedure.
2. Discuss the procedure.
3. Discuss possible safety issues.
4. Demonstrate proper lab techniques.
5. Allow groups of 3–5 students to perform procedures as you and the rest observe. After the first group completes the procedure to your satisfaction, rotate the rest of the class through in groups of 3–5 students. Students should be allowed to do lab procedures until they feel comfortable doing them. (This can easily take four or five times doing the procedure before they are comfortable with it.)
6. After each student has finished the procedure, make sure the area is cleaned and any waste is disposed of properly.
7. Test your students on the lab and safety procedures.

Even though your students have read about the lab procedures and you have discussed them, do not assume students are able to perform these without supervision. Direct supervision is a must for your and your students' safety.

To help build confidence and develop skills, I choose a student to demonstrate a procedure a week or so after we have studied it. At the end of the year, everyone has had a chance to do a demonstration two or three times.

The following safety suggestions are from *Clinical Procedures for Medical Assistants,* Third Edition.

Carefully handle and store glassware to prevent breakage as follows:

1. Carefully arrange glassware in storage cabinet, to prevent breakage.
2. Carefully remove glassware from storage cabinets.
3. If glassware does break, dispose of it in a special container, to protect trash handlers from being cut.

The medical assistant should handle all chemical reagents carefully by adhering to the following:

1. Make sure all reagent bottles are clearly and properly labeled.
2. If a label becomes loose, reattach it immediately.
3. Recap reagent bottles immediately after using, to prevent spills.
4. Do not pipet reagents by mouth, to avoid ingesting hazardous chemicals.

Laboratory specimens should be handled carefully as follows:

1. Follow the CDC (Centers for Disease Control) recommended precautions when collecting and handling laboratory specimens.
2. Wash hands frequently before and after handling specimens. The hands should be washed immediately if the medical assistant accidentally touches some of the material contained in the specimen.
3. Avoid hand-to-mouth contact while working with biological specimens.
4. Do not pipet any specimen by mouth (e.g., serum, plasma, blood).
5. Immediately clean up any specimen spilled on the work table and cleanse the table with a disinfectant.
6. Properly dispose of all contaminated needles, syringes, specimen containers, and infectious waste.
7. Cover any break in the skin, such as a cut or scratch, with a bandage.
8. Make sure all specimen containers are tightly capped, to prevent leakage.

Handle all laboratory equipment and supplies properly and with care as indicated by the manufacturer. For example, when using a centrifuge, wait until it comes to a complete stop before opening it.

Lab procedures are an excellent learning experience for your students as long as you keep safety as number one on your list. Most students enjoy the hands-on experience, and when you work with a group of 3–5 students, you can get to know them better.

Remember—have fun, do it with safety in mind, and enjoy yourself.

☞ FOLLOWING INFECTION CONTROL PROCEDURES

What Is Infection Control?

Infection is the contamination with and establishment of a disease-producing substance, germs, or bacteria into a susceptible host. So, infection control is the regulation, direction, and, ultimately, prevention of a disease-producing substance from contaminating and establishing itself in a susceptible host.

There are different types of infections. A community-acquired infection is an infection a person develops from exposure to microorganisms found among the general public. Nosocomial infections are infections that were not present or incubating prior to a patient's being admitted to the hospital. They are infections that develop while in the hospital or infections produced by microorganisms that are acquired during hospitalization. Nosocomial infections occur not only in patients but also in anyone else in the hospital, including staff, visitors, and volunteers.

In 1958, the American Hospital Association recommended the formation of infection control committees, although few hospitals formed such a committee voluntarily. Until 1970, the main focus and infection control efforts of hospitals that had established a committee were directed primarily toward routine microbiologic culturing of the air and the environment, such as floors, walls, and other surfaces. In 1970, the first International Conference on Nosocomial Infections convened. It represented the catalyst for change by bringing together people who worked in the field of nosocomial infections to share their experience and knowledge in reducing infections. From this conference came two messages: one was the need for surveillance of nosocomial infections; the second was that only rarely is the environment the cause of infections and microbiological sampling is not needed to determine if a shelf is clean. Even the shelf will have its own normal flora, and therefore, who is to determine what or how much is normal?

Until 1976, no regulations or standards for infection control programs existed, and programs were voluntary. In 1976, infection control became a requirement by the Joint Commission on Accreditation of Healthcare Organizations for hospitals seeking accreditation. Now hospitals based their priorities on their own infection problems, on patient risks, and on the resources available.

Why Is Infection Control Important?

The results of a study conducted by the Centers for Disease Control (CDC) Study on the Efficacy of Nosocomial Infection Control indicated that a well-organized infection surveillance and control program in hospitals could expect to prevent approximately one third of all nosocomial infections (Hughes and Jarvis, 1985). Preventable infections varied with various type or site of infection (urinary, surgical wound, penumonia, bloodstream, etc.).

It is estimated that 5.5% of all patients, or 5½ of every 100 patients, will acquire an infection while in the hospital (Hughes and Jarvis, 1985). Nosocomial infections result in morbidity, prolonged hospital stay, increased costs for the hospital and patient, inconvenience for the patient, and pain for the patient and can even result in mortality. In these days of diagnosis-related group (DRG) reimbursement and the high cost of hospitalization, neither party can afford such possibly preventable additional expenses.

Are Some Infections Preventable?

Depending on the type of infection or the site of infection (urinary, surgical wound, pneumonia, bloodstream, etc.), it is estimated that from 22% to 35% of such infections can be prevented (Hughes and Jarvis, 1985). A nonpreventable infection is one that will occur despite all possible precautions' being taken to avoid the infection, for example, a person whose immune response is suppressed and who develops an infection from microorganisms from his or her own flora. A preventable infection then would imply that by altering some event related to the infection, the infection would have been prevented. For example, nurses who do not wash their hands between handling a urine collection device and examining a surgical dressing on the same patient, could transmit gram-negative organisms to the wound. Could handwashing have prevented this infection?

The liability for nosocomial infections may be assessed to the hospital, physicians, and health care providers. As people become more conscious of treatment complications, including infections, the number of awards from health care providers for nosocomial infections has increased in the past few years.

How Are Infections Spread?

Infections occur when an infectious agent comes into contact with a susceptible host. This contact is called transmission. Six factors, called links, must be present for an infection to develop. The interrelation of these factors is called the chain of infection.

The first link in the chain is the **infectious agent.** An infectious agent may be a virus, bacterium, fungal protozoan, or rickettsia but must be present for any infection to occur. The infectious agent has a home, also called a **reservoir**, which is the second link. This is where the infectious agent lives, grows, and multiplies, and it may be quite specific for a particular agent. A reservoir can be skin, water, dirt, body surface openings, or any and all bodily fluids. The infectious agent may also come from a source that may be either the same as the reservoir or a contaminant of an animate or inanimate object from the reservoir. The third link in the chain is a portal of exit, for example, in humans, any bodily opening.

Infectious agents *must* have a way to travel as a means of transmission. Contrary to some opinions, microorganisms do *not* walk, run, jump, hop, skip, or crawl from place to place. Well, at least not on their own. They remain perfectly happy in their reservoir just living and multiplying. Movement of organisms, the fourth chain link, can occur by one of the following four means of transmission: contact spread, common vehicle, airborne, or vectorborne.

With contact spread, the victim has contact with the source. This contact may be direct contact, meaning person-to-person spread, for example, respiratory therapists' not washing their hands between collecting a sputum specimen on one patient and performing oral suctioning on the next patient. Contact spread may be indirect contact in which an intermediate object — most often inanimate, such as an endoscope contaminated by not properly disinfecting or sterilizing it between patients — becomes the source of transmission. Droplet transmission is the third type of contact spread, occuring by means of large droplets that can be spread over only a few feet, such as by coughing or sneezing. Because the droplets are so large and heavy, they do not travel more than two or three feet.

Common-vehicle spread consists of a contaminated inanimate vehicle, which can include food, blood, blood products, diagnostic reagents, and medications, such as developing hepatitis B from a needlestick, acquired from improperly recapping a syringe used on a patient. Airborne transmission describes airborne spread of microorganisms over great distances, more than a few feet. These microorganisms are contained in droplet nuclei or dust particles and can stay airborne for prolonged periods of time, sometimes up to one or two days. Aspergillosis and legionellosis are examples of this means of transmission. Vectorborne spread rarely occurs as a means of transmission in the hospital setting.

The fifth link in the chain is a place of entry. Entrances for an organism include the skin, mucous membranes, and respiratory, gastrointestinal, and urinary tracts. Organisms called leptospires can penetrate the skin, but few other organisms are able to. Other organisms cannot gain access through the skin unless there is a breach in the skin's integrity. Organisms gain access through body openings, such as by ingestion of contaminated enteral feeding, by poor technique or contaminated equipment during Foley catheterization, or by intravenous cannulation. The organism must overcome the body's natural defenses, such as the skin, tears, cilia, mucous secretions of the respiratory tract, and acid secretions of the gestrointestinal tract to gain entrance to the body.

The final link in the chain is the person at risk. Two different hosts can be infected with the same organism and will respond differently to the impending infection depending on their individual immune system's response.

Who Can Get Infections?

Break the chain of infection! Hippocrates centuries ago said, "First do no harm." The application to health care today is so relevant. Maintenance of sound personal hygiene is every individual's responsibility in the control of infections and doing no harm. This includes no harm to yourself, family, friends, coworkers, and any other people you may contact during the course of the day. Handwashing with soap and water represents the single most important way to break that chain and prevent the spread of infection.

Organisms on your hands are described as transient and resident. Resident organisms are organisms that are necessary for healthy skin because they inhibit the growth of "bad" organisms. Transient organisms come and go on your hands. They are usually the ones that can cause illness or infection. This is why handwashing, as Ignaz Semmelweis proved by decreasing the death rate from puerperal fever, is so effective and so important. It helps to remove transient organisms. Most cold or flu viruses infect people because people have not washed their hands, and they then touch their eyes or nose with contaminated hands. Few viruses infect by droplet spread of the organism from an infected person's sneeze or cough.

Health care personnel with direct patient contact are more likely to be a link in the chain of infection. The goals of infection control are to prevent health care workers from acquiring organisms from patients and to prevent health care workers from transferring organisms to patients.

Why Are Barrier Precautions Important?

As early as the 1700s, infection precautions were used to control the spread of disease. "Fever hospitals" were established during yellow fever epidemics and closed when the epidemic was over. People with communicable diseases were quarantined, or placed in buildings separate from other hospitalized patients. The first published recommendations for isolating patients with communicable diseases were published in 1877. By the 1950s, tuberculosis hospitals began to close, and patients needing isolation precautions were placed in single isolation rooms in the general hospital. Procedures called barrier nursing were designed in 1910 to protect health care workers from acquiring infectious organisms from patients with communicable diseases.

In June 1981 in Los Angeles, a group of five previously healthy homosexual men sought medical treatment for an unusual illness normally associated with a defective immune system. Shortly thereafter came reports of a rare cancer, previously occurring in the elderly and now occurring in young homosexual men. Earlier cases had been identified as far back as 1978. These early reports constituted the first glimpse of what now is known as human immunodeficiency virus (HIV) disease.

By 1983, epidemiology quickly proved this disease to be spread through blood or blood products, sexual contact, and perinatal events. This mode of transportation or spread was the same as for other bloodborne pathogens, such as hepatitis B, hepatitis non-A non-B, and now hepatitis C. But hepatitis B, until then, had never earned the respect the disease deserved until HIV disease.

HIV disease changed the world of the health care worker/system. Other bloodborne organisms, until then, had been treated with a rather cavalier attitude despite the devastating illness and outcome that many of them could cause.

Now HIV disease was causing the delivery of health care to be viewed in a different fashion. Originally out of fear of the unknown or the AFRAIDS (anxiety and fear of AIDS), care was delivered, but through research and education, care delivery developed to a level consisting of what should have been common sense all along. HIV disease prompted the rethinking of old barrier use practices by reinforcing the reasons for, stressing wider application of, and demonstrating the need for better application of the barrier techniques.

In 1983, the CDC published "Guidelines for Isolation Precautions in Hospitals," in its Morbidity and Mortality Weekly Report. This document contained a section entitled Blood and Body Fluid Precautions that recommended protection against the blood and body fluids of people known or suspected to be infected with bloodborne pathogens.

As more became known about HIV disease and together with what was already known about other bloodborne pathogens, it became clearer that persons may be infected with the disease, not exhibit signs or symptoms of the disease, yet be infectious to others who may contact their blood or body fluids. In August 1987, the CDC published "Recommendations for Prevention of HIV Transmission in Health-Care Settings," which, in contrast to the 1983 publication, now recommended that blood and body fluid precautions be consistently used on *all* patients regardless of whether the patient is known to have or suspected of having a bloodborne disease.

Using blood and body fluid precautions on *all* patients is referred to as universal blood and body fluid precautions or universal precautions. The blood and body fluids of anyone are considered potentially infectious not only for HIV, because equally important are hepatitis B and all other bloodborne pathogens. The practice of universal precautions is intended to provide for handlers of body fluids protection from parenteral, mucous membrane, and nonintact skin exposures.

Acquired immune deficiency syndrome (AIDS) — HIV disease — is probably the most serious health issue to face this nation in the twentieth century. The disease has produced feelings of fear and helplessness and poses a unique challenge for both the general public and the medical profession. Few people will find their life untouched by the disease. Difficult decisions lie ahead involving individual patient care and public policy.

Some states have passed laws addressing the AIDS and HIV disease issues in regard to how they affect the public health and welfare. In 1988, the state of Florida passed the Omnibus AIDS Act, which is based on the knowledge that the spread of bloodborne illnesses can be controlled by an informed public. Knowing the facts about HIV disease and other bloodborne illnesses can prevent their spread. Education of those at risk of infection and of those with infection (to prevent them from infecting others) is the only and the best weapon available in this battle.

What Are the Implications for the VHO Teacher?

Infection control becomes an important matter not only in the health care setting but also in schools, in industry, and in our homes with our family and friends. Whether the infection is a disease as devastating as HIV disease and hepatitis B or of lesser consequences as salmonellosis, the flu, or the common cold, the elements of good infection control apply. Knowledge and understanding of handwashing are relevant to everyone's daily activities to prevent acquiring infections ourselves and to prevent the spread of our own germs to those around us. Handling or coming into contact with body fluids, if part of health occupation teachers' job or part of their home or social life, requires using some type of barrier between the handler and the "wet stuff," followed by scrupulous handwashing.

☞ PLANNING SIMULATIONS

Laboratory settings provide the student with a simulated real-world environment in which learned theories are applied and procedures are practiced in controlled situations. Students need a place to practice skills until competent to safely perform the procedures in a real-world setting. The student laboratory is a proving ground where mistakes can be made and corrected without the risk of injuring patients.

Students come to the laboratory excited, anxious, and apprehensive. Be absolutely sure they thoroughly understand the safety rules and requirements before they attempt the first exercise. Point out unusual safety concerns throughout the laboratory sessions. Always be aware of safety concerns when working with students in the laboratory.

Plan for safety. Have a fire blanket and fire extinguisher near the exit. Depending on the type and size of laboratory training being conducted, several fire extinguishers may be needed. Request the type of extinguisher that is designed to be used on the types of fires most likely to occur in your laboratory setting, for example, type A for paper and clothing, type B for inflammable liquids and gases, type C for electrical fires. Oftentimes, schools purchase combination fire extinguishers that are capable of extinguishing a variety of fires.

Early in the term you will want to conduct a safety inventory of the student laboratory. Have the necessary equipment in functioning order, starting with eye washes. Either purchase safety goggles, pipette bulbs, pipette mouthpieces, and stethoscopes, or arrange with the bookstore or administrator to stock these items for incoming students. Provide a place in the student laboratory where students can hang up their laboratory coats and store their books and supplies. Plan traffic flow to determine if a different arrangement of workstations would be better; if so, request physical plant or janitorial assistance, if needed, to accomplish the rearrangement.

Have a working idea of the general number and content of laboratory exercises to plan. Outline the exercises, accommodating the school calendar in the plan. Determine the days available for laboratory exercises. Review your instructional content outline. Make a list of possible laboratory exercises that could be created to correlate with the theory being taught. Count the exercises you have listed, and compare them to the number of laboratory hours available. Usually you will have many more exercises than time allotted. Therefore, you must list the items in order of priority. Priority should be based on the importance of the skill; the critical nature of the skill; availability of supplies, equipment, and appropriate specimens for the exercise; the likelihood of students' being unable to be involved with this exercise in the clinical sites due to its rarity; costs involved; time required to complete the exercise; and complexity of the skill. Once you have decided which exercises will be conducted, design a plan for using laboratory sessions efficiently.

Throughout your career, you will be making contact with salespeople, manufacturers, and suppliers. Develop a file of business cards or a database system of information on your computer. Toll-free numbers are extremely valuable as you prepare equipment and supply requests. And many companies provide educational assistance in the form of videos, demonstrations, literature, and samples.

Make sure the laboratory is clean, orderly, and in good repair. Refrigerators and sinks should be cleaned. Disinfectants, soaps, hand towels, and linens should be purchased if needed. Clean-up kits for chemical spills should be requested. Computerized equipment should be plugged into surge protectors. Lighting should be adequate to perform all planned exercises.

Determine if any of your incoming students have physical disabilities that would require special planning, assistance, or modifications. If so, each exercise must be carefully examined to plan for such accommodations.

The amount of time, thought, and effort put into the planning of laboratory simulations will determine the competence level your students are able to achieve prior to entering the clinical sites. Remember—your management skills are manifested in the functioning of your student laboratory. Your students and your administrators will regard your laboratory as the most visible evidence of your competence.

☞ ASSESSING STUDENT PERFORMANCE

Performance Instruments

Appropriate assessment of student competencies requires instruments very different from the paper-and-pencil tests used to evaluate theory comprehension. Skill assessment is a result of observation and judgment on the part of the evaluator. To reduce subjectivity, an evaluation instrument should be developed that can be used by all students for assessment of a specific competency. For example, one assessment instrument for checking vital signs is used to evaluate each student's skill in this area.

Basically, these instruments are designed to measure one of two outcomes: process or product. Two types of instruments may be developed depending on the assessment needs: rating scale or checklist.

First, let's discuss the checklist type of instrument. A checklist is simply that; yes, I saw it, or no, I did not. In other words, a checklist involves an all-or-nothing response, namely, yes or no, satisfactory or unsatisfactory, acceptable or unacceptable. When you make a list of things to do, you check off each item as you do it. The same is true for assessing a student's skill; each step is checked off as to whether it is satisfactory or not. An example of a checklist is included as Figure 3-1 from the Illinois health occupations instructor booklet "Communication Skills: Physician's Orders and Use of Telephones, Call Signals, and Intercoms."

Notice that the duty area and specific task are stated at the top of the instrument, along with identification information. It is very important that a complete, detailed performance objective be stated that clearly identifies the task to be accomplished and the criterion level at which it is to be

Duty Area A: Communicating Information   Student _____

Task #13: Call patient/staff using intercom   Date _____

Instructor _____   Final Score _____

Representative Occupations: Professional Nurse (associate degree), Practical Nurse (L.P.N.), Nurse Assistant, Geriatric Aide

Performance Objective: Given an intercom, pen/pencil, and message pad, the student will be able to call patient/staff using the intercom. All steps in the instructor's checklist must be completed to the instructor's satisfaction. All signals must be responded to within two minutes, messages must be written, and initiated calls must be implemented within two minutes.

Equipment and Supplies Needed: Intercom system, pen/pencil, message pad

Scale: S = Satisfactory   U = Unsatisfactory   NA = Not Applicable

Steps:	First Try		Second Try	
	S	U	S	U

1. Acknowledged the signal.
2. Activated the equipment.
3. Identified yourself.
4. Offered assistance.
5. Identified the patient.
6. Recorded name, room number, time, and written message on a form.
7. Located the person assigned to the patient via the intercom
8. Relayed the message accurately to the assigned person quickly.

IF THE ASSIGNED PERSON IS OFF THE UNIT OR OTHERWISE UNAVAILABLE:

9. Summoned another qualified person.
10. Sought assistance of the supervisor if needed.
11. Reported back to the patient promptly via the intercom.

Instructor's Comments:

_____   _____   _____
Student's Signature   Date   Evaluator's Signature

Figure 3-1: *An example of a performance checklist.*

performed. A list of equipment and supplies needed for the skill is also suggested.

It is also important that all steps in the process be listed in the order in which they are performed, so that the evaluation is smooth and orderly. At the bottom of all performance evaluation instruments, there should be a place for the signatures of the evaluator and the student, as well as a place for the date. The signatures should be obtained at the time the evaluator reviews the results with the student. This provides evidence that the student is fully aware of the outcome of the assessment.

Notice that this checklist allows a student two attempts to perform the skill at a satisfactory level. If the student does not meet the performance criterion on the first attempt, he or she should practice the skill until proficient for a second observation. Policies must be established that describe the outcome of not passing a skill performance evaluation.

Some policy statements require students to repeat the entire course or laboratory. Other policies simply record a failure for that skill on the competency profile for the occupation. In many of the health occupations, a student will not be allowed to go to a clinical site until all necessary skills have been satisfactorily performed at the required criterion level in the student laboratory. All signed performance evaluation instruments should be placed in the student's program file and kept until the student graduates or for two or three years after dropping out of the program.

Next, we will look at the rating scale. A rating scale instrument provides a range of possible evaluation levels, for example, 1-5, poor to good. Rating scales are especially appropriate whenever you want to determine the level of skill shown in performing each step of a task. By contrast, a checklist shows only whether or not the step was performed satisfactorily. The rating scale, on the other hand, allows the evaluator to differentiate among students based on the degree or level at which skills were performed. Figure 3-2 is an example of a descriptive rating scale. Notice that the rating is based on a brief description of the quality of the skill at each level.

Compare this form with Figure 3-3, which is an example of a numerical rating scale that requires that a standard adjective be assigned to each number on the scale and that the scale be used consistently throughout the form. For example, the number 1 might represent poor skills, and the number 5 represents outstanding skills. Information on how the rating scale is interpreted must be clearly stated on the paper.

The previous figures (3-1, 3-2, and 3-3) are examples of the performance evaluation tools that are used while each step of a performance is observed and assessed. Whenever a process is important in terms of how it is performed, a performance assessment tool should be used. However, if the product is most important, regardless of how the process was performed, then you should use

PARKLAND COLLEGE, DENTAL ASSISTING: EVALUATION OF CLINICAL PRACTICE

STUDENT: _____ DATE OF SERVICE: _____

DOCTOR: _____ FINAL SCORE: _____

Performance Objective: To demonstrate knowledge and use of chairside equipment and techniques with a final score of 10 or better.

1	2	3	4

Ability

1. **Perform chairside functions effectively and efficiently; degree of manual dexterity.**

No dexterity; no ability at chairside assisting.	Good dexterity; shows continual improvement in chairside assisting.	Demonstrates good ability at chairside; works with efficiency and little aid.	Excellent chairside assistance; needs no aid or direction during normal procedures.

2. **Knowledge of instruments, equipment, and supplies; ease of adaptation to individual office circumstances.**

Demonstrates little knowledge of equipment and supplies.	Usually recognizes equipment and materials; needs a little help adapting.	Recognizes instruments and equipment; rarely needs assistance in adaptation.	Always recognizes equipment and supplies; adapts readily to office circumstances.

3. **Care of instruments, equipment, and supplies; sterilization technique.**

Careless with instruments, equipment, and supplies; Poor sterilization technique.	Usually careful with instruments, equipment, and supplies; needs direction in office sterilization routine.	Careful with instruments and supplies; rarely needs direction in sterilization routine.	Always careful; needs no direction in sterilization technique.

4. **Assisting technique during moisture procedure.**

Demonstrates little knowledge of moisture control technique or injures oral tissue.	Demonstrates continual improvement in technique; still requires direction from operator.	Usually keeps operating field clear; seldom obstructs view or injures tissue.	Always keeps operating field clear; never injures tissue.

Student's Signature _____ Date _____ Evaluator's Signature _____

Figure 3-2: *An example of a descriptive rating scale.*

PERFORMANCE RATING SCALE

_____
Student's Name (print)

OBJECTIVE: Perform an oral peripheral exam.*

DIRECTIONS: Evaluate each of the following steps based on a scale of 1–5.

5 = excellent
4 = good
3 = average
2 = poor
1 = failure

PERFORMANCE	ACCEPTABLE			UNACCEPTABLE	
	5	4	3	2	1
1. Explained exam procedures to client?	5	4	3	2	1
2. Noted normalities and/or abnormalities of head and face on chart?	5	4	3	2	1
3. Examined lips and charted findings?	5	4	3	2	1
4. Examined interior of mouth and recorded findings on chart to include:					
a. teeth?	5	4	3	2	1
b. tongue?	5	4	3	2	1
c. hard palate?	5	4	3	2	1
d. soft palate?	5	4	3	2	1
e. uvula?	5	4	3	2	1
f. velopharyngeal closure?	5	4	3	2	1
g. fauces?	5	4	3	2	1
5. Examined nasal cavities and noted findings on chart?	5	4	3	2	1
6. Examined breathing mechanisms and charted observations?	5	4	3	2	1

*Minimum passing score = 3 or better for each step.

_____   _____   _____
Student's Signature   Date   Evaluator's Signature

Figure 3-3: *An example of a numerical rating scale.*

a product evaluation tool. An example in health occupations is found in medical records, where the product is critically important, but the process consists basically of the standard typing or word processing procedure. A product checklist from the Illinois instructor booklet entitled "Recording Patient Data: Using Medical Abbreviations, Measurement Conversions, and Medical Forms" is shown in Figure 3-4. You will notice it incorporates all the

---

Duty Area A: Communicating Information   Student _____

Task #2: Record Patient Data   Date _____

Instructor _____   Final Score _____

Representative Occupations: All Health Occupations

Performance Objective: Given a patient, medical forms, clipboard, and pen/typewriter, patient data should be recorded with all characteristics in the instructor's checklist incorporated at a 100% satisfactory rating.

Equipment and Supplies Needed: Blue or black ink pen/typewriter, clipboard, medical forms for the patient's medical record

PRODUCT CHECKLIST

Scale: Y = Yes   N = No   NA = Not Applicable

Attempt:	First Try		Second	
Characteristics:	Y	N	Y	N

1. The information was written in ink or typed.
2. The information was printed.
3. The information was written legibly.
4. The information was spelled correctly.
5. The proper form was used.
6. The information was recorded under the proper headings.
7. Correct medical terminology was used.
8. Correct medical abbreviations were used.
9. Medical terminology was consistent.
10. Words were used accurately.
11. The form was signed with the health care worker's name and position.
12. Errors were corrected.

Instructor's Comments:

Student's Signature   Date   Evaluator's Signature

Figure 3-4: *An example of a product checklist.*

components of a checklist, but you are evaluating only the final product. A product rating scale is shown in Figure 3-5. As with other rating scales, a range of evaluation levels is possible. In most cases, the quality of the product is a clear indicator as to the accuracy of the process. One example of this is a radiograph development process. The product (a radiograph) can be evaluated on a rating scale to determine the competence level of the developer.

Tips and rules for developing your own evaluation tools are included at the end of this section. They are guidelines to help you get started. Much more can be learned concerning evaluation, but for now, you have enough information to make a good start.

TIPS

1. Student should have the product or performance evaluation tool throughout the learning process.

PRODUCT RATING SCALE

Duty Area: Illustrating Anatomical Organs

Student's Name _____

Instructor's Name _____

Task: Draw a kidney

Date _____

Final score _____

Performance Objective: Draw a human kidney in a 5" × 6" space. The kidney should be a longitudinal dissection that is anatomically correct and includes a closeup inset of a nephron.

Rating Scale   1 = poor   2 = fair   3 = good

Characteristics	Rating		
1. Drawing is correct size.	1	2	3
2. Drawing is anatomically correct.	1	2	3
3. Inset is large enough to see detail.	1	2	3
4. Labeling of parts is clear.	1	2	3
5. Each part is proportionately sized.	1	2	3

Comments:

_____   _____   _____
Student's Signature   Date   Evaluator's Signature

Figure 3-5: *An example of a product rating scale.*

2. Be sure each item can be evaluated as stated.
3. Determine in advance how retesting will be conducted (under different conditions or after a period of time or both).
4. State on the evaluation tool any special restrictions, cautions, time limits, equipment.

RULES FOR DEVELOPING PERFORMANCE EVALUATION TOOLS

1. Should be based on steps in task analysis.
2. Use past tense verb (performance must occur prior to evaluation).
3. Each item must be observable and measurable.
4. Checklists have only two possible responses (yes/no, pass/fail, satisfactory/unsatisfactory).
5. Rating scales have 3–5 levels of performance.
6. One distinct step per item.
7. Clear, concise items.
8. Complex items should be categorized into subitems.
9. List items in sequential order.
10. Include safety requirements.
11. Put the objective (with criterion) on the evaluation sheet.
12. Include lines for teacher and student signatures and the date.

RULES FOR DEVELOPING PRODUCT EVALUATION TOOLS

1. Include only critical characteristics of the finished product.
2. Use present tense verbs.
3. Do not use repetitious words and phrases.
4. Include exact criterion requirement.
5. May use either a rating scale or a checklist, depending on which is more appropriate.
6. Include lines for signatures of teacher and student and for the date.

☞ ORDERING SUPPLIES

An instructor cannot successfully teach in a VHO program without conducting lab sessions, so when you do, you must have the appropriate supplies and equipment on hand. Obtaining these supplies takes some time and preparation.

The things you must do consist of finding out if your program has a budget and how much it is, if you are responsible for calling or sending in orders, and whether or not you are limited on the dollar amount for your purchase orders. (If a purchase order is over a certain amount, then it will usually have to be approved by the school board.)

If your program does have a budget (and most do), you will have to do some planning so that your money will last all year. If there are other health programs at your school, you may be able to share the cost of supplies. Buying in larger quantities may be a little less expensive.

When filling out your purchase order, make sure that you list the correct company you are ordering from, the catalog number, and the price. This is especially important when you have a purchasing agent placing the order. If the purchase order has not been completed properly, it will cause delays on your order.

After you learn the purchasing protocol, sit down with your textbooks and go through them to determine what supplies you will need for what labs and approximately when you will be needing them. Make a list of what you need and how much it will cost per unit and per case. If you have enough storage area, buying by the case may be your best bet as long as there is no expiration date on a product. For example:

Text: Clinical Procedures for Medical Assistants

Chapter 1   Medical Asepsis and Infection Control

Item	Quantity	Price	Cat.#
1. Autoclave-distilled water	1 gallon	$ .89	45795
2. Cold sterilization, Cidex	gal./case	50.81	5975
3. Hand soap, liquid	1 gallon	16.40	78138
4. Examination gloves	2,000 gloves/case	195.50	123754

This should be done for each chapter in the textbook.

Decide if students will be able to share supplies or if each will need individual items.

Ordering supplies does take time, but with a little effort you should be able to make it through the year. This is also a good time to do an inventory.

☞ ACQUIRING EQUIPMENT AND TOOLS

You should have completed an inventory of all equipment and tools currently in your student laboratory. All of these must be in good working condition, or you must report equipment problems in a memorandum to your administrator. Immediate repair should be requested, if the equipment is up-to-date enough that repair would be cost-effective. Keep in mind that medical equipment repair is usually very costly. You may be asked to bid the repair job or to do without the equipment for a while. Several alternative solutions are possible.

First, if your local community college or area vocational-technical school has an electronics technology or biomedical equipment technology program, contact the program director to determine if the program's students can repair your equipment. You will be asked to pay for all parts, which can be expensive. But, generally, these programs can provide you with a list of replacement parts, and you will be responsible for contacting the suppliers for prices, unless it is a common part, say, a resistor. Once you have obtained the list, meet with your administrator, present the list, and explain the savings you will enjoy by using a student program to make the repairs. If the costs are still too high, then ask your administrator what course of action you should pursue: develop specifications for bidding on a new piece of equipment, fill out paperwork to have equipment removed from your inventory, or attempt to borrow the equipment from another program, school, or clinical site.

In many instances, health care facility administrators have a graveyard storeroom of equipment no longer in use. Sometimes this equipment will be much newer than yours but either too slow or out-of-date for the needs of the facility. Public-owned health care facilities administrators are usually thrilled to transfer their outdated equipment to another public-owned institution, such as a school. They are also glad to donate outdated supplies. However, you must initiate the suggestion. Simply meet with the appropriate official to determine if there is any available stored equipment. If so, you will probably then have to arrange to meet with the top administrator. Volunteer to inspect the storeroom yourself, pick out what you want, transport it, and repair it. If agreement is reached, action will be required from the health facility's board of trustees before the process can begin. You may have to agree to take many pieces of equipment in order to get what you want, because this is a golden opportunity for the health facility to unload unwanted items. In this way, you can salvage many good parts from the unwanted items. Also, your Health Occupations Students of America group can have a competition to come up with creative decorations, furniture, and so forth from what remains. For example, a bed pan makes an eye-catching flower pot.

A second alternative is to share equipment with another program, preferably in your building. You would need to correlate your needs with the faculty in the other program. The equipment, though, would be the responsibility of the program listing it on its inventory.

A third alternative is to borrow equipment from a health care facility for the few hours you would need it. Obviously, this tactic would work only for rarely used equipment items and would require the full knowledge and permission of officials at the health care facility. On occasion, medical equipment suppliers will provide you with a demonstration model for a period of time, in the hope you will purchase one in the near future.

Of course, the best situation is the one where you can repair your equipment or buy new equipment. Do some comparison shopping. Consult your business card file and call those toll-free numbers. Ask for catalogs. Call the manufacturers of your current equipment and request service prices. There is a manufacturer's equipment tag on teach piece of equipment, which gives pertinent information you would need (i.e., model number, serial number, wattage, etc.). It is a metal tag usually located on the back or bottom of the equipment.

If you are allowed to purchase new equipment, then a specification must be written for bidding. Most schools try to let equipment bids out only once a year. Carefully develop your equipment specifications. List things like table, floor, or hand-held model; size, speed, and wattage requirements; load or weight capacity; operator and repair manuals; optional cycles, color, or gauges; and safety requirements. The best way to determine these items is to carefully review all available models from the product information and medical equipment catalogs you have collected from manufacturers.

Once bids are received, school boards usually accept the lowest one unless you convince them that the product will not handle your needs or is not cost-effective in the long run (e.g., reagents may be very expensive for that model.) Otherwise, suppliers should contact you regarding an appropriate date for installation. Once the item has been installed, you should read the operator's manual and thoroughly check each operational function.

Check with manufacturers to determine maintenance needs and schedules for your equipment. Sometimes we forget to have professional cleaning done on our old faithful equipment, such as microscopes, dental chairs, centrifuges, sterilizers, typewriters, and dictaphones. Most equipment that is regularly used should be professionally cleaned and serviced once a year. A variety of students using the equipment all year long increases maintenance needs.

Also, an inventory of all small or low-cost tools should be carried out. Such tools can usually be replaced or repaired without taking bids. If not, be sure to include these items in your equipment or supply requests or in your annual maintenance contracts, if the tools are mechanical.

Carefully review every planned laboratory situation, and make a list of all the tools and equipment needed for each exercise. Multiply that by the expected number of students in order to determine the number of individual-use tools. Check the capacity of group-use equipment to determine its adequacy. You may need to stagger exercises or assign half of the students a different exercise, then switch exercises on the next laboratory day.

Acquiring adequate equipment that is well maintained is an ongoing process that often requires several years of slow, steady persistence. The payoff, though, can be marvelous. You will have a student laboratory that is envied by all.

References

Bennett, J. V., and P. S. Brachman (eds.) (1986). *Hospital Infections* (2nd ed.). Boston: Little, Brown.

Hughes, J. and W. Jarvis (1985). "Epidemiology of Nonsocomial Infections." In E. Lennette, A. Balows, W. Hausler Jr., H. J.

Shadomy (eds.). *Manual of Clinical Microbiology* (4th ed.) (pp. 99–104). Washington: American Society for Microbiology.

U.S. Department of Health and Human Services Public Health Service Centers for Disease Control (June 1988). "Update: Universal Precautions for Prevention of Transmission of Human Immunodeficiency Virus, Hepatitis B Virus, and Other Bloodborne Pathogens in Health-Care Settings." *MMWR* 37(24), 377–82, 387–88.

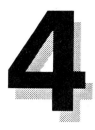

Clinical Instruction: Teaching the Job

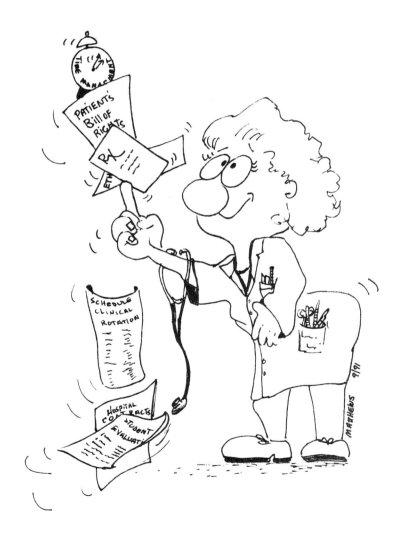

The unique aspect of a VHO teacher's role consists of clinical instruction. Whereas most teachers spend their teaching time in the classroom with their students, health occupations education teachers divide their time between the classroom, a simulation laboratory, and the clinical agency. While in the clinical agency, the teacher is a "guest," taking advantage of the actual situation rather than a simulation situation. Teaching moments become often just that — a moment. Learning to take advantage of that moment and turn it into a teaching moment spotlights the best of teachers.

In some programs, the teacher is responsible for the actual instruction and supervision of students in the clinical setting; in others, the teacher only facilitates the clinical experience, and another individual is designated as the clinical instructor. In either case, the instructor is responsible for the welfare of the students as well as the welfare of the individuals whom the students care for. This responsibility can be overwhelming for a new teacher. Being responsible for 12–15 students, sometimes spread throughout a clinical agency, always behind closed doors or privacy curtains, constitutes a real challenge for the VHO teacher.

This chapter is designed to discuss your role as a clinical instructor and to offer you some foundation for the role and responsibility that you undertake as a supervisor of clinical instruction.

☞ PLANNING CLINICAL EXPERIENCES

Clinical experiences for health occupations education students must be planned and sequenced the same as classroom instruction is. There must be objectives for each experience that identify what students are to learn, how they will learn it, and to what level of competency. Often, as teachers, we find planning and sequencing instruction a very difficult task because we cannot always guarantee that all of the experiences we desire for our students will be available as we need them. Nor can we guarantee that all students will have the same experience, that it will be a normal experience, or that it will be an experience that can ever be duplicated. In addition, we sometimes neglect to write objectives for the clinical experiences we require of our students. Yet it makes sense to agree that clinical experience for students must be planned and sequenced.

Learning theory dictates that the best learning occurs when classroom instruction is followed by the opportunity to put theory into practice. In reality, this cannot happen for every student in health occupations. In reality, the instructor plans, one student experiences, and the instructor facilitates the learning of others using a variety of teaching techniques. In writing learning objectives for students, health occupations education teachers have learned to be very creative. For example, instead of having a student care for an individual following gallbladder surgery, the objective can be for the student to care for a postoperative patient or to follow a patient from surgery to recovery. These objectives and skills are generic, offering a planned, meaningful experience for more than just one student. Students can then compare the recovery of postoperative patients either among ones they cared for or among those cared for by their classmates. The health occupations teacher has followed learning theory, has provided experiences for more than one student, and has planned the clinical instruction.

CLINICAL SUPERVISION OF STUDENTS

Who is responsible for the clinical supervision of students? Although types of clinical instruction may vary, the teacher is ultimately responsible for supervision of students because it is the teacher who will submit their grades.

Use of Clinical Instructors

In some health occupations education programs, a clinical instructor is hired to instruct students in the clinical area. Such instructors may be currently employed by the clinical agency or they may work part-time at the school, called on only when students are in the clinical setting. In this situation, the classroom teacher has a coordinator's role, making necessary arrangements, seeing that the clinical instructor is knowledgeable about the learning objectives, and working with the clinical instructor in evaluating students' performance.

In other health occupations education programs, the clinical instructor may be an employer, such as a dentist or physician. In this situation, the classroom teacher works cooperatively with the clinical instructor, placing the student in the experience and making frequent checks to see if the student is performing satisfactorily. In this situation, the classroom teacher must have good relationships with clinical instructors because they may not be available immediately if a problem arises. In evaluating students, both individuals are involved, but it is the educator who is more knowledgeable about the process and ultimately evaluates the student.

In still other situations, the classroom instructor is also the clinical instructor, supervising a number of students in a cooperating clinical agency. Here the teacher must work closely with the clinical agency, alerting staff to the arrival of students, the skill level of students, the learning objectives, and the evaluation process. The instructor often is responsible for the assignment of students but must work closely with the individual in charge. The individuals involved must use their skills to the highest level, making sure that students undergo the necessary planned experiences. During clinical experiences, the teacher relies on information from the agency staff to keep posted regarding changes in the condition of patients and new procedures. Agency staff may also assist in the supervision of students assigned to care for the patients under their responsibility. However, the teacher is ultimately responsible for the performance evaluation of all of the students.

Clinical supervision of students represents an integral part of the role of the health occupations teacher. Developing a high level of comfort in this role is one of the most difficult skills to acquire as a health occupations education teacher. Be assured that over time, the needed clinical supervision skills will develop.

☞ MAKING CLINICAL PRACTICE RELEVANT

Learning theory dictates that learning is best when it builds from the simple to the complex and from the easy to the difficult and that experiential learning is best when correlated with didactic learning. Your job as a clinical instructor is to make that experiential learning relevant for students. When all beginning students are at an inexperienced level, where do you begin?

With clinical experiences, as with classroom experiences, you must begin with objectives. In the case of clinical objectives, these must be individualized for each student, and each patient must be assessed for applicability to those objectives. Usually, objectives for the clinical setting will give relevance to the learning experiences for your students.

Clinical objectives can be in each of the domains — cognitive, psychomotor, or affective. They are usually activity oriented but can be written at the application level of cognitive because the students will be applying to an actual situation the knowledge they have learned in class. Each clinical activity should have at least one objective, usually more. This helps students to know why they are in the clinical setting and what they are supposed to learn.

Clinical experience dictates that in the beginning, students perform simple skills. Often they have been able to practice those skills in a simulation laboratory prior to performing them in the actual clinical setting. In the beginning, you as the instructor will want to find an organizational tool to be able to keep track of all of your students. This could be as simple as using index cards (have each student complete one with necessary information for you) or limiting what students can do until you are sure they can do it unsupervised. Some skills can be safely performed so as to be evaluated in a summative way; other skills require your direct observation. In nursing, for example, a student recording the intake of a meal does not require your direct observation and would not represent a critical situation if it were not exact. Taking a blood pressure, however, requires your direct supervision because you need to hear the sounds at the same time as the student to be sure they are hearing them correctly. After students develop some essential early skills, you will be able to concentrate on more advanced skills and then higher-level objectives, such as synthesis and analysis, helping them to actually put the knowledge from class to the test.

Evaluating student performance: The most difficult aspect of clinical supervision after you get the assignments down is the evaluation. Evaluating student performance could be compared to evaluating the performance of subordinates if you were in a management or supervisory role before becoming a teacher. Evaluation is done in a formative manner or several glimpses, and summative, which summarizes many formative observations. Students should be evaluated against the standards of the profession but should be given gradual opportunities to achieve those standards. If they can perform at the standards of the profession as a beginning student, they should not have to complete the educational program.

☞ ANSWERING THE ASSERTION: HEY, THAT'S NOT THE WAY WE LEARNED IT!

This section will discuss what to do when a student moans, "That's not the way we learned it," reasons for this lamentation and how to troubleshoot it ahead of time, and how to establish the link between the ideal and reality.

In the classroom, students are frequently led to believe there is only one way to do things. This is of course not true, and if your students have a very narrow mind-set, then they are being set up for frustration and failure. In our teaching it is sometimes a pitfall we fall into because of the use of the textbook case. Remember—your classroom and laboratory settings are tightly controlled environments until your student is out in the clinical setting. Therefore the basic examples that your student learns from constitute the textbook case.

Of course, you will augment each learning situation with personal experiences to illustrate and emphasize certain points. Such war stories serve more than just to liven up a lecture or discussion. They show that indeed in some instance, things were not the way you learned them. This is an excellent opportunity to give students an insight into the clinical setting, what you expected, what really happened, and how you handled it. If you handled it well, good, and if you did not but learned how to handle it in the future, even better. Students need to realize that when confronted with an unusual or unexpected situation, they have the skills and knowledge to handle it.

"Hey, that's not the way we learned it" very often points up the uncomfortable situation we are faced with when we do not know what to do, at least not initially. At this point you need to review the critical thinking skills of your students. They have the information needed. Do they know how to take that information to a higher level of problem solving? Students may be rather slow at this unless you have been practicing with them and demonstrating how they can attain a higher order of thinking.

If you are teaching a skill, you can still demand critical thinking from your students. Build on the skill they are performing for you, and throw in some alternative situations.

EXAMPLE: In learning CPR, students must have basic assessment and performance skills. While performing CPR on a baby, I call out, "Oh, no, the baby is throwing up!" Immediately students must respond. What are they going to do? Turn the head to the side. Clear the mouth. How far down? Reassess the airway or begin ventilation again? Higher order of thinking. In real life, this is going to happen. But in practice and in class, the situation is often not given.

The student needs to know that, even though it is not part of the lecture, as you are performing the Heimlich maneuver, the victim is often throwing up on your foot. So what do you do? By continually putting your students in the position of expecting the unexpected, they start to think globally and to look at the whole picture with its possibilities and probabilities.

The other component in "that's not the way we learned it" is the belief that there is only one way to do something. Again, that is often not the case. As you are teaching, broaden your students' horizons by including different methods or at least mentioning other ways of achieving the same goal.

EXAMPLE: How does one tie shoe laces? Each one of us has our own way of tying shoes. Whether you double-knot or double-bow, is one method more secure than the other? You probably could argue that one is better than the other. In reality, the way you tie a shoe is based on the way you were taught and which is easiest for you. Remind your students that we assimilate what we are taught with what aptitudes and abilities we have.

Reality Versus the Ideal

Very often as we teach the textbook scenario, we forget to remind students that there may not be, say, enough linens because of cost or equipment breakdowns or because they were simply not put away. The student needs to think, what is most important? Do I have to have this in order to complete my task? Will my job or patient care be compromised because of what I do or do not do? This is a very important component in the relationship between reality and the ideal. There may be legitimate reasons why a task cannot be completed the way one learned it. What will be compromised if it is not done? In the beginning, your students lack the sophistication to know if this is acceptable or not. Again, they need the skills to reevaluate a situation, incorporate the legalities if applicable, and implement their higher-order-of-thinking skills.

The student needs to consider each situation as it arises and make a decision based on knowledge, expertise, and what is available.

There is no doubt that students will run into the individual who says, "Oh, you learned it that way in class, but we don't do that here." Aha, the dilemma for the student. Assure students that whether or not they choose to follow that advice is totally up to them. They have the knowledge, they know what is expected of them, and they now have a new piece of information requiring them to either take a stand or do as the Romans do. It should be a conscious decision. Your students will need practice with these scenarios. Role playing helps students identify these problems when they arise and gives them confidence in their choices.

In order to troubleshoot this possible problem, which can occur at any time, you need to be realistic about your teaching. True, everything you teach is important, but many things can be modified. Therefore, it becomes paramount that you identify what cannot be changed. That must be written in stone for your students. But also be advised, do not do so unless it is really important. Sometimes, we as teachers think some things cannot be compromised. We are wrong. How do you know whether it is right or wrong? Check with your community, your advisory board, and the like. This issue will be discussed further in the chapter on curriculum development.

☞ EVALUATING STUDENT PERFORMANCE

One key to good evaluation is a good instrument. A good instrument is one that is simple to use, appropriate in its definition of the areas to be evaluated, and objective in its administration. Whereas the optimum situation would eliminate subjectivity in a student performance evaluation, such is not realistic. No matter how hard you try, because you are a caring professional, subjectivity enters the process. As an educated health professional, you are knowledgeable about the role of the health professional you are preparing, and your judgment as to level of performance — satisfactory or unsatisfactory — is critical to the education of others for your discipline.

A simple instrument is one that is easy to understand and one that considers all aspects of performance appropriate for the level of the student. Too often, when evaluating students in the beginning of their experiences, we utilize an instrument designed to be used at the end of the course work. There is nothing wrong with having several instruments, each used at different points in the program. Beginning skills and behaviors should have more value for the student just starting out, but as students progress through the program, their beginning skills and behaviors are expected to become routine and consequently assumed to be there, and the evaluation should focus on other areas.

An instrument that is appropriate in its definition of area to be evaluated is one that describes the performance and the acceptable level. It should reflect the psychomotor skills appropriate for the term as well as the application of classroom knowledge. It should be shared with the student at the beginning of the term so that expectations are known.

An instrument that is objective is one that allows the evaluator either to rate the described skill as satisfactory or unsatisfactory or to rate it on a grading scale using letter grades (A, B, C) or points (e.g., 93–100 equals an A). An instrument that gives the evaluator an even distribution of choices, 4 instead of 5 for instance, forces the evaluator to make a choice rather than selecting the middle. Some evaluation tools add an N.O. category for any performance that was not observed.

The second key to a good evaluation consists of the formative evaluations collected prior to the summative evaluations. The more formative evaluations there are, the easier it is for you as a teacher to see patterns of behavior. Optimally, you need to look for patterns that show improvement and consistency of behavior. When the patterns are positive, the summative evaluation will be positive. When the patterns are erratic, the clinical instructor should intervene with strategies to help the student improve to an acceptable level. If the patterns show no attainment in achievement of the acceptable level, the student may need to be dismissed from the program. In any evaluation situation, however, the student has a right to due process. Due process means that the student knew the standards of expectation, was informed the standards were not being achieved, was given instruction or interventions to help meet the standard, and had reasonable opportunity to do so. Due process does not mean the student is given several opportunities to cause harm to an individual.

Clinical evaluation requires that the instructor gather as much data as possible with which to make an appropriate judgment. This translates to copious notes, made as often as necessary, but at least daily, especially in the beginning. Use of a tape recorder to dictate notes is one way to keep up with this process. Using the cards that students turned in that identify their needs is another way to keep up. Notes can be put on the card immediately after a procedure is completed and later translated into the appropriate evaluation. A clipboard, carried by the instructor is another way. Whichever way you choose, the key is to keep good notes as an activity is occurring, because it is often too difficult to reconstruct each instance for every student at the end of the day. As you become more skilled as a clinical instructor, you will become more skilled as a clinical evaluator as well.

☞ DEVELOPING AFFILIATION AGREEMENTS

Official relationships with managers and administrators are necessary and important for creating formal contracts that admit your students into an agency.

Agency staff members are the key people you will want to know on a personal level. Staff will have many perceptions about your students, the most prominent being that your students will take time away from their very busy days. Your job is to convince and show staff that students will in fact help them.

Your first responsibility is to the students. No matter how much expertise you have in any clinical field, students come first. Staff will be cooperative when they know that you will look after students. Acknowledgment to staff that you support their clinical knowledge allows them to share their knowledge with students.

Getting to know the staff is important. Find out how long they have worked, what they do best, how they may help your students meet learning goals, and what they like best about their job. This information must be obtained sometime before students appear in their area. Even though you have made the necessary formal arrangements, you must informally contact people in the clinical area. Managers and supervisors often forget to tell staff about the formal arrangements. Leave written material that indicates who and how many are coming and how long they will be there. Be sure to include your name and a means of contacting you. Update students' schedules frequently, and call if last-minute changes occur. If you worked in any of these clinical areas prior to teaching, you have the advantage of knowing some of the staff.

Concentrate on your students. Staff will be grateful that they do not need to watch your students. They will learn to trust you to take care of the students. Make frequent rounds and talk to staff. Ask specific questions such as "What procedures are scheduled?" "Is there something students could help with?" Listen to the answers, and include students in any appropriate conversations so they know that you and the staff are coordinating and supervising their experiences. Instructors have three groups of clientele: staff, patients, and students. You will need to attend to the needs of all of these groups while your students are having clinical experiences.

Offer immediate feedback to students when appropriate, but remember to counsel students in private about significant problems. When problems occur, face them early and head-on. Find the source and listen to all sides before commenting. Determine who will help you solve the problem, and contact that person. Take action to solve the problem, then give the feedback to the clinical staff and students involved.

Even though staff are very important for students to obtain good experiences, the supervisors and managers will have a great deal of influence on the fate of your clinical privileges. Take time to meet with supervisors and keep them informed of students' progress, emphasize positive experiences, and relate the success stories of former students.

Learn to manage student criticism of the facility. Often when students learn new skills, they see all its applications in strictly black-and-white terms. They are unable to see that unique adaptations of rules and procedures are made by experienced staff. They do not understand that the patient's or client's needs require adjustments in some techniques. A good approach to their criticisms is to discuss the concern openly with them and try to have them generate possible reasons for the action observed. Generating ideas is a preliminary step to enhancing critical thinking skills, too. If the violation is of a serious nature, you should take responsibility to approach the staff member, relate the incident observed, and ask for suggestions on how to handle the student reactions after the incident. Be sure that you indicate both your support for the individual and your responsibility for students by using a nonconfrontational approach.

Remind students that their purpose is to learn some skills about a health career, not to provide critiques of the institution. No institution is perfect, and you must make the decision about how much discrepancy between ideal and real situations can be tolerated.

Your personality is your best asset. Be open and listen to staff. Be a resource for staff with the same clinical background as yours. The most important student objectives are not always the most important staff objectives. Do not give the impression that you cannot or will not do difficult jobs. Observe how to be helpful. Your first responsibility is to the students, but when you see a job that you or students could do that does not compromise learning, volunteer to do it. A helping attitude shows staff that students can provide tangible work and help for them. Once staff know that students can be a help to them, staff may be more willing to work with students and offer them good opportunities.

There will always be one or two staff members who will not agree that you or your students are worth their time. Spend your time with and turn your efforts to helpful staff. If one staff member is causing many problems, it may be worthwhile to find out in a private conversation exactly what the problems are. Often these staff members are more unhappy with their particular work situation, and students are an easy target on whom to vent their frustrations.

Staff are the gatekeepers of clinical opportunities. You are dependent on staff to allow students to obtain good experiences. Staff can find those extra areas that may make the difference between a mediocre and an excellent experience. Treasure their expertise, give them credit for knowledge, and always keep them informed about students.

Letting the clinical staff know about your students — where they are in their program, what they should be able to do skillwise, what objectives you have for their learning experiences — will give the staff the information they need both to suggest assignments for students and to help you learn about procedures you would like your students to experience. Informing the clinical staff about your schedule will allow them to prepare for the students, which could be very supportive.

At the end of the year or semester, write an official summary report, and send it through formal channels at the institution. Send a personal note of thanks to units or particular staff members who worked with students during the year.

When staff start regarding student contact as an opportunity to share knowledge and skills, you will know that your efforts at developing staff relationships have succeeded.

When you are in a clinical agency with your students, you are often a guest in that agency, as your salary is not paid by the clinical agency but by your school district. Establishing, developing, and nurturing agency relationships will be critical if you are to succeed in obtaining the best learning opportunities for your students. Even though your students may be, for example, respiratory care students, it is helpful to have good working relationships with other agency departments as well. The medical laboratory, nursing, and occupational and physical therapy departments may have experiences to offer your students.

It is characteristic of health care professionals to be very supportive of students; they want to help. We as educators should not take unfair advantage of our colleagues but should try to involve them as much as necessary in the task of providing appropriate experiences for our students. These colleagues can provide us with that extra set of eyes that we don't have.

☞ RECRUITING AND ORIENTING CLINICAL FACULTY

A valuable component of any health occupations program is the selection of faculty and assistant instructors. Personal interviews should be conducted by the lead teacher. The prospective faculty needs to be informed of the guidelines and how they should be implemented. Sharing the philosophy of the instructor with this person explains the overall content as it relates to the student, and in this manner, the teacher can evaluate in a professional manner.

The teacher should set guidelines according to the state department of education or college competencies. In program reviews, which are conducted on a regular basis, these competencies must be included and taught to students.

The teacher conveys the knowledge to all the members of the group in the required areas that must be covered in the program. The instructors should be invited to sit in on classroom teaching to give them a better understanding of what the student is learning. This should assist them in following through to see that students successfully complete the performance of these skills. The teacher has the responsibility to direct and implement a course of action for the assistant instructors to follow. In this way the certainty of students' acquiring the necessary knowledge and skills continues to be under the supervision of the lead teacher. The assistant instructor must also be capable of relating this to students. Each member of the assisting faculty should participate in scheduled meetings with the instructor in which guidelines are presented so that all the teaching methods will be consistent. It is recommended that the assistant instructor keep in close touch with the teacher, and a specific time for the report should be designated. Good communication between all parties enables the teacher to follow the progress of students.

The evaluation process is completed by the use of a form prepared by the teacher and containing the necessary competency skills that students must complete. This is done during the clinical or practical period of the program. Certain competencies are taught, and each student is observed by the individual assistant instructor. In the performance of these skills, the level of learning is elevated, and confidence is developed by the student. This is an important component, because the assistant instructor must be able to impart constant supportive teaching to the student. The end result of such supervision is that the student develops individual knowledge and self-confidence in the new learning opportunity, which enables the student to progress at a reasonable pace and still feel comfortable with the training received. The assistant instructor should, at this time, develop a rapport with the student so that either may initiate personal conferences.

The advantage of a vocational program continues to be its flexible scheduling, one that has options for a student to receive training and still be able to accommodate a job. This is most appreciated by students because working is sometimes a necessity.

The importance of the evaluation process completed by the assistant instructors cannot be overstated, because the teacher is ultimately responsible for the success of the program. Being well informed is an essential attribute that a competent teacher must have.

The principal instructor has the responsibility to interview assistants for the teaching staff. Such instructors are informed of the curriculum, the agenda, and the department of education guidelines that are required. The assistant instructors are familiarized with the skills and competencies taught to the students in the classroom. Meetings are scheduled to confer with assistant personnel in order to facilitate consistency in the program.

The assistants are requested to maintain close contact with the teacher for the purpose of following the progress of the students. At this time, any necessary conferences with particular students are scheduled. The supervision required is explained, and the assistant is included in the evaluation of each student at the end of the program. The teacher prepares an evaluation form listing the various competencies that must be accomplished by the student and used for evaluation by the assistant or clinical instructors.

☞ PLACING STUDENTS IN THEIR FIRST JOB

Another basic component of a health occupations program is preparing students for a future job opportunity. At the very beginning of a course, the areas of interview skills, knowledge of ethical behavior during a job placement conference, reliability, and commitment to an employer are emphasized to students.

The student who has been well prepared in a health occupations program promises to be a better employee. The background education that the student receives ensures a more competent caregiver. Teaching students how to participate in a job interview can be done effectively by the use of videos, visual example, and role play with explanation. Students should be aware of proper dress, be ready to answer pertinent questions from an employer, have a desirable attitude, and ask some previously prepared questions about the prospective job offering.

One important aspect the student must remember is to read and understand all rules and regulations given and to be certain what the job responsibilities are before signing any application. Each job description is unique depending on the place of employment and placement of the health care worker, which varies from one area to another.

The conduct displayed to an employer will have a bearing on receiving an offer. The student should be advised to have several references ready if a request for them is made. Remind students that permission must be obtained from people before giving their name as a reference.

Reliability, dependability, and competence in the new job cannot be overstated, and students should be made aware that a record of employment is long lasting and their job reference requests may be reviewed during the work experience.

A beneficial exposure during class is an open house, when various employers in the community come to the classroom at designated times to inform students of job opportunities in their field. At this time, students may request a job application and may schedule an appointment for an interview with the employer of choice.

In the health care field, commitment to a place of employment is extremely vital, as the employee is responsible for numerous tasks and must be dependable, or an employer is placed in the situation of substituting for both. This creates a hardship and is usually noted on the employment record. The same situation occurs if there is a history of tardiness. The student should keep this in mind when applying to and being placed in the first job.

If the student has a sense of self-discipline and has been attentive in class, the same assertiveness will remain when employed. The groundwork has been laid in class for the continued practice of being reliable and capable. When employment practice is included as part of the curriculum in a health occupations program, it enables the student to understand the significance of the learned resources taught. The training received is valuable in preparing students for the work force, which is appreciated by employers in the various areas in which students will work. It will make a favorable impression and will generate a referral source for future potential applicants.

Health occupations programs that include preparation for the student to enter the work force through clinical experiences provide the ability to conduct personal interviews. Reliability and competence are qualities a health care worker must have and are observed by potential employers in clinical rotations. The instructor assists the student in awareness and understanding of the rules and regulations in the various work areas.

Exposure to the employers in the community is offered to the student for the benefit of explanation of duties and responsibilities in each organization. The student is made aware of how important the individual work record can be and how the practices can follow the health care giver through all job experiences.

5
The Learners: Knowing the Students

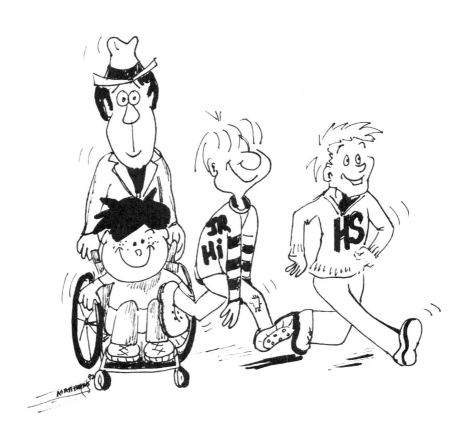

☞ CHARACTERIZING MIDDLE SCHOOL STUDENTS

Parents grow watchful as their children mature through the elementary grades. They know that changes will come with the transition from childhood to adolescence. Many names have been used to describe this group: transescents, preadolescents, in-between ages, young adolescents (McEwin and Thomason, 1989). A child between the ages of 10 and 14 may undergo a smooth, gradual, and relatively serene transition from childhood or may experience tantrums, tears, and trauma. It's hard to forecast the emotional climate that will surround a given child's entry into adolescence.

One thing is certain — early adolescents are experiencing change. In fact, physical changes are more dramatic during these years than at any other time in the life cycle, with the exception of infancy (Van Hoose and Strahan, 1987). The rate at which the transition will occur is difficult to predict. Some children change overnight, and others enter early adolescence slowly and over an extended period of time.

We can expect identity to be an issue during early adolescence for several reasons. First, changes brought on by biological maturation demand a reassessment of who one is and how these changes relate to other aspects of the self. Second, the acquisition of new thinking processes enables young adolescents to reflect on how they are seen by others. Third, adolescents achieve changes in autonomy. With these changes come experiences in new arenas, and their performance in these new arenas gives young adolescents additional information about themselves (Benson, Williams, and Johnson, 1987).

Fortunately, in recent years, interest in the education and welfare of this age group has increased significantly. This interest has intensified for at least two major reasons. First is the recognition that there is a serious lack of specialized knowledge about this stage of development. A second major factor is the growing recognition of a widespread increase in the problems experienced by large numbers of early adolescents, e.g., increased pregnancy and suicide rates and tragically high levels of illicit drug and alcohol use (Carnegie Council, 1989).

The remainder of this section will briefly address some of the major characteristics of early adolescents, including their physical, social, and intellectual development. It is not a comprehensive treatment of the topic but rather is included to serve both as a reminder for those already knowledgeable about early adolescence and as an introduction for those who have not had the opportunity to study this fascinating stage of human development.

Physical Development

Young adolescents are concerned about their physical and sexual development or lack thereof, and often this concern becomes a central theme in their life. As young adolescents make their way through the many physical changes, they believe that someone is always watching them or that they are always on stage. Because young adolescents think they are always being watched, they become engaged in mirror checking. They are drawn to mirrors like metal to a magnet and are constantly checking themselves out (Van Hoose and Strahan, 1987). Due to the increased interest in oneself during this time of development, privacy at home, in their room, or in some other place becomes quite important. After all, being on stage day after day is stressful, and a young adolescent may want to close the door in order to eliminate the imaginary audience for at least a little while.

We have already said that growth during this part of the life cycle is second only to that which takes place in infancy. Additionally, growth does not take place evenly, and certain body parts, most notably the extremities, develop early and more rapidly. Young adolescents become embarrassed about their decreased ability to walk or reach out, because simple movements often lead to falls, spills, or other undesirable outcomes due to rapid growth. The average gain in height of young adolescents is from 2 to 4 inches per year; the average weight gain per year is 8–10 pounds. From the age of 10 to 15, this means that the average young adolescent may gain 10–20 inches in height and 40–50 pounds in weight (Van Hoose and Strahan, 1987).

The pituitary gland generates increases in the hormones that serve as a catalyst for more rapid growth. Huge quantities of adrenalin are released in the body. This hormonal secretion, which can be compared to an electrical power surge, makes adolescents squirm, move, stretch, and, perhaps, yell at the top of their lungs. Observations confirm that young adolescents continually compare themselves to others. If they are bigger or smaller, shorter or taller than what they perceive to be the norm, they worry about themselves. If they deviate from the norm, they think that something is wrong. Middle-grade students spend a lot of time worrying about their physical differences—both at home and at school during classes.

Social Development

Emotions begin to play a key role in the life of the young adolescent. Young adolescents become more idealistic and are frustrated when their ideals do not materialize. The range of the emotions felt is of greater width but more closely resembles those of childhood than those of late adolescence. At times, emotions may be volatile, and that is when they can reach remarkable highs and lows, e.g., jealousy, spite, envy. Fortunately, emotions are more easily forgotten during this time period.

It is not uncommon for such youth to lose themselves in anger, love, or fear as they experiment with the emergence of more adultlike feelings. They often criticize themselves and others unrealistically, which may lead to feelings of uncertainty, anger, and frustration. Anger is short-lived but is common among this age group.

It is also during this stage that feelings about parents, teachers, peers, and others begin to undergo significant changes. Interpersonal relationships take on a new perspective as the peer group gains in importance and adults are looked at from new perspectives. The new perspectives include the recognition that even the most trusted and loved adults are not perfect and cannot always be depended on (McEwin and Thomason, 1989).

Early adolescents are searching for self-identity amid confused sex-role models, a changing environment, and the impact of puberty. They experience not only exceptionally turbulent emotions but also a tremendous flexibility in self-concept. Fear, which often manifests itself in early adolescence, may emerge in the form of worries. Questions these youth may be dealing with include: Am I normal? Does anyone like me? What if I fail in school? What if I don't make the team? Fears related to areas such as death and religion are also sources of uncertainty. The fear of being ostracized or ridiculed by peers is a powerful force and at times wields so much influence that early adolescents may compromise their own personal convictions rather than defy the peer group (McEwin and Thomason, 1989).

Young people are often coerced by parents, schools, and the media to emulate adults. These sources, which sometimes encourage young people to grow up, to be more like adults, and therefore to do all that adults do but at a younger and younger age, detract from the experiences of young adolescence. When this tendency occurs throughout young adolescence, then by the end of their high school years, some young people have already experienced all that life has to offer. This includes boy-girl relationships that start in the elementary years, that lead to dating and beginning intimacy in the middle years, and culminate in adult-level sexual intimacy in the late middle years or high school years. Some people think it is cute to get boys and girls together to ensure that they will know how to relate to the opposite sex. Such early experiences lead young people to the point of feeling that they have done it all and that nothing exciting is left to try.

Adolescent students should be encouraged to do what feels natural at their age, such as having same-sex friendships, as opposed to encouraging them to engage in adultlike relationships. There will be interest by girls in members of the opposite sex because girls mature earlier socially. However, this interest can be kept on a casual friendship level in most cases if parents and teachers provide proper guidance.

Boys are also interested in and puzzled by girls. They would certainly prefer, in most cases, to view and love them from afar. If given the opportunity, girls will spend most of their time with girls and boys with boys, and this is perfectly natural (Van Hoose and Strahan, 1987). Social development concerns are dominant in the life of young adolescents. They crave guidance in social skills so that they will be less likely to be embarrassed and more likely to be accepted by their peers and significant adults. Though they may reject some guidance from parents and teachers, they do accept a great deal of input. It is our duty to provide sensitive input and structured programs that anticipate and fulfill the needs of young adolescents.

Intellectual Development

During the time of young adolescence, students begin to develop the power of abstract thinking. They begin to think of the world around them and themselves in new ways. For the first time, young adolescents can "think about thinking" — which often confuses them. This is shaped by interactions between their experiences and their new powers of reasoning, so reflexive thinking becomes especially important. Van Hoose and Strahan (1987) reported that Piaget's 1977 book *The Science of Education and Psychology of the Child* indicates that mental development occurs in four distinct phases. Each child passes through the stages in the same sequence, but by varying rates.

The logical operations of each stage develop from the operations of the previous stage. Within this framework, the early adolescent period is a time of transition from the concrete operations stage to the formal operations stage and may begin as early as the eleventh year of life. The concrete stage is a very conceptual one in which information is organized around categories that are generalized from one instance to another. The formal stage is characterized by formal thought and utilizes the components of logic and reasoning in decision making. This process constitutes the beginning of adult thought.

It should be fully realized that the cognitive development of early adolescents is highly variable among individuals. In fact, only approximately one third of eighth-grade students can consistently demonstrate formal reasoning. Many early adolescents are still limited in their reasoning to immediate or past experiences and have difficulty handling problems with more than two simultaneous dimensions or relations. Others have negotiated the transition between the real and the impossible and are able to hypothesize contrary-to-fact possibilities. As in other areas of early adolescent development, wide diversity exists and should be carefully considered when planning learning experiences.

☞ DESCRIBING HIGH SCHOOL STUDENTS

Adolescence represents the transitional period between childhood and maturity. This phase of life presents many challenges as the high school student is learning to formulate mature values, develop adult relationships, and improve cognitive competencies such as abstract thinking. One minute their parents and teachers are requiring them to act like mature adults, and the next minute treating them like little children. The adolescents themselves fluctuate from logical thinking and rational behavior to childlike dependency, ignoring responsibility and desiring to have needs met by someone else. Rebellion and even delinquency may occur as a young person attempts to establish autonomy and self-identity.

Peer pressure continues to be a major influencing factor in the life of adolescents, and peer groups become even more structured during high school. However, during later adolescence, individuals with high self-esteem tend to be able to make judgments on behavior that are based on their beliefs, and they are not as strongly influenced by peers. A major question then becomes how to assist high school students in developing positive self-esteem.

Friendships with others of the same sex and boy-girl relationships tend to occupy much of an adolescent's time. The need to be accepted is characterized by dressing alike (same brands) and using the same expressions in their speech. The "valley girls" and different gangs are current examples that most people have been exposed to by the media.

High but realistic expectations need to be established. If expectations are set very low for students, they will achieve only to that level of expectation and no further. High expectations encourage students to reach a little higher. Always give praise for work accomplished on setting a goal or on a goal met. Also, let them know it is all right to reevaluate a goal.

A good sense of humor makes instruction fun for all parties involved. More learning and retention of ideas occur when students are enjoying what is happening during the instructional process. A point to keep in mind is that humor should never be used at any person's expense.

Because of the tendency toward rebellion, being firm and correcting behavior immediately are important. Helping the student maintain self-respect and accepting the student but not the misbehavior are critical to a good teacher-student relationship. Treating students with equality and consistency is very important to adolescents.

You may find that this age group requires that a thorough orientation and enthusiastic motivation be provided by the instructor. It is important for the teacher to role model desired attitudes and behaviors. Among some groups, social skills are lacking, and expressions such as "please" and "thank you" are not normally used. Teachers must understand that they must use the language and phrases expected of students. The teacher should regularly use "Yes, ma'am" or Yes, sir" out of respect to students if they expect the same treatment in return. Respect from students is one of the most important classroom tools you may acquire. Respect is gained through establishing fair and consistent expectations and treating each student as a consumer requiring a high-quality education.

☞ ASSISTING SPECIAL NEEDS STUDENTS

Agencies that receive federal funds must not discriminate on the basis of a disability. Most education agencies receive such funds. Federal funding for vocational programs targets services for the economically disadvantaged and the physically or emotionally challenged.

Many individuals with special needs can be successful in a vocational health occupation. The goal is to match each individual's capabilities and desires with the cognitive, affective, and psychomotor skills required in an occupation. There are various ways that teachers can help disadvantaged individuals and those with disabilities to be successful in a health occupation.

Special Needs Populations

Special needs populations are those groups of individuals with identified disabilities or economic disadvantages who require special assistance to be successful in an educational program. The Individuals with Disabilities Education Act of 1990, which replaces the Education for all Handicapped Children Act, the Carl Perkins Vocational Education Act of 1984 and its 1990 amendments, and Section 504 of the Rehabilitation Act of 1974, are federal laws addressing education for special needs populations.

P.L. 101–476 identifies eleven categories of handicapping conditions. These are:

- Head injuries
- Hearing impaired, including deaf
- Mentally retarded
- Multihandicapped
- Orthopedically impaired
- Other health impaired
- Limited functioning due to chronic or acute health problems such as asthma, heart conditions, diabetes, and leukemia
- Seriously emotionally disturbed
- Specific learning disability
- Speech or language impaired
- Autism
- Visually impaired, including blind

The Carl Perkins Amendments identify a prorated amount of funds based on the number of students who are economically disadvantaged or disabled. Local educational agencies receiving these funds from a designated state agency must identify the number of individuals within each of the special populations, address assessment of needs, and coordinate activities with Job Training Partnership Act (JTPA) agencies. The JTPA programs provide a stipend and funding for the training of economically disadvantaged adults.

Secondary Programs and Special Needs Populations

The vocational teacher can effect a major change in the life of a disadvantaged student. Pride in accomplishment, the financial rewards of employability, and improved self-esteem are just a few of the benefits of a vocational program for a young person from, for example, a family receiving welfare benefits. Such students are generally socially disadvantaged and may have a lower reading and comprehension level as well as deficiencies in math. They may not have had the opportunity to experience many of the activities that would improve their social graces and increase their chances at interviewing well for a job.

Disabled students, formerly called handicapped students, are now generally referred to in the schools as identified students. The majority of students with disabilities will have been diagnosed by the time they are in high school and are applying to a health occupations program. Identified students must have an Individualized Education Plan (IEP), which is a written plan that is developed with the child, parents, academic teachers, administrators, and any health personnel that may be involved in providing care or treatment for the student. If a secondary school student has an interest in a health occupation and could benefit from the program, the IEP can be written to include the vocational program. The first step, however, is to assess a student's cognitive, affective, and psychomotor skills to determine if he or she could indeed benefit from the program.

A student with a disabling condition may not have the ability to complete an entire program or to progress at the level and pace expected of nondisabled students. The specific program objectives for this student are incorporated into the IEP to match the student's abilities. For example, an identified student may be required to define fifteen medical terms instead of a hundred. Vocational teachers must be involved in writing the IEP because they know the competencies needed for an occupation and will be responsible for assisting the student in acquiring those skills.

Some states have special skills olympics for identified students in all of the vocational areas. Some of the best hospital bed making is performed by special needs health occupations students!

Postsecondary/Adult Programs and Special Needs Populations

Disadvantaged students may be going through your program with the help of JTPA or other federal loan assistance. These students may have many obstacles to overcome in order to participate in the program. Unreliable or nonexistent transportation, inadequate nutrition, poor hygiene, and poor stress-coping skills are just a few of the problems they may have to face. Of course, you will also have disadvantaged students who will not have problems in the program. Working closely with counselors is important to help students identify community resources for help, such as the Lions Club for eyeglasses and church groups for clothing. You must have the same expectations of disadvantaged students that you have of other students, but you may need to work a little harder to help them get any needed additional assistance.

Students must not be excluded from your program merely because they have a disabling condition. Any exclusion must be based on inability to acquire the necessary competencies for employment. Individual assessment provides information on the skills a student may or may not be able to acquire. The school will have to determine what level is necessary for safe functioning. As an example, an individual is not denied admission because of a hearing impairment. Hearing level is compared to the level needed for performing skills such as taking blood pressures. Applicants are denied admission only if they do not have the capability of performing the skills required.

A more difficult assessment has to do with individuals who have been confined or treated for mental health problems. In these cases, the stress of the program must be considered and a professional decision based on the circumstances of each individual. Be fair and consistent with your decisions about admitting any particular student, whether disabled, disadvantaged, or not.

Curriculum Adjustments for Special Needs Populations

First, know your own limitations. You cannot be everything to everyone! Identify the resources that are available to help you with your students. Are curriculum adjustments, such as lowering the reading level of the materials or providing supplemental worksheets, needed? If so, does your school have a resource center with teachers who can help a student with reading or math? For high school special needs students, do you need to have tests written at the third-grade reading level or the fifth or the eighth? Adjustments cannot be made unless students have been adequately assessed by their home high school or an adult education program.

Is someone available to help you write learning activity packets (LAPS) that would let a student progress through the program at his or her own rate or to reinforce your lectures? LAPS are individualized modules that can be used to supplement a classroom presentation for a slower learner, challenge a gifted student, or be used in place of the classroom lecture/presentation entirely. LAPS contain a pretest, the specific objectives for the unit of instruction, an introduction, the steps to be completed in order to learn the material, the information to be learned, worksheets or crossword puzzles or other activities to reinforce the information, and a posttest. The section with the information to be learned may be self-contained or a referral. Self-contained LAPS have all of the reading material included. Referral LAPS refer the student to chapters in a textbook. Videos to be watched, computer programs to be completed, or instructions for lab practice are also listed in LAPS.

In addition to curriculum adjustments, special adaptive equipment may be needed for a student with a disability. The classroom must be barrier free for a student with a disability. Are the aisles between desks wide enough for a wheelchair? Are any adjustments required for student safety? An example of a safety adjustment would be making sure the fire extinguisher was positioned low enough on the wall to be accessible to a student confined to a wheelchair.

Teaching Techniques

A variety of teaching methods should be used each day. Use visuals with lectures, include time for discussions, ask frequent questions of students to determine if they are understanding the information, and allow time for lab practice as soon after the lecture as possible. Start with an introduction, and close with a summary. In using gaming techniques such as jeopardy or baseball, make sure all students can participate in some manner. Do not allow any student, whether gifted or identified, to dominate the class or the teacher's time. A well-planned lesson will allow all students to progress in the program.

All students in your program need job-seeking skills. Special needs students may require even more help. Techniques include role-playing, asking individuals from a health agency to come to class and interview students in a mock job interview, or scheduling students to go to a health agency for a mock interview. The students then receive feedback, which helps improve their interviewing skills.

Flexibility is a must for the vocational health occupations teacher. If a student with a disability cannot perform a procedure exactly the same way as a nonlimited student, is there another way you can teach the procedure that does not violate or omit any principles that are important? Be flexible and creative, and the success of your students will be your reward.

Summary

Vocational health occupations programs may not discriminate against students who are disadvantaged or have a disability. Admission to programs should be based on a student's ability to succeed in the program and become gainfully employed. Students in secondary school who are identified as having a disability must have an IEP developed for them. Secondary and postsecondary/adult programs must be fair and consistent in decisions relating to the admissibility of all applicants.

All students in the program will benefit from a variety of teaching techniques. Special curriculum adjustments such as LAPS will allow for differences among students. Disadvantaged students and students with disabilities may have had limited life experiences, and their job-seeking skills may require additional time to be developed

☞ DESCRIBING ADULT STUDENTS

What do we know about the adult learner? Why might an adult enter a vocational health occupations program? Are adult motives different from those of middle school or high school students?

Differences

A student is somewhat different as an adult and yet in many ways similar to a student in middle school or high school. The first difference for most adults is that they are in school by choice; they are "wannabees." The adult has decided for reasons of a career change or a career upgrade to enter your program. That is a big hurdle. Some adults have not had many successes in their life, and being accepted into a program may be the first big success that they attain.

Because the adult who chooses to come into your program can also leave at any time, whatever you do as a teacher of adults is important in maintaining their self-respect, self-esteem, and interest in the program. The teachers that adult learners have had could have been as long ago as thirty or forty years, and adult students may have misconceptions or misperceptions about what a teacher should be. You will be asking of them different responsibilities than were asked of them when they were in high school thirty years ago. Now this does not mean that all adult learners in your program are going to be above the age of 60, for that is probably not the case. There are misperceptions about adults as learners whether the adults are 18 or 78. On the other hand, the adult learner is a person; just because a person is 28 or 58 does not mean that the skills expected by teachers are in place.

Adult students have life skills, and they come to you and your program with a family already grown in many cases and with plenty of other life responsibilities. Some of these adults have taken care of or are taking care of a relative, and maybe this is their primary interest in entering a vocational health occupations program. They will bring you something already written on their slate; they do not come to you with a tabula rasa, a blank slate, nor do the middle school and high school students come to their teachers with a blank slate either, for they all have something written on their life slate.

Responsibilities

Adult learners — the ones who likely have responsibilities in life already with their own family — may be working at one or two jobs to maintain an income and to pay for rent, transportation, and food. They have the singular purpose of getting through the program to get a better job and earn a better living.

Let's look for a moment at some of the obstacles the adult learner may have had to overcome just to get to the first day of class. One of them may be transportation. For adults, especially those with children and a spouse, access to transportation may be the deciding factor to even enter the program. One of the first questions may be "Will my old jalopy be able to make it to all the different clinical sites around the city? How many miles will I have to drive? What about parking? Will I have to pay to park at school? What about getting the car to my spouse at the end of the day?"

Another major concern of the adult deciding to enroll in your program is the cost. Adults say to themselves that they want to be involved in vocational health occupation to be what they can be, to be a success in a health occupation field. "What will it cost me in terms of time, travel, tuition, books, uniforms, supplies, and equipment?" Those questions must be answered so that adult learners can evaluate their ability to meet those economic demands.

They will bring these questions to you before the first day or on the first day of class; even though they have been admitted, they will start thinking of the economic realities involved in the program. Whether it is a short-term program or two years long, a lot of costs are involved, and although the first question may be their acceptance into the program, the second may be related to the costs of completing the program. Another demanding factor may be the job or jobs the person may have to put on hold or even quit before entering a health occupations program.

There are probably a thousand questions in the mind of the adult learner on entering the program. It is hoped that you will have answered most of them and identified before the first day of class in a preadvisement session conducted by either you, the counseling staff, or other people in the school program the types of financial assistance available. Let's look at some concerns the adult learner will have, other than financial ones, in deciding to enter and complete the program.

Let's look first at those deciding to enter the program. Adult learners may not have had many or any successes in school. The memory of school could be very painful. In high school, they may have been advised not to go to college or could not afford to go to college. As a result, they did not pursue the career they were interested in during high school. In many cases, this time was interrupted for jobs and raising a family.

Now it is time for Dad or Mom to go back to school. Maybe there is an empty nest; maybe the children are still at home but Mom or Dad has decided anyway to pursue the dream of being a health occupations practitioner. They may have decided to make a sacrifice and do something they would especially like to do right now. The adult student is really to be admired because it takes a lot of personal fortitude to make such decisions and complete the program.

Environment

Another challenge for the adult learner is that of the environment. Whether it be an adult center, vocational technical center, technical college, or community college, it is a postsecondary formal education setting. Rules and regulations are a little different from high school but in some respects not a lot different. In some areas, the responsibility is great while the school and the environment are developed to train learners to assume responsibility.

The environment, the room, the classroom — how are they arranged? Are they arranged for adult learners to be accepted? What about the size of the chairs? The chairs need to be regular size for adults and comfortable enough to be in for a long period of time. An adult learner or even a younger student who needs to be near the front because of a hearing impairment or for visual reasons must be accommodated. Where are the restrooms? Are there lockers or places for adult learners to keep things so that they have a place away from home that is theirs in which to put things? Is coffee permitted? Describe the environment. Is it physically acceptable? How are the seats arranged? How are the lab facilities arranged? Are they geared for the adult learner?

All students should be treated with respect and dignity. Adult learners are definitely here by choice. Maybe they will not show up the next day because the chair was not comfortable or because they were asked to sit in the chair for four hours at a time. Maybe the scheduling and the environment were not arranged for the convenience of the adult learner.

Accept adult learners as responsible people and treat them respectfully; they will react accordingly to you.

References

Benson, P., D. Williams and A. Johnson (1987). *The Quick Silver Years: The Hopes and Fears of Early Adolescents* (1st ed.). San Francisco: Harper and Row.

Carnegie Council on Adolescent Development (1989). *Turning Points: Preparing American Youth for the 21st Century: The Report of the Task Force on Education of Young Adolescents.* Washington: author.

McEwin, K., and J. Thomason (1989). *Why They Are, How We Teach: Early Adolescents and Their Teachers.* Columbus, Ohio: National Middle School Association.

Van Hoose, J., and D. Strahan (1987). *Promoting Harmony in the Middle Grades.* Columbus, Ohio: North Carolina League of Middle Schools.

Student Relations: Charting Unknown Territory

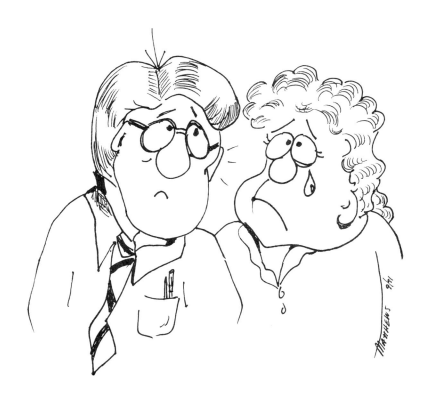

CONFERENCING AND ADVISEMENT

Conferencing and advisement are important aspects in the learning experience of the health occupations student. Proper scrutiny of one's readiness and suitability is essential to the successful educational process.

This section will consider the student's process from the initial application for a health-related program through the entire educational phase of the program. Care is given to include the counselor, the health occupations instructional personnel, and the student in the assessment and implementation of effective counseling and career alternatives.

The Initial Process

The counselor is the main communications anchor for the prospective student in a health occupations program. The counselor helps to determine whether all the puzzle pieces will mesh cohesively for success during the academic experience and in the health care industry upon completion of the program.

Returning to school is a giant step for many. Some individuals continuing with their educational pursuits may not have gained the necessary skills sufficient to handle the demands associated with a health occupations curriculum. Therefore, the evaluation of the prospective student's goals, preparation, and skills must be critically analyzed. Attention should be given to understand and assist the student in an honest and caring manner.

Important facts to consider include basic needs that are often overlooked by the counselor as well as by health occupations faculty. The following are of importance in determining readiness and appropriateness for a health-related program.

- Attitude
- Motivational factors
- Mental, emotional, and physical capabilities
- Academic skills
- Financial resources
- Study skills
- Child care needs
- Transportation
- Work schedule
- Support of significant others
- Other external forces

How then is it determined that an applicant should seriously consider entering a health occupations program? This is accomplished by a counselor's initial interaction with the individual. Thus, a counselor must be perceptive enough to support the selection of an appropriate program. Understand, however, that it is not the counselor's responsibility to select a program, but rather to assist in identifying strengths and weaknesses associated with the appropriateness of the program for the applicant. The counselor should carefully consider all factors to ensure that an applicant is genuinely satisfied that all preparation is thoroughly evaluated.

The initial step is assessment of the applicant's basic academic skills. Academic readiness is of primary importance and should signal whether the applicant has the necessary background to understand the theoretical aspects of the program. A thorough understanding of the instructional content in the classroom will greatly affect the carryover of knowledge to its application in the clinical setting. Remedial services should be offered to the applicant who does not demonstrate the required academic aptitude for program success. Because most health-related programs require a tremendous amount of intense learning, it is the responsibility of the counselor to suggest that academic readiness be achieved first. In some instances, the applicant's manual dexterity is of importance for program success. For example, an applicant interested in a surgical technology program must be able to handle surgical instruments with skill and speed.

An application for entry into a program is completed by the applicant and used as a counseling tool by the counselor. The application will contain certain information necessary to properly assess an applicant's readiness and appropriateness for a health-related program. Suspicion of a problem should be dealt with immediately. Indication of a compromising medical condition may require a letter of support from the attending physician. This not only protects the student but also safeguards the training facility from liability.

Financial resources are often of primary consideration for the applicant. Though sometimes funds are limited, the counselor will have an available reservoir of resources for the program applicant. The public library is another source of financial information. The Pell Grant Program is an excellent resource for the student enrolled in a long-term program. Information about it is available through the school counselor or the financial aid administrator at a participating school.

If an applicant has not been properly oriented toward good study habits, it is advisable that the counselor suggest available resources for assistance in this area. The school's media center probably has tapes, filmstrips, and other materials that can provide instruction on studying.

The applicant will also be advised by the counselor concerning the amount of time and preparation required for a successful experience while in the program. Therefore, before-school and after-school daily work schedules are of primary consideration and must be examined carefully.

Child care and family support are essential for the applicant who has children. Because it is important that the student maintain a wholesome and healthy attitude, preplanning will ensure adequate arrangments during the day.

The applicant should be aware of bus schedules, car pools, and the like if there is no available transportation to and from the training facility. Absenteeism and tardiness are usually grounds for dismissal. The health care professional must always demonstrate a sense of dependability and responsibility, and the time to learn this is during the training period.

Another important area of consideration is the applicant's mental, emotional, and physical capabilities. It is essential that students possess the skills necessary to display a wholesome and healthy attitude in caring for those in need of primary care assistance.

Often overlooked is the motivating factor associated with one's decision to explore a health-related program. Motivation is important to the applicant's ability to overcome obstacles that may interfere with the training experience. A motivated student will seek answers to problems and move in a more productive manner to correct or overcome a situation. The end result will be a positive outcome. Motivation and determination are recognized by the counselor as signs that the applicant may be successful in a program. The motivation of an individual is reflected by personal needs or desires at any given opportunity. Not all interested applicants will be suited for a health-related career. If it is determined through a critical analysis of an applicant that he or she is not suited for a program, the counselor can suggest and assist with alternatives better suited to the applicant's strengths.

One might argue that everyone has the right to choose and pursue an education based on interests and goals. Others might assert that entry into a health-related program should involve scrutiny of one's values and skills. The latter represents a more mature approach because it heightens the awareness of the individual's strengths and weaknesses as they relate to program success. In addition, it provides the necessary information to critically evaluate the worth of the choice first determined.

Before the conclusion of the interview, the counselor will offer a brochure giving information on program expectations and referral agencies that might further assist the applicant through the educational process. An orientation at the training facility and to the program constitutes an added stimulus that often will make a difference in developing a self-confident student.

An applicant who has the skills needed to make a decision and stick to that decision is usually motivated to the level of believing in success in the career selected. One must not, however, mistake applicants who continue to explore options as ones who are not in control of their life. This method of discrimination might suggest a positive sign that the ultimate goal is adequately determined because it has been thoroughly analyzed.

If the initial advisement session with the counselor has consisted of a comprehensive positive assessment of the applicant's readiness for a health-related program, the applicant is now prepared to explore a successful career as a health occupations professional.

The Instructor as a Conferencing Agent

Conferencing and advisement extends far beyond the counselor's office. The involvement of the health occupations instructor is of utmost importance in identifying a student's strengths and weaknesses. Because the student will spend a great deal of time with the instructor, it is essential that there develop an open and trusting relationship.

The instructor is the first line of communication after entry into a program; your attitude has a direct effect on the student, whether negative or positive. Mixed messages should always be avoided. Remember that students' behavior displayed in the classroom will ultimately reflect in their success or failure. Students should feel compelled to express concerns to the teacher if the teacher has in fact provided an avenue for open and positive communication.

The steps to consider in determining the appropriateness of a referral should follow the pattern described previously. The instructor is the first communicator when a problem exists in the classroom. Often a problem or concern can be resolved at this level. If further counseling or advisement is needed, the counselor is then notified and given proper referral and supporting documentation. It may be necessary for both the instructor and the counselor to be present during the conferencing process.

The instructor will be able to verbally express the assessment of information shared during the conferencing session. It is desirable that a solution to all concerns be effected at this level.

Involvement of an administrator in the conferencing session is considered as a last effort. If the student has been properly oriented initially and the instructor and counselor have provided an atmosphere in which the student has the opportunity to explore options, then the inclusion of an administrator is almost always un-necessary.

Exploration of choices constitutes a learning experience for the student. It provides an avenue to better discriminate between situations upon the completion of a program. It also shows the student the need to become assertive concerning relationships. Remember that the student is in a developmental stage, and the health professional must allow the student the opportunity to explore — to become self-actualized.

Research has identified several different approaches to advisement and counseling of individuals. One approach that is significant in identifying when counseling is needed requires that the instructor become acquainted with the student in such a way as to be able to recognize any change in the behavior of a student. Should this become apparent, the instructor will explore the situation and immediately involve the counselor. Understand, however, that the counselor cannot always assist in finding a reasonable solution. In this instance, the counselor should be prepared to refer the student to an outside agency that will, ultimately, assist in the resolution of the problem.

Another approach might suggest that the student become involved in a counseling group on a regular basis. This approach offers the student basic support from peers. However, it must first be established that there is a need for group interaction based on identified deficits.

A third approach used is to identify potential problems and seek solutions to avoid their occurrence. For example, a student with the necessary academic preparation to successfully understand the information being given has been observed to have poor study habits. The student is given instruction on proper study skills so as to assist with better organization of the class materials and thus improve the ability to communicate effectively on class tests.

The developmental approach is aimed primarily at assisting the student with the normal growth and development that are necessary for career achievement. This approach is a way of ensuring that the likelihood of success in the program is predictable. Group activities are planned on a regular basis to address situations that often exist among health occupations students. This technique is accomplished by either the instructor or the counselor or both acting as the facilitator. Developmental counseling also includes the sharing of additional resource information that may be of further use to the student.

Behavior modification is important in assisting the student to avoid problems by gaining more control in making better and more suitable decisions and responses. The instructor might suggest to the student who lacks sufficient study habits that the student set aside a certain time each day to devote only to the preparation of classroom assignments. The same amount of time each day is designated as study time. Such a habit, if observed, will have a direct impact on improvement in class presentations and written assignments, thus improving desire and motivation to learn.

It is important to remember that the student may desire to talk freely with a counselor or instructor in order to share concerns or experiences that will have no relation to the educational pursuit. The educator must be able to listen and understand what the student is communicating and assist the student in finding a workable solution or alternative. The counselor or instructor may be the only source of information or support for that student. However, the most important role of the classroom instructor is to become familiar with each student and establish a warm and caring environment that will allow the student to feel comfortable enough to interact with the instructor and other students without inhibition. In other words, an accepting attitude on the part of the instructor should be maintained throughout the entire educational experience.

Summary

Making a career decision involves many variables that are often overlooked in determining a suitable educational program for the prospective health occupations student. The student must understand and accept the various phases of initial advisement conferencing. This involves, but is not limited to, academic assessment, an understanding of the individual's own interests and values, the individual's ability and readiness for a health-related program, and the individual's acceptance of the final results of the conferencing. The counselor must be genuinely involved to ensure the best possible results or alternatives associated with the advisement process.

The health occupations instructor plays a vital role in how students perceive their role in the learning process. The instructor must display a warm, caring, and helpful attitude to facilitate a successful educational experience for students.

☞ ADAPTING TO THE CHANGING WORK FORCE

When the twenty-first century begins, will we be ready to meet the educational and work place challenges that will face us? Many of the challenges to be faced by health occupations educators are related to changes both in the populations that will be entering the work force for the first time or participating in postsecondary technical education/training and in current workers who will need to be retrained as requirements of the work place change. Consider the following facts according to the reports of the Workforce 2000 committee.

- Service industries will create most of the new jobs over the next thirteen years, in which 80% of the workers are female and earn low wages.
- The work force is growing more slowly as well as becoming older more female, and more disadvantaged.
- Only 15% of new entrants into the labor force will be native white males compared to 47% in 1990.
- Approximately 83% of all new workers will be nonwhite, women, and immigrants.

- About 27% of all adult workers now hold low-wage jobs — and 67% of them are women.
- Women, especially women of color, are more likely to be low-wage workers.
- About 50% of black women's families are at or near the poverty level despite their earnings from low-wage jobs.
- New and emerging jobs will require higher skill levels than today, including those in the health field.
- Health and business services in Florida will account for almost half of all service jobs.
- Six of the ten fastest-growing occupations in Florida are in health services.

Do these facts have implications for you, a health occupations teacher? You bet they do! You will have a student population that may be very different from today's. The job market will continue to change — nothing new, but still worthy of your constant monitoring so as to keep your program up-to-date. The implications for you include administrative areas such as student recruitment, admissions, and placement. Instructional implications include your attitudes toward and awareness of nontraditional students, instructional activities, student-teacher interactions, gender-free language, and the selection and development of instructional materials. The clinical portions of your programs will also be affected in areas such as site selection, scheduling, and assignments. The changing work force will have an effect on you and your health occupations program.

The Florida Department of Labor and Employment Security predicts that Florida's labor force is expected to grow to almost 8 million workers by the year 2000. This rate of growth will add an annual average of 447,000 new jobs to Florida's economy. By the year 2000, women and the elderly will make up the additional workers.

Many of the new jobs available will be in Florida's fastest-growing occupations, which are high-paying and high-skilled jobs. Three of the ten fastest-growing occupations are in computer-related fields. Over 2 million new jobs will be created in the Florida job market by the next century. A possible gap between prepared workers and job openings could exist. To fill the gap, women, members of minorities, youth, the elderly, the handicapped, and immigrants will assume a more prominent role in the work force. And these groups are now appearing at the door of the vocational education classroom.

Recruitment of nontraditional students, such as male students for health occupations programs, brings diversity to your classroom and enlarges the pool of workers traditionally available for the myriad of jobs in health-related fields.

The following strategies will assist you in recruiting males for your programs.

- Examine your own attitude toward males in your program and in health-related occupations.
- Help students to make informed occupational choices based on their own interests, abilities, and goals by conducting career days, individual advising, and visits to your program.
- Provide accurate employment information on salaries, working conditions, the labor market outlook, and the placement rate of graduates of your programs.
- Develop a variety of recruitment materials (schoolwide or program specific) such as audiovisual presentations, brochures, posters, and pamphlets that contain pictures of males and females as well as descriptions that are free of the pronouns he and she when referring to students in the program.
- Encourage hands-on visits to your program so prospective students can learn about health occupations and experience directly some aspect of the program. Be sure your classroom is inviting to males by depicting males on bulletin boards, in photographs, and on posters.
- Use role models (males working in health-related occupations) during recruitment activities on campus or at high schools and as speakers at community groups.
- Select current male students or male graduates to speak to prospective students or serve as tour guides in your program area.

Retention of nontraditional students in vocational education programs represents a concern for administrators and teachers. Frequently students leave a program for valid reasons; more frequently, however, students leave without the teacher's having an opportunity to assist in the decision making.

Retaining nontraditional students presents a challenge for teachers. The major barrier to retaining nontraditional students is their perception that they "do not belong."

The following strategies will assist you in retaining nontraditional students in your program.

- Enroll a minimum of two or more nontraditional students; retention rates increase when there is more than one nontraditional student in the class.
- Examine your own biases and eliminate them from your behavior in the classroom; the teacher's attitude is critical to the other students' acceptance of nontraditional students.

- Use instructional materials that depict males, females, members of minorities, and handicapped people in various work roles.
- Enforce fair and consistent discipline, dress standards, safety regulations, achievement expectations, and grading procedures for all students.
- Offer mentoring or shadowing experiences in which students can experience hands-on field training with workers in the community who are already in nontraditional occupations.
- Invite nontraditional role models working in the field (including graduates of the program) to speak to your classes.
- Sponsor tours to hospitals, businesses, and industries to observe people working at nontraditional jobs.
- Encourage nontraditional students to participate in extracurricular activities such as HOSA, and support those interested in leadership positions.

Significant contributions that increase the quality of vocational programs are made by members of the community who serve on program advisory committees. While advisory committees constitute a topic covered in depth in another section of this book, a separate point can be made here. When selecting members, attempt to achieve a balance of males, females, members of minorities, and handicapped persons (or advocates for the handicapped). Placing on the committee people who are in nontraditional occupations such as a nurse who is male provides visibility and role models for students considering nontraditional vocational education programs. These same members can also provide insights into the needs of these populations, which will assist you in program management and instruction.

Classroom Instruction

Some of the students in your health occupations program will be nontraditional females (older, single parents, teen parents, the disadvantaged, or even handicapped in some way), and some will be males in a program that has been filled traditionally with females. These students are part of the changing work force described earlier. Although they are different from the traditional students in your health occupations program, they will need the same good teaching techniques you use with traditional students. At times you will also need to adapt or apply teaching techniques to meet the unique needs of the nontraditional students in your program.

Most health occupations students have opportunities during their program to see and hear guest speakers (generally practicing professionals in the occupational area), take field trips, and, on occasion, work in a job-shadowing situation or with a mentor. It is important to provide opportunities for your students to interact with and have exposure to nontraditional workers whenever possible. This might include inviting as guest speakers to your program male nurses and nontraditional female workers who can serve as positive role models for your students. You may also carefully select sites for field trips to enable your students to observe work environments free from stereotypes related to gender, age, race, ethnic origin, and handicaps.

In terms of student-teacher interaction, numerous studies in the past five years have found significant differences in the way teachers interact with female students and with male students in the classroom. Many of the differences are based on expectations that teachers hold for males and females in general based on sex-role stereotypes. Results of the studies indicate the following.

- At all educational levels, teachers tend to interact with male students more than female students.
- Teachers tend to interact more with white males than with minority males. Teachers interact the least with minority females.
- Male students receive more praise, encouragement, and criticism from teachers than females do.
- Females are given less wait time to answer a question in class than males are.
- Males generally receive harsher discipline than females for similar behavior.
- Teachers tend to "do" for females, but they "show" males and let them do for themselves.
- Teachers generally take males' career choices more seriously than females'.
- Females are usually criticized for calling out in class; males are not.

This research summary indicates that teachers interact with students differently based on gender and gender expectations. Although teachers for the most part are unaware of the above behaviors, the research does indicate a need for them to monitor their interaction with students.

The choice of print and nonprint curriculum materials for instruction usually centers on the content. Obviously content is critical when selecting textbooks, audiovisual aids, and other instructional materials. However, also important are the other messages that the materials send. Language as well as photographs, drawings, and other visual presentations should be critiqued during the process of selecting materials. Bulletin boards and exhibits or displays used at career fairs or other schoolwide events should portray your program as accessible to males, females, and members of minorities.

The following are items to check when reviewing textbooks and other materials for purchase.

- Are males, females, and members of minorities shown in all occupations, not just those traditionally held by males and females?
- Are both males and females shown in a variety of occupational levels and responsibilities?
- Are sex-free occupational titles used as found in the *Dictionary of Occupational Titles?*
- Are nontraditional students or workers depicted?
- Are members of minorities included in photographs and drawings?
- Are the pronouns he and she used in the materials when referring to persons in a specific occupation?
- Are males and females shown to be capable of similar emotions and abilities, such as nurturing, leadership, and decision making?
- If roles at home are depicted, are males and females shown in a variety of roles?
- Does the material give you the impression that males, females, and members of minorities are capable of working in a variety of occupations and in leadership positions and that occupations are not limited on the basis of sex or race?

Language usage has a powerful impact on students' perception of what is appropriate for males and females. The use of the pronoun he when referring to physicians, and she when referring to nurses gives the impression that certain occupations are more appropriate for males or for females. To avoid stereotyping in language usage, the following are recommended guidelines.

- Use plural pronouns whenever possible so as to avoid using he and she.
- When discussing unspecified persons in occupations, avoid using he and she.
- Use occupational titles such as police officer instead of policeman and supervisor or manager instead of foreman.
- Avoid reinforcing racial, sex-role, or ethnic stereotypes.
- Include the contributions of women in studies of science, math, and history.
- Avoid placing emphasis on women's clothing and grooming; males are also interested in their personal appearance.

- Acknowledge that males and females can have the same characteristics, such as being caring, kind, aggressive, assertive, intelligent, etc.
- Use parallel terms when referring to men and women of the same status, such as Dr. David Brown and Dr. Susan Green.
- Describe people in comparable terms: do not describe women in terms of their appearance while men are being described in terms of accomplishments.

Clinical Instruction

Of prime importance to the success of any health occupations program is the clinical experience portion. The clinical sites where students gain practical experience and have opportunities to apply the knowledge and skills learned in your program can go a long way toward serving the needs of each student (including the nontraditional ones), the school, and the community. Selection of clinical sites as well as units within sites, in addition to coordination with the personnel at the site are important for the success of the nontraditional male and female students in your program.

Teachers who place students in work situations during training/education programs or at the completion of training must follow the mandates in Title IX regarding treatment of males and females. The following are guidelines when performing job or clinical placement activities.

- All decisions concerning student employment and job placement must be made in a manner that ensures that discrimination based on sex does not occur.
- Students who have completed the perequisites should be admitted to enter work-study, cooperative courses, job placement, and apprentice training programs regardless of their sex. They must also receive equal treatment with regard to task assignment, number of hours worked, responsibility levels, and pay.
- Employers with whom the district places students must provide written assurance that students will be accepted, assigned to jobs, and otherwise treated without regard to sex.
- Teachers should encourage employers to request students on the basis of ability, not on the basis of the sex of the student.
- Students participating in cooperative education, work-study, job placement, and apprentice training programs must not be discriminated against by employers or prospective employers on the basis of sex.
- Teachers must not refer or assign students to an employer who is known to discriminate against persons on the basis of sex.

Civil Rights Legislation and Teachers

The Carl D. Perkins Vocational and Applied Technology Education Act of 1990 requires all vocational programs to serve students who traditionally have been underserved by vocational education. Fulfilling the intent of the Perkins Act involves considering the unique needs that females, members of racial and cultural minorities, handicapped and disadvantaged students, and single parents bring to the classroom. A major goal of vocational education is to provide equal educational opportunities for all students. Educators, including teachers, administrators, and counselors, have the responsibility of ensuring that all students have equal access to programs, services, and activities regardless of their sex, race, color, national origin, or handicap. Several laws have been passed that affect teachers in the classroom as they interact with their students.

Title IX of the Education Amendments of 1972 constituted a landmark piece of legislation that mandates that males and females cannot be treated differently or separately in the educational environment. Issues such as vocational education, facilities, admissions and recruitment, pregnant students, marital status of students, athletics, and physical education are addressed in Title IX.

Teachers should be especially aware of the areas in which Title IX prohibits discrimination on the basis of sex. Some are:

- admission and recruitment of students
- use of facilities
- access to course offerings
- access to vocational education programs
- guidance and counseling services
- marital and parental status of students
- employment and job placement of students
- financial assistance
- sexual harassment

Title VI of the Civil Rights Act of 1964 mandates that educational programs receiving federal financial assistance may not discriminate on the basis of race, color, or national origin. The areas of concern under the mandates of Title VI are basically the same ones listed in Title IX.

Section 504 of the Rehabilitation Act of 1973 addresses the education of handicapped students. Briefly stated, Section 504 mandates that, solely by reason of a handicap, a student cannot be denied access to vocational education programs, services, activities, or facilities. The passage of this law had an enormous impact on policies of schools and colleges in terms of handicapped students. The law mandates that new construction must conform to standards of accessibility for handicapped persons. In addition, school districts and colleges may be required to provide related aids and services for handicapped students.

References

Blake, Duane L. (1979). *Dynamics of Human Relations in Vocational Education.* Cranston, R.I.: Carroll Press.

Herman, Sonya J. (1978). *Becoming Assertive: A Guide for Nurses.* New York: Van Nostrand.

Lewis, Edwin C. (1970). *The Psychology of Counseling.* New York: Holt, Rinehart and Winston.

Myrick, Robert D. (1987). *Developmental Guidance and Counseling: A Practical Approach.* Minneapolis: Educational Media Corporation.

7
Program Survival: Marketing the Program

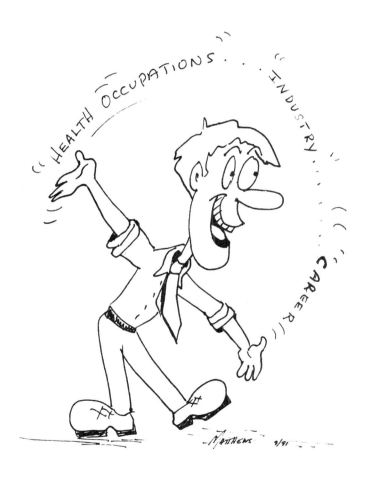

This chapter offers assistance to the health occupations teacher in methods of recruiting students, marketing the program, and developing partnerships with the health care industry. The recruiting process requires effective advertising and sufficient referral from various job areas to keep up with the number of students enrolled and later placed in employment. Marketing the program is essential for survival and must have adequate partnerships with and the support of the health care industry and community to incorporate classroom teaching and practice learned skills.

RECRUITING STUDENTS

The highlight of vocational education is the availability of courses that are offered to the individual person regardless of age or status in life. The opportunity afforded cannot be measured because it means something different to each person. The vocational education teacher can use these facts to set up recruiting guidelines for the students. The first question that a health occupations teacher ask is "How can I develop good recruiting techniques?" Fortunately, the demand is continually present for health care people in the workplace, and this represents an asset for the teacher. The recruiting methods need to make a significant impression so students will really want to take the vocational program offered. This is an opportune time to show students some of the offerings the program will include — a varied and interesting curriculum that can be absorbed in the number of hours allowed, taking a busy life-style into consideration. Normally, the vocational program charges a reasonable tuition — something the average person can afford.

Counseling

The teacher can guide prospective students through personal counseling that outlines the benefits offered by the program, explaining to recruits how the program can promote and improve their capabilities. It is important to instill enthusiasm and motivate students to become aware of their own potential.

The health occupations instructor must believe in the product and constantly develop new incentives for students. This will create in the individual a desire to pursue the advantage that vocational education offers. During the recruitment process, the teacher should indicate what students can contribute and what the program can do for students.

Community

The teacher can begin by learning more about the school and the area where courses are taught. Reviewing what jobs are available for students can be fundamental in setting up recruitment. Visits should be made to all of the facilities or agencies that employ students. Use this information as groundwork for what might be the needs of the community.

The very fact that the teacher is spreading the word about the program stimulates active interest within the community. It will be these very people who may refer a student to the teacher and thus accelerate the recruiting process. This enables the instructor to keep the various employment areas aware of what the vocational program has to offer, which represents an advantage to the success of the program.

Advertising is a way of presenting the information about the program to the community. This can be done in many ways, in newspapers, on radio, and in bulletins placed in all of the facilities to enhance recruitment. It should be made known in the advertisement that the health occupations program offers a learning process that can be incorporated with maintaining a job as well as attending class. Average adults need to do both and still feel they are accomplishing something of value. For those who have been left out of educational opportunities, vocational education opens many doors to learn a trade or vocation.

The other form of advertising comes from the student who has successfully completed the program. The knowledge and competence displayed by graduates speak for themselves. The community administrative personnel are aware of the end product and will be interested, supportive of the program, and instrumental in passing the word to other influential persons. The quality of the program must be maintained in order to ensure the continued success of graduates. Other practitioners in the community will be aware of what students have learned once graduates are in the workplace. This stimulates interest and an eagerness to hire competent people. The teacher can be a significant factor in giving students the knowledge and capability they would otherwise never have acquired.

Recruiting techniques are very important due to the need in the job market for health occupation workers. Vocational education makes these techniques much easier, because the tuition and availability of courses are most attractive to the average person.

Maintaining community contact in the areas that will offer referrals to the health occupations program can be accomplished by the instructor. Informing applicants of what is offered in the program stimulates interest and makes recruiting easier.

Advertising plays an important role in making the public aware of what is offered. Student referral can be developed from the success of the program and the capability of graduates.

MARKETING THE PROGRAM

Once you have a good program in place, students will usually register for your classes and you won't have to recruit very hard. If you find yourself having to recruit, try some advertising activities and make sure the counselors know about your program.

One of the most visible ways to advertise is to use posters. Have your students create the posters as a club project. You could also ask an art teacher if some of the art students would like to make posters depicting class and HOSA activities for a graded project. Place these posters all over the school two to three weeks prior to registration. Suggestions for posters could include:

- health occupations education courses being offered
- job placement possibilities
- advantages of taking a health occupations education course (more prepared for college, getting a job, hands-on experience, better idea if you want to enter health field)
- advantages of joining HOSA (leadership training, looks good on the résumé, another activity to list on scholarship forms, friendships)
- HOSA activities (homecoming, competition, leadership workshops, running for office, community programs)

Advertising throughout the academic year in the school and in local newspapers helps make parents and students aware of health occupations programs. The local HOSA reporter should submit an article each month to the instructor. It is then edited and sent to the newspapers. If the article warrants a picture, ask the newspapers if they can send a photographer to the school. The instructor can take pictures and send them with the article. Items to include in articles are:

- election of officers (include pictures)
- involvement in activities (homecoming, Christmas project, community projects, etc.)
- winners of competitive events (include pictures)

If a new course is going to be offered during the upcoming school year, announcements should be made on the public address system and a special article submitted to the school paper. Current students are informed about the new course so they can tell friends. Word of mouth is a good way to recruit students.

Every program should have an updated brochure for distribution to students who might be interested in a health occupations course. The brochure can be made available to students prior to or during the time they register for courses for the next semester. Brochures should also be left with counselors, who can distribute them to new students. The brochure should include the following for each course offered.

- course description
- prerequisites for the course
- length of course
- purpose of course
- who can take the course

Creating a slide presentation or video can be a lot of work, but it can pay off in the long run. Students like to see what goes on in courses they are going to take. If you make it look good, they will want to take the course. If a camcorder is not available at your school, see if a student has one you may borrow. Write out the script, and practice it several times before taping. This will cut down on the borrow time you and will produce a more professional tape. Make the finished product available to counselors, and show it at every opportunity.

Counselors are key people to get to know if you want students to take your classes. Arrange a meeting with them and discuss why students should take health occupations courses. Tell them that such courses help students:

- Gain knowledge and hands-on experience in the field they are considering entering.
- Investigate a field they are considering entering.
- Gain employment.
- Gain leadership skills through HOSA.

Discuss prerequisites, if any, for each course. Also tell counselors what types of students should take each class.

Through advertising and working with counselors, you will be on your way to enrolling students in health occupations courses and guiding young minds to pursue a career in the health care industry.

☞ USING ADVISORY COMMITTEES

Both the stability and growth of a health occupations program are enhanced by organizing competent administrative personnel into an advisory/technical committee. The welfare and productivity of a class that graduates qualified health care workers are of great interest to employers in the community.

The health occupations teacher begins by making visits in the area and holding conferences with the various directors, owners, and managers of health care establishments. Information is given regarding the program curriculum offered and acquainting officials with the benefits that the curriculum offers their organization. This understanding may encourage them to participate on an advisory committee.

The purpose of the committee is to oversee the program, evaluate it, and offer recommendations. The expertise expressed collectively by the participants can be a positive and creative force in maintaining the caliber of students graduating from the program. The reinforcement that the program gains by the cooperation of health care members in the area is invaluable in continuing the superiority of the program. The recommendations given are useful for the principal instructor to incorporate into the curriculum each school year.

Regular meetings are scheduled, usually quarterly, for the committee to meet, and an agenda is outlined by the instructor. Included in the group are the director of adult and vocational education and the coordinator of adult education. The agenda is composed of current events taking place in the program and any recent directives from the department of education or health and rehabilitative services. The instructor gives members a copy of the current curriculum for their information and consideration. In this way, everyone on the committee is apprised of the training that students receive.

The meeting is conducted appropriately, and minutes are taken to document the business conducted. Even though this committee cannot create rules, it can offer constructive suggestions for the continued success of the program. The recommended size of the group is 12–15 people.

One option is to involve a graduate of the program as a member of the committee. This person should be a practitioner who has been in the work force and has supportive information to offer. The position offers prestige, and it stimulates interest among former graduates to know that one of their peers is a member of such an influential group.

The health care giver shares opinions and actual job experiences that can be of value for improvement in the health care program. Each school year, a different graduate should be selected and invited to sit on the committee. The purpose of this is to gather new ideas and suggestions from another perspective. Therefore, activities involved in the committee are constantly renewing and modifying based on trends in health care.

Another function of the committee is to form a network with the members for the useful exchange of pertinent information regarding the caregivers in the community. This kind of interaction keeps everyone aware, as the health care field is growing in major proportions. The group serves as a common ground where all employers can meet.

The final purpose of having an advisory/technical committee is the members' participation in the graduation ceremony of each class. The students are given an impressive commencement and reception, furnished by dues paid by the committee members. It is meaningful to graduates to see the members in attendance and gives them a feeling of pride to know that employers care enough to be there and join in to congratulate their accomplishment. Following the ceremony, the employers present students with gifts to honor the occasion. Every graduation year, the advisory committee votes for an outstanding health care giver, and an award is presented to the recipient and to the employer. Considerable pride is taken in receiving such an award.

Each health occupations program needs a supportive group such as the one described in this section. The gathering of professionals is an asset to any vocational education class. The combined effort of the members of this group, who give their time voluntarily, is commendable. And the contribution that a committee of this stature can make is essential to maintain high quality in a health care program. Recognizing an outstanding health care giver and the associated publicity promote a positive image in the health care community.

DEVELOPING PARTNERSHIPS WITH THE HEALTH CARE INDUSTRY

The demand for health care employees continues to grow for a variety of reasons, including the growth in size of the elderly population, increasing hospital acuity, the AIDS/HIV epidemic, and innovations in medical technology. Of the top twenty jobs in the year 2000, ten are in health care. In addition, those pursuing a career in health care are finding that the educational and technical preparation requirements are increasing.[1]

The health care community is now looking beyond its previously established recruitment efforts and is pursuing partnerships with education agencies beginning at the elementary school level and continuing on through university preparation.[2]

Concurrently many efforts are being made at the local, state, and national levels to fund new, experimental school-based health care community and education partnership endeavors. Many of those initiating the new efforts have little experience with the parameters, requirements, and protocols of these unique partnerships.

---

[1]Workforce 2000: Competing in a Seller's Market: Is Corporate America Prepared? 1990.

[2]The Allied Health Fields: Problems and Opportunities, September 21, 1990.

Establishing partnership requires a planned, organized approach that includes both identification of the education program needs and identification of services that the education partner can offer that will be of benefit to the health care partner.

Partnerships can support programs that are exploratory in nature, provide entry-level or technical-level skills, and prepare students for entering a university to study for a professional-level career. The amount of preparation necessary will be directly correlated to the level of skill-specific training included in the course of study.

The content of this section, developed by experienced health care community and education representatives, is designed to offer a step-by-step guide that will assist in creating the partnership.

Partnerships (Figure 7-1) should result in the opportunity for students to see the occupational result of their education, motivating them to expand and meet their education and career goals; teachers' experiencing a relationship with the health care community that helps them to establish relevancy in their curriculum; and an adequate number of well-prepared and motivated health care employees to continue to meet national health care needs.

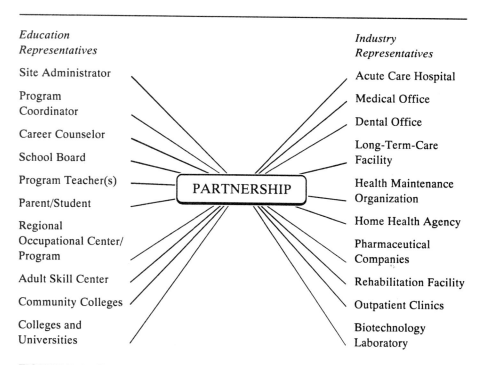

FIGURE 7-1: *Recommended Partnership Membership*

Establishing the Health Care Community Partnership

There are specific suggested steps necessary for ensuring that the health care community partner will agree that this is a worthwhile partnership. Like educators, those working in health care often are overburdened with unmanageable workloads and lots of paperwork. They need to understand that the benefits of the partnership will equal the effort required.

A motivated, knowledgeable, and committed school site program coordinator is essential to establishing the partnership. This individual contacts officials at the health care sites and seeks their commitment. The coordinator should be familiar with the health care community, its chain of command, and its nomenclature.

The following are recommendations to help secure the interest of the health care community partner.

1. Identify local education agencies.
   Include all appropriate education agencies in the planning process for the partnership. This ensures coordinated use of the health care facilities and results in an articulated program for the students. On occasion, health care providers feel as though they must choose between one education agency and another if facility use planning is not cooperatively coordinated.

   Education agencies that have been in the health careers student training business for many years will be able to submarine the new program if they are not included in the planning and assured that their program is not being duplicated.

   Education agencies to consider include:

   - Regional occupational centers/programs
   - Vocational schools
   - Adult skill centers
   - Community colleges
   - Colleges and universities

2. Identify local health care sites.
   Identify by name all potential health care partners that might be interested in participating. Contact appropriate health care associations such as the National Association of Health Care Recruitment to receive information about the local affiliate. Visit the local EDD office to determine those sites that have the largest projected and current employment needs. Scan the local newspapers for those agencies/facilities that are advertising for health care employees. Look in the yellow pages for a listing of health care providers. Titles might include:

- Acute care hospitals (general hospitals, university hospitals)
- Long-term-care and intermediate-care facilities (convalescent hospitals, nursing homes)
- Health Maintenance Organizations (HMOs)
- Outpatient clinics (urgent care, pre-op care, diagnostic and treatment centers)
- Home health agencies (visiting nurses, homemakers)
- Biotechnology laboratories
- Pharmaceutical firms
- Physical therapy and sports medicine offices
- Private medical offices and laboratories
- Private dental offices and laboratories
- Rehabilitation centers
- Public health agencies

3. Obtain initial site contact, Figure 7-2.

    The initial site contact is crucial to establishing the partnership. The person contacted should be familiar with the employment needs and training opportunities within the facility, clinic, or independent practice office.

    At large facilities or clinics, initial contact should be with the human resource department manager, personnel director, or recruitment manager. A second choice might be the director of educational services.

    In independent practice offices, small clinics, and labs, the office manager would most likely be the first contact.

4. Survey the identified potential partners and education agencies, Figures 7-3, 7-4, and 7-5.

    Help confirm the employee needs by occupation at each health care site, determine the many training programs in the general community that may already be using the facilities, determine the interest of all of those surveyed, and establish the name of a site contact person. Identify any issues that may need to be considered for training purposes.

5. Establish a forum to discuss health care training needs.

    The forum will provide the opportunity to share the goals of the program, ascertain health care partnership interest, and orient the school site personnel to the needs and resources of the health care partner based on the results of the survey.

FACILITY:

Name _____

Address _____

City _____ Zip _____

CONTACT PERSON:

Name _____

Title _____ Phone _____

RESOURCES AND SERVICES AVAILABLE:

Title
_____

Description
_____

Title
_____

Description
_____

Title
_____

Description
_____

FIGURE 7-2: *Local Contact Form*

DATE

Dear :

The State Department of Education, __ Unit, is working in concert with the __ School District to determine the need for a Health Careers Academy. The academy is tentatively planned for the ___ High School site.

Part of the needs assessment will include the collection of baseline data in relationship to current and projected health care industry hiring patterns. The data will be utilized to determine the academy's course parameters and content. It is anticipated that the academy will encourage students to consider the health care industry as a career option and that those enrolling in the academy will be prepared academically to continue their education at the level commensurate with their career choice.

A team of health careers consultants will be assisting in the data collection process. I am requesting the assistance of your staff in providing the data in an interview format with the assigned health careers consultant. The interview should take no more than one hour. *Name* is the consultant assigned to *place. Mr./Mrs.* will contact your office within the next week to schedule the interview.

Thank you for considering this request. I am anticipating a successful outcome that will result in an increase in the number of well-qualified health care providers. Should you have questions regarding the academy or the data collection process, please feel free to contact me.

Sincerely,

FIGURE 7-3: *Sample Form Letter*

Committees to establish support for the program by area of interest should be formed at the forum, with next-step efforts and short-term goals identified.

6. Form an advisory committee, Figure 7-6.
   The advisory committee should include those forum participants who seemed most interested in supporting the program. The roles of the committee will include identifying new health care trends; reviewing course curricula, facilities, and equipment; promoting the program; recruiting students; and supporting health care community partnerships. The committee also assists the instructional staff in developing short-range and long-range goals to ensure that the course remains current and relevant with industry practices.

   The advisory committee, through the development of short-and long-term goals, will help identify the immediate program needs that can be met through the health care community partnership.

7. Provide ongoing information for the health care community.
   Continue to share successes and additional needs of the program with

Name of agency _____

Contact person _____

Daytime phone _____

Consultant _____

SUGGESTED QUESTIONS
Health Care Agencies

1. Do you have employee shortages?
   If yes, in what specific areas? (nursing: RN, VN, aides/therapist, etc.)

2. Have the shortages increased/decreased?

3. What are your plans for addressing the shortages?

4. Are you considering new categories of workers?
   Are you considering changing job description for the current job titles?

5. Does your facility have plans for growth/expansion?
   If so, in what departments or types of services?

6. Are your new employees well prepared for their job?

7. If a ___ Academy were created, what courses/content would you like included?

FIGURE 7-4: *Sample*

Name of agency _____

Contact person _____

Daytime phone _____

SUGGESTED QUESTIONS
Education Agencies

1. What courses do you offer?
2. Do you plan to add/delete?
3. What is the status of enrollments (increased/decreased)?
4. Are students prepared to enter courses/programs?

   If no, what are their predominant areas of weakness (academic/attitude/language/behavior)?

5. If a ___ Academy were created, what courses/content would you like included?

FIGURE 7-5

Advisory Committee Responsibilities:

- Adopt curriculum
- Provide mentors
- Secure field trip and training sites
- Identify guest speakers
- Recruit students
- Monitor training
- Offer skill demonstrations showing relevancy to curriculum
- Promote recognition events
  - Brush-in Day
  - Good Health Day
  - Blood pressure clinics, etc.

FIGURE 7-6: *Implementation Plan*

the health care partners. Let them know their support is helping the program in general and students specifically to meet the goals that have been established by the advisory committee. Sharing can occur through a regularly scheduled news bulletin that can be managed by either the school site coordinator or one of the health care partners.

Identifying Resources and Services That Health Care Community Partner Offers

Often educators have the perception that the health care community has lots of available funds and can provide all kinds of financial support for the program and students when, in fact, the health care community often has the same kind of fiscal constraints as education. However, the health care community is well aware of the growing need for health care workers and is willing in most instances to provide a variety of resources and services that will result in an increase in the number of potential employee candidates. Some of the resources and services are listed below. It is likely that additional services and resources will be identified as partnerships are formed and expanded.

(Examples are listed in alphabetical order and do not imply priority.)

- Clinical rotations
  Clinical rotation experiences are short term but do provide hands-on activities. They are intended to give students a more intense view of the occupations they are considering. These experiences can be in the form of job shadowing or actual assigned short-term work. Clinical rotations are intended for students enrolled in exploratory and core courses.

- Educational materials
  Many health care facilities can offer lending library privileges to their vast array of patient education, recruitment, and scientific materials. Most libraries have audio, video, and printed materials available. This is a very good resource for introductory and core courses.
- Equipment and supplies
  Many health care partners replace equipment with newer models or wish to dispose of infrequently used items. Such equipment, as well as office products and promotional items, can be made available to the school program if the health care partner is aware they would be of use. An equipment and supply procurement committee might be formed at the initial forum to help link excess property with program needs.
- Grants/loans/scholarships
  There are a variety of grants, loans, and scholarships that can be made available to students as they continue their education. Often the awards are in specific career areas such as nursing or physical therapy. The health care partner can help locate these awards and provide information for students who are interested. This, too, might be a committee assignment from the forum meeting.
- Health care site tours
  A site tour gives students the opportunity to get a firsthand view of the health care environment and its culture, its job responsibilities, and the variety of careers available.
  Prior to a site tour, it is advisable to prepare a set of questions for the students to respond to or case studies to be developed based on their observations.
- Meeting rooms
  On occasion, meeting rooms are available at some facilities. It is a good place to convene meetings for partnership purposes because the health care professional staff are more available.
- Mentors
  Mentors provide the one-on-one support needed by many students to successfully complete the course work required to meet their education and career goals. Mentors role-model appropriate health care professionalism and the ethical behavior necessary for employees in the industry. Mentors check with their assigned student on a regularly scheduled basis to ascertain whether the student is completing schoolwork related to the career path. They offer, as needed, inspiration and motivation to help students continue to pursue their career

path. The mentor can assist the student with selecting and completing a project related to the career goal.

Many students fail to recognize their own capabilities, and a professional outside source can help them build their self-esteem and realize their potential for success. Once students become motivated, they often become excellent health care employees.

- Mobile units (rotating occupational labs)
Mobile units can be used to provide (1) hands-on opportunities for students who are unable to leave the high school campus due to travel restrictions and students who live in rural communities that do not offer the breadth of experiences that are available in more urban settings and (2) services that serve the community while allowing hands-on experiences for students.

The mobile units may be cosponsored by university medical or dental schools.

- Networking
A networking committee can establish a written or electronic system for information exchange. Job announcements, new training sites, student successes, student awards, new health care partnerships, new course information, and curriculum revision approval are only a few of the ideas that can be shared through networking.

- Publicity
The health care partners can provide in-house and community media publicity to build program and student support. Such support can increase the number of partnership opportunities and scholarship, grant, and loan awards for the students.

- Recruitment
Health care partners are usually members of professional organizations and service groups that are in a position to promote student enrollments. The partners are also able to provide employment opportunities for students completing their training or for those seeking part-time employment while continuing their education.

- Speakers
Health care professionals can offer career information relative to their area of specialization. The information might include education and training requirements, career benefits and responsibilities, working conditions, and job outlook.

Other speakers might include information on student scholarships and grants, advanced education opportunities, trends in health care, and bioethical issues.

In seeking speakers, be certain to outline what you would like the presentation to address.

- Summer/off-track jobs
  Many health care partners are able to provide summer/off-track employment for students. They can assist in the selection and coordination of student and facilities assignments.

- Teacher support
  Many of the teachers in the new career path programs have academic credentials and lack health care professional experience. An on-loan professional to assist the teacher as new health care applied academic concepts are introduced would be of significant benefit to both the teacher and the student.

- Training sites
  Training sites provide hands-on experience consistent with the students' course of instruction. Students are assigned to a training site once they have achieved, through classroom and lab experiences, competence in the skills that will be performed. The skills are then performed on-site under the combined supervision of the course instructor and the designated health care professional.

  These experiences normally extend on a regularly scheduled program the entire time the student is enrolled in the occupationally specific training program. In most instances, this training occurs during the last year of high school. Health care facilities in general do not allow hands-on experiences for students under the age of 16 years.

- Volunteer/community service
  There are a variety of opportunities for students to experience health care through volunteer and community service. It gives students a sense of working in the health care environment and at the same time provides a service for the health care partner by adding the extra pair of hands often needed in the facilities. The experiences help students focus on a career that is most consistent with their personal goals.

  In-facility professional development for teachers to orient them to the health care environment will help teachers determine student on-site assignments and understand the culture and ethics unique to health care.

Identifying Resources and Services That Education Partners Offers

Employers are more concerned with education and training issues than ever before. They also expect more from education and training than in the past. In order to establish a successful partnership, it is necessary to determine what benefit health care partners will receive and how their expectations can be met. Some of the resources and services that may be presented as the partnership is formulated are listed.

(Examples are listed in alphabetical order and do not imply priority.)

- Affirmative action/equal employment opportunity goal achievement
  Health care employers are required to meet AA/EEO goals. Since the student population often mirrors the community, potential employees selected from health careers courses can fulfill these employment goals.
- Employee recruitment
  Health care employee recruitment can occur in a setting where students are preparing to work in the industry and being informed of the benefits, opportunities, and requirements of working in health care.
- Networking opportunities
  Networking opportunities promoted by the education partner such as shared informal lunch meetings with health care partners can result in trend information sharing, issues identification and resolution, resource sharing, and the creation of partnership events.
- No-cost or low-cost training
  No-cost or low-cost training for entry and technical-level workers allows many students to prepare for employment in health care. This training results in a substantial number of candidates to fill entry-level positions.

  The public-sponsored training guarantees a return on tax dollars by providing service for the community through the health care employment of the graduates.
- Performance-based curriculum
  Performance-based curriculum and assessment ensure relevant learning experiences that result in job proficiency. The health care partner can feel certain that a skilled work force is being prepared.
- Public relations
  Publicity of the partnership demonstrates the health care community's commitment to community support and involvement.
- Student volunteers
  Student volunteers offer no-pay health care services within facilities, for example, a personnel office, for a specified time period. This allows the student the opportunity to observe firsthand the employment potential that exists in the health care field, and the health

career partner has the opportunity to observe firsthand the reliability and interest on the part of the students.

- Teacher volunteers
Teachers can consider volunteering to work in various departments, clinics, and private practices, including but not limited to their area of expertise. This not only provides a support service for the health care partner but also helps keep teachers' skills current with industry practices.

- Training expertise
Industry-experienced teachers can ensure that student graduates are well prepared to enter the health care work force and that the training provided meets the needs of the health care partner. Graduates are competent in their specialty areas.

    Teachers can also offer continuing education and professional development for health care employees as needed in coordination with course work presented to students. This is particularly useful when vendors are demonstrating new products for student information.

- Volunteers for special events
Students can serve as volunteers to support the health care partner in community service and outreach. Activities in which students might participate include: job fairs, blood pressure and other screening clinics, brush-ins (dental care), Good Health Day, adopt-a-grandparent at a long-term-care or adult day care facility, Meals on Wheels, hot-line phone response, telethon assistance, and assistance with setting up or judging state competitive events for Health Occupations Students of America.

Describing the Partnership Proposal

As the partnership is established, it may be beneficial to prepare a proposal that can be presented to the health care partner for review and consideration. The proposal should make clear the education partner's interest in meeting the health care partner's needs and should give the health care partner a concept of the education partner's expectations. A second benefit to the education partner is the clarification of partnership goals as the proposal is developed.

The proposal might include at least the following:

- Program purpose and description
Describe the purposes of the program, namely, whether it is to inform the student of health care career opportunities or provide exploratory experiences or occupationally specific training. Identify

when the course is offered (days and hours), where the classroom and laboratory instruction occurs, students' average age group, and estimated number of students enrolled annually.

- General purpose of partnership
  Describe the kinds of services and resources that the health care partner could provide that would be of most benefit to the students in the course. List the proposed responsibilities of both partners, for example, who determines the topic for guest speakers, how clinic rotation stations are determined, and who assigns the students.

  Describe the services and resources that the education partner is willing and able to offer for the benefit of the health care partner. Include the responsibilities for each partner.

- Goals, timelines, and evaluation
  List both the goals of the program and the goals of the partnership. Include projected timelines for each of the activities that are required to meet the goals and evaluation procedures that will be used to determine if the outcomes have been met.

Keep in mind that the proposal is only a working document. The health care partners will have the option to decline any of the suggested services and resources and will also have the opportunity to add suggestions that may not have been considered.

Adhering to Legal Requirements for Health Care Site Use

Health care is a unique industry in that it is restricted by both legal and ethical rules and regulations. There is a high level of confidentiality required due to the sensitive nature of the information that is gathered and available. Patient safety is utmost in the mind of those providing health care, and the legal and ethical parameters are designed to protect patients. To protect the health care client and the student, the following should be adhered to. Policies may differ from state to state and facility to facility. The following are intended simply as a guide.

- Affiliation agreement, Figure 7-7.
  The agreement is necessary for both exploratory and occupationally specific training programs. The agreement should include student liability, education agency responsibilities, and health care facility responsibilities. This is a legal document and can be developed by either the facility's legal department or the education agency's legal department at the county office.

  The agreement must be signed by representatives of the education and health care partners. If there are union issues to be considered, they may be included in the agreement as well.

THIS AGREEMENT is entered into this day of , 19, by and between County Office of Education, hereinafter referred to as "County," and (Name) (Address) hereinafter referred to as "Company."

WITNESSETH:

WHEREAS, Company desires to provide for the instruction of students to gain employment skills by means of program of on-site training; and

WHEREAS, Company is in sympathy with the educational objectives of providing training for the students of County.

NOW, THEREFORE, IT IS HEREBY AGREED as follows:

1. Company shall provide training stations which will provide for said students furnished by the County who are eligible to participate in the training program and who are qualified and acceptable to Company as determined by its PERSONNEL MANAGER the opportunity to expand the competencies developed in the classroom instruction portion of their training. Company may reject students who are not qualified or are otherwise not acceptable and may reject the training of any student when it determines that no suitable training station is available.

2. Company may terminate the training of any student hereunder if the student does not perform satisfactorily or if Company determines at any time that no suitable training station is available. Company will advise County prior to taking such actions.

3. Company *shall not compensate students* for any activities related to the training provided hereunder, and students performing training activities for Company hereunder shall not be considered employees of Company.

4. County, pursuant to the provisions of Education Code Section 5992, agrees to secure, upon written request, a Certificate of Insurance showing public liability and property damage insurance for County with limits of _____ for one person injured in one accident, and _____ for any one occurrence regardless of number of persons injured, and _____ property damage for any one occurrence.

5. The County Office of Education will provide coverage under the policies of the Schools Insurance Authority for Liability and Worker's Compensation Liability for medical benefits for students during the training activities.

6. County shall hold harmless the Company, its officers, agents, and employees for any claim for damages or loss, and any claim for wages, benefits or other compensation resulting form the acts or omissions of County, its officers, agents, employees, and students with respect to the program.

7. County shall:

   a. Assign students performing training activities hereunder to training stations providing experiences consistent with the purpose of the training program.

   b. Instruct students as to Company's rules and regulations to be adhered to while performing training activities hereunder.

   c. In cooperation with Company provide a written plan of training activities for each individual student placed in training at the Company which ensures that said student may realize maximum training benefits.

   d. Verify that the training activities set forth in each individual student's plan of training are in occupations for which there is a local job market.

   e. Make suggestions on training site safety to see that the requirements of the law are met and that health, safety, and welfare of students are not endangered.

FIGURE 7-7: *Sample Affiliation Agreement* (continues)

8. Company shall:
   a. Provide County with a written performance rating on each student performing training activities hereunder. Said performance rating shall be accomplished on forms furnished to Company by County.
   b. Consult the County instructor-supervisor assigned to each student regarding problems which may arise pertaining to student's training performance and behavior.
   c. Permit the County instructor-supervisor of each student to observe the student while performing training activities hereunder.
   d. Maintain accurate records of the student's attendance at the training station.

9. Company shall not utilize the services of any student pursuant to this agreement to displace or replace any Company employee, to impair existing contracts for services, or to fill any vacant position.

10. No student shall be denied participation in the program either by County or by Company because of race, age, color, religion, sex, national origin, or handicap.

11. All laws or rules applicable to minors in employment relationships are applicable to students participating in the training program pursuant to this Agreement.

Either party may terminate this Agreement upon delivering to the other party thirty (30) days' written notice of intent to terminate. Notwithstanding such termination, this Agreement may remain in full force and effect as long as assigned students are performing training activities.

IN WITNESS WHEREOF, the parties hereto have executed this Agreement as of the day and year first above written.

_____   _____
Superintendent   (Company Name)
_____ County Schools   _____
                                            (Street)
By: _____
    Assistant Superintendent   (City and Zip code)
                                            By: _____
                                            (Signature)

"COUNTY"   "COMPANY"

Approved by County Board of Education
in regular meeting held _____

Approved as to form by County Counsel.

— —

FOR INSTRUCTOR'S USE ONLY (Instructor must complete the following information.)

Instructor Information   *Company Contact Information*

Course Title: Company Contact Name:
_____   _____

Instructor: Department:
_____   _____

Instructor's Telephone #:   Company Contact Telephone #:
_____   _____

FIGURE 7-7: *Sample Affiliation Agreement (continued)*

Dear:

Please be advised that Worker's Compensation is provided through the Schools Insurance Authority. Worker's Compensation coverage under the authority program is the same as under the State Compensation Insurance Fund.

Pursuant to Education Code 51769, the school district or county superintendent of schools under which the supervision, work experience, or occupational training classes are held, shall be considered the employer, unless such persons during such training are paid a cash wage or salary by a private employer or unless such private employer elects to provide Worker's Compensation Insurance.

Employers who participate in the vocational training program by providing training experiences and do not pay a cash wage or salary to provide Worker's Compensation Insurance are not liable for Worker's Compensation for the youths being trained.

Yours truly,

FIGURE 7-8: *Sample Letter Worker's Compensation Authority*

Note: It is suggested that a sample agreement be shared at the first partnership meeting.

- Liability, Figure 7-8.
  The education partner is responsible for providing proof of liability coverage for students training in a health care facility. The students may be covered through district insurance. If not, the coverage may be purchased through a private insurance company. Often there are reduced rates for groups of students. The health care partner may be able to direct the education representative to a company that provides the reduced insurance. A university that offers health care education may also have the information available.

- Parental consent, Figure 7-9.
  Parental consent forms should be kept on file for minors participating in an on-site training experience. These forms should be signed by the parent, student, and teacher.

- Training plan, Figure 7-10.
  A training plan is necessary for students involved in occupationally specific on-site training. The training plan will include tasks that are within the students' scope of preparation and provide an outline for the on-site trainer that lists the work that can be expected of the student trainee.
  Note: A sample training plan should also be shared at the initial meeting.

Dear Parent:

Your son or daughter has enrolled in the following class:

_____

The content of this course may include discussion, descriptions, and/or illustrations of human reproductive organs and their functions and processes. Under Section 8506 of the California Education Code, a parent may withdraw a child from this class by a written request. Any written or audiovisual materials to be used in this class pertaining to reproductive organs and their functions and processes are available for inspection by the parent or guardian by arrangement with the _____ . The curriculum and materials are continuously being reviewed and revised by an Advisory Committee that consists of professional and lay members. If you wish to inspect these materials, please contact _____ to make the necessary arrangements.

Sincerely,

Date: _____

Parent's or Guardian's Signature: _____

Student's Name: _____

Teacher's Signature: _____

FIGURE 7-9: *Sample Letter Parental Consent*

- Scope of practice
  Students should have a clear understanding of what they are and are not permitted to do consistent with scope-of- practice rules and regulations.

  Students also need to be prepared to feel empowered to say, "I am not trained to do----," regardless of who is making the request. Understanding scope-of practice-parameters will support their empowerment.

- Health clearance, Figures 7-11 and 7-12
  To ensure that students are free from communicable disease and are protected from disease they may come in contact with, they are required to provide health clearance confirmation that may include:

  — Tuberculosis testing (purified protein derivative) or chest X ray

  — Vaccinations

  — Measles, mumps, rubella vaccination

HOSPITAL/COMMUNITY HEALTH SERVICES
EMERGENCY ROOM AIDE

INSTRUCTIONS: Please fill in the date and the time spent on each activity daily. When form is complete, submit to instructor.

TRAINING PLAN FOR: _____

Competencies:	Instruction at School	Rcvd. Site	Performance Level	Est.	Act. Hrs.	Date Done	Ver. by
General Clerical							
1. Take and relay phone messages			1 2 3 4				
2. Deliver charts, specimens, etc.			1 2 3 4				
3. Stamp requisitions.			1 2 3 4				
4. File department forms.			1 2 3 4				
5. Operate duplicator, addressograph.			1 2 3 4				
Patient Care							
1. Measure and record temp., pulse, respiration, height, and weight.			1 2 3 4				
2. Measure and record blood pressure.			1 2 3 4				
3. Admit patients to treatment rooms.			1 2 3 4				
4. Assist doctor/nurse in examination.			1 2 3 4				
Transportation							
1. Assist in transporting selected patients in beds, gurneys, and wheelchairs.			1 2 3 4				

COMMENTS:

FIGURE 7-10

This report/examination is being requested to satisfy the agreement for affiliation between the _____ program and the affiliate and is necessary to meet the objectives for the _____ class.

Name _____ Age _____

Do you consider this person free of infectious disease and physically and emotionally able to perform the duties of the above class?

_____
_____
_____
_____
_____
_____

_____   _____
Physician's Signature   Date of Examination

FIGURE 7-11: *Sample Physician's Report*

 — Polio vaccine

 — Diphteria, pertussis, tetanus vaccination

 — Health questionnaire

 — Physical examination

In some instances the cost of the exams and immunizations may be covered by the health care partner.

- Identification badge
  Most health care facilities require a picture identification badge. The cost of the badge may be covered by the health care training site. Such badges may not be necessary for students in private offices and clinics.
- Security clearance
  Some health care sites have a patient population or information that is highly sensitive in nature. These sites may require a security clearance for students participating in training experiences.
- Oath of confidentiality
  An oath of confidentiality should be signed by each student and kept on file before the student participates in exploratory or training experiences at a health care site.

_____

Name _____

Address _____

_____

Have you ever had a positive tuberculin skin test?

      Yes   No

_____   _____

Date of Testing   Site

_____   _____

Name   Dosage/Solution

_____

Nurse's Signature

— —

_____   _____

Date of Reading   mm Induration

_____

Nurse's Signature

FIGURE 7-12: *Sample Certificate of Skin Testing*

- Oath of loyalty

  Some health care sites may require that students sign an oath of loyalty that essentially states they will uphold the mission of the institution.

- Radiation monitoring

  Monitoring may be required for students training in areas where radiation exposure is possible. This will include dental offices, some dental labs, radiation therapy offices or clinics, and diagnostic imaging areas in hospitals.

- Accident procedure

  A written procedure for accidental injury or other incidents that may befall students must be established and shared with each health care training site. An information sheet for each student should also be on file at the health care site and should include whom to contact, an emergency phone number, the teacher's name and phone, insurance information, and an "authorization to treat a minor" form (parental release).

Fulfilling the Expected Health Care Professional Image

Health care is a competitive business. At the same time, the services offered are often in the most stressful of circumstances. All providers, whether employed or voluntary, must present an image that exudes professionalism and inspires confidence in the recipients of the services provided.

"Of the negative perceptions (expressed by potential industry partners), many were based on a single bad experience. A number of the employers interviewed recounted 'horror stories' involving administrative delays, faculty resistance, or sensitivity to employers needs."[3]

Critical components for consideration as both the teacher and student prepare to enter the health care setting are as follows:

- Professional attire
  Professional business dress is expected. An example might be the attire one would wear for a job interview. A second option would be clinical attire that could consist of a health care uniform or lab coat. If this option is appropriate, the name of the school/program should be prominently displayed on the uniform or lab coat. Closed-toe shoes are always required for safety and sanitary purposes. Name tags must be worn at all times.

- Professional behavior
  In the highly sensitive health care environment, all employees, trainees, and volunteers are expected to demonstrate ethical behavior, use good judgment, and act responsibly.

- Effective communication skills
  Presentations, both formal and informal, should be organized, well prepared, and succinct.

  Meetings should be scheduled well in advance, agendas prepared, and information disseminated in a timely manner.

  Language used should be simple and understood by all concerned. Avoid educational jargon.

  Written communication must be in an appropriate format, such as memos, letters, forms, or proposals, and either typewritten or word processed.

  Confidentiality continues to be a primary requirement for all who enter the health care setting. In large facilities, there are designated areas for educational staff, trainees, and volunteers. The designated areas must not be violated, as injury, contamination to a patient, the educational staff, a trainee, or a volunteer could be the result.

---

[3] A Community College Guide To Working With Employers in the Bay Area, September 1988.

- Health care site policy
  An important issue is to check with the health care site to determine if it has specific policies or procedures regarding professional dress, behavior, or designated areas that are peculiar to that site. The first contact for this information might be the human resources department.

☞ ENSURING PROGRAM ACCREDITATION COMPLIANCE THROUGH QUALITY AUDIT MECHANISMS

The American Medical Association defines accreditation as "a process of external peer review in which a private, nongovernmental agency or association grants public recognition to an institution or specialized program of study that meets certain established qualifications and educational standards, as determined through initial and subsequent periodic evaluations." (CAHEA, 1983)

The standards of program evaluation are specified in the Essentials. The extent to which an educational program satisfies the standards specified in the Essentials determines its accreditation status.

Unfortunately, interest regarding accreditation concerns is often directly related to the proximity of an on-site evaluation. It is the responsibility of the program administration and faculty, however, to ensure continuing compliance with the standards of accreditation. The implementation and maintenance of quality audit mechanisms facilitate meeting this responsibility.

Quality Audit Mechanisms

Quality audit mechanisms include those internal and external processes associated with the formative evaluation of an educational program. The focus for formative evaluation is on the monitoring methods that ensure the maintenance of open communication within the program. External measures provide data from sources outside the program, including graduate and employer follow-up studies and information gained from the review of the program by accreditation agencies. These methods of evaluation are characteristic of the goal based or behavior objective model of program evaluation. The purpose of this chapter is to describe the goal-based model of evaluation and illustrate the application of specific measurement procedures as quality audit mechanisms.

Goal-based evaluation: According to Tyler, "Evaluation is essentially the process of determining to what the educational objectives are actually being realized by the program of curriculum and instruction" (Tyler, 1949).

This perspective is indicative of the goal-based model of evaluation. The evaluation process involves collecting evidence to measure the extent to which the stated program goals are being achieved. Tyler advocates defining these goals in behavioral terms. Objectives were refined over the years to include domains (cognitive, psychomotor and affective) and in writing of behavioral objectives. The competency-based approach to instruction is founded on using behavioral objectives as the basis for both instruction and evaluation.

Internal programmatic evaluation: Internal goal-based evaluation provides a mechanism for quality control. This is accomplished through methods that stimulate dialogue among the groups of people involved in the educational program.

According to the "Essentials and Guidelines of an Accredited Educational Program for the Radiographer," as an example, structured and documented channels of communication among all aspects of an educational program shall be provided. The implementation and maintenance of an advisory committee represents a mechanism not only to satisfy the requirements of this standard but also for formative program evaluation. Emphasis should be placed on the necessity to maintain the operation of the advisory committee. Without attention, the advisory committee may become nominal rather than functional. Including representation from the agencies that employ program graduates provides an opportunity to ensure that the program is meeting the changing needs of the community. In addition, the advisory committee should serve as an internal mechanism of curriculum validation.

As participants in the learning process, students represent a valuable resource for the formative evaluation of the educational program. Frequently, institutional policy requires that students evaluate courses and instructors. The appropriate use of the information obtained by this process depends on the purpose of the evaluation. An instrument designed to assess teacher effectiveness may be too limited in scope to measure aspects of program-level evaluation. For example, institutional concerns may not address the integration of didactic and clinical instruction. In addition to the formal evaluation of classroom instruction, students should have the opportunity to evaluate the quality of the instruction in the clinical setting. This may be accomplished through the use of a clinical evaluation instrument that provides information regarding the availability and nature of clinical supervision, the enforcement of clinical education policies, the quantity and variety of examinations available, and the students' perception of the attitude of the staff regarding their participation in the instructional process.

A third internal quality audit mechanism involves the process of student counseling and advisement. Regularly scheduled advisement meetings provide an opportunity for students and faculty to share ideas regarding the quality of the educational program. Information obtained in the process of advisement should be documented and discussed by the faculty.

Both didactic and clinical faculty members should participate in the formative evaluation process. Commonly, the opportunity for this involvement is provided by regularly scheduled faculty meetings. Articulation among clinical faculty should be accomplished through a clinical education committee chaired by a clinical coordinator, who should also serve as the communication link between the didactic and clinical faculties.

In order to ensure continuing compliance of the program with accreditation standards, it is recommended that all faculty participate in an ongoing process of internal review. Documentation of this review may be accomplished by using the program evaluation guidelines developed and published by the accrediting or approval agencies. This type of instrument is often used to ensure consistency and standardization of reporting in the evaluation of programs. The guide may consist of a checklist indicating the degree to which the program is in compliance. As deficiencies in the instructional system are identified, corrective action can be taken before the effectiveness of the program is impaired.

External programmatic evaluation: Goal-based evaluation methods should measure the extent to which the program graduates achieve the terminal competencies of the program. Quality audit mechanisms that accomplish this evaluation function include both graduate and employer follow-up studies.

These studies may be conducted by either phone, personal interview, or mail survey. There is more underreporting on self- administered questionnaires than on personal interviews. Additional considerations when selecting a study procedure include the type, quantity, and sources of data required and the time and resources available.

The graduate follow-up study may be conducted on an annual basis or in phases. The initial study should be completed no later than one year after graduation. According to Norton, this initial study is undertaken to obtain data such as employment status, job title, and further education and to gain the graduates' insight into the instructional program. Subsequent studies provide information regarding career mobility and continuing professional development. After one year, the extended time elapsed after graduation decreases the probability of collecting valid data regarding graduates' perception of the program.

Information regarding the abilities of graduates may be obtained from the employer follow-up study. The scope of each interview or survey should involve the general performance of several graduates rather than the ability of a single individual. The results of both the graduate and employer follow-up studies should be correlated with data obtained from other measures of program effectiveness.

The formative evaluation data from quality audit mechanisms is derived from the desire to hold all aspects of the instructional program accountable for achieving specified goals. External methods provide data from sources outside the program, and effective communication within the program provides the basis for a process of internal quality control.

References

R. W. Tyler. *Basic Principles of Curriculum and Instruction.* Chicago, 1949, p. 105.

Essentials and Guidelines of an Accredited Educational Program for the Radiographer, 1983, p. 3.

Sudman, S., and N. Bradburn. *Asking Questions.* San Francisco, 1982.

Norton, R., et al. *Establish a Student Placement Service and Coordinate Follow-up Studies.* Columbus, Ohio, 1980.

8
Curriculum Development: What the Instructor Will Teach

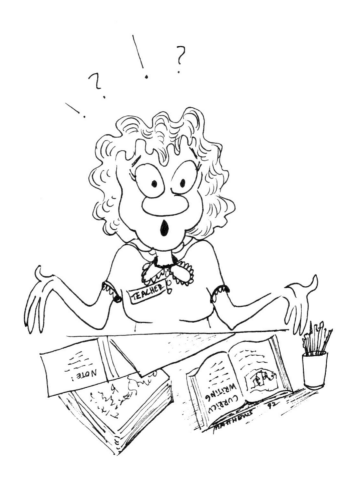

IDENTIFYING THE CURRICULUM

In an earlier section entitled "The Transition: From Clinician to Educator!" the author informed you that the subject matter you will teach is, in most health occupations education programs, related to the job in which you were previously employed. This is true; however, an essential question for you to resolve before accepting a teaching position is "What am I specifically expected to teach, and are there materials already available?" In education, this is referred to as a curriculum.

Definitions

The term curriculum may be defined in both a broad and narrow sense. Its Latin derivation means to run a course or a race. This definition implies that before one can accomplish such a feat, one must know some essential information.

In its broadest sense, curriculum refers to a body of knowledge or a group of learning experiences that students need to successfully acquire or achieve while preparing, for example, to be a health clinician. In most educational settings, this knowledge or group of learning experiencs is conveniently divided into preidentified subject matter or courses and referred to as a program. Consider all the courses or subjects you completed to become a health clinician. The scope and sequence of these subjects or courses, including their many learning experiences, composed an entire curriculum or health occupations program, Figure 8-1.

In a more narrow application, the term curriculum may be defined as a written plan for what students are expected to learn. This plan is not unlike a road map or a route to be taken while pursuing a health occupation. Refer to the previous illustration, and visualize a plan for completing preparation for a health occupation. Do you see certain courses taken before others? Do you see time frames in quarters/semesters/years?

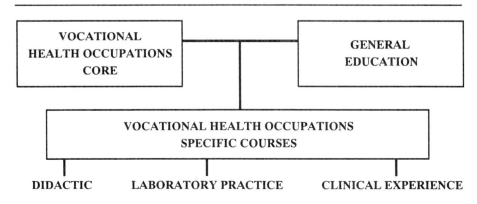

FIGURE 8-1

Although the above definitions are general in nature, and there are many others, these should suffice for your initial use. It is important to be familiar with how a curriculum is identified. Otherwise, you may mistakenly proceed on the wrong path while preparing your students for a health occupation. To discover how specific curriculum is identified, two approaches will be shared. The first is the process in which curriculum has been identified and developed; the second is used when no curriculum has yet been identified or developed. Each requires similar, yet different, responsibilities for you, the teacher.

Refer to the Latin meaning of curriculum: to run a course or race. Think of all the questions to which you would desire answers if you were asked to participate in this activity. Perhaps the following would come to mind:

- What is the name of the course or race?
- Who determined a need for it?
- What is its purpose?
- Who can participate?
- Where does the course or race begin?
- What route needs to be taken?
- How much time is allowed?
- Is there an entry fee?
- What is needed to participate?
- Where does the course or race end?

Interestingly, these questions are similar to the ones an effective teacher must answer in order to identify an appropriate curriculum for any health occupations education program. Since curriculum is also defined as a written plan, you must initially lay out that plan and work to achieve it. Be aware, however, that there are many available resources to help you. Do not try to "reinvent the wheel."

☞ STEPS FOR IDENTIFYING CURRICULUM

Identifying an appropriate health occupations education curriculum and establishing a plan for its implementation or its use are not difficult, but they do involve several steps. Overall, it takes qualified people—both professional health clinicians and educators; planning and implementation time; and an adequate budget to support the entire process.

Scenario: There is a critical shortage of both nursing and allied health care workers. Rumor has it that local hospitals and long-term-health-care facilities are in dire need of a particular health occupations education program. You have been employed by an education institution to give leadership in determining the need for such a program and to identify an appropriate curriculum if the need is justified.

Where do you begin? How do you complete this task? The following are suggestions.

STEP 1 • *Conduct a Needs Assessment*

Even though the above scenario implies there is a need, how great a need must be determined. Surely you would not want to unnecessarily start any health occupations education program that duplicates what is already existing nearby or that would serve a population of only one or two students. Conducting a needs assessment involves either or both a written and oral survey of the community. The same kind of questions could be used while conducting a telephone or on-site visitation survey. Important to this process is documenting the results.

In addition to assessing community health agencies, it is essential to determine potential student interests and aptitudes. Though health agencies may have a need, there can be no education program without students. Surveying high school students or adults, talking with school counselors, using local news media, town meeting announcements, and the like are effective approaches.

Scenario: Preliminary information from your assessments seems to prove a need for the health occupations education program desired. You are now ready to initiate the next step.

STEP 2 • *Organize an Advisory Committee*

While conducting the needs assessment, you probably met with interested and supportive educators, local citizens, health clinicians, and potential students. These are the categories of individuals you will need for advice and direction in this program. In addition, it is likely that state departments of education have specialists who may assist. In essence, each of these individuals can become invaluable in the entire curriculum process.

A total number of ten representatives is recommended for the committee. Make selections that will give balance to male, female, and racid populations. It is also suggested that the chairperson be a health industry representative. Such leadership has, in most cases, the most to gain by ensuring that the education program come into existence. You should serve as secretary, at least during the beginning phases of the committee's work.

During the initial meetings of the committee, agendas that permit discussions and decisions on at least the following items should be included:

- Assessment results
- Budgets
- Staffing
- Training of staff
- Occupations analysis
- Curriculum identification/development

- Instructional materials
- Equipment and supplies
- Facilities
- Credential requirements
- Accreditation/program evaluation requirements
- Clinical practicums/internships
- Articulation/matriculation
- Institutional scheduling
- Student recruitment
- Program marketing

A comprehensive implementation plan is strongly encouraged. It should include, in detail, the following areas:

- Goals
- Objectives
- Strategies for implementation
- Resources needed (fiscal and human)
- Assignments to committee members
- Deadlines for completion

Obviously, all of the above needs adequate time to take place. It is suggested that at minimum a year's time frame be used to develop and implement the plan.

Following the program's implementation, the original advisory committee members may be placed on rotating terms of tenure. Continued guidance from this group is considered essential throughout the duration of any health occupations education program.

Scenario: With a comprehensive curriculum plan in place, you are ready to embark on its implementation. Important to your role is appropriate identification of the health occupations education curriculum. Notice that the next step may not be necessary to implement if you have been employed to teach in an already existing curriculum. The information covered in the step, however, is worthy of your consideration. Having a thorough knowledge of the curriculum's scope and sequence and of your role as a teacher within it better equips you to effectively and efficiently execute it.

STEP 3 • *Create a Curriculum Design/Model*

What is it a student needs to know, value, and be able to perform in order to prepare for a health occupation? This is perhaps the most critical question related to identifying an appropriate curriculum.

The decision about an appropriate curriculum design or model should not be made by a single person. Involvement of selected advisory committee members, educators, professional health clinicians, and others, who have expertise in curriculum and the technological area is especially helpful. This also affords accountability to financial supporters, such as taxpayers and grant-giving institutions.

Discussions and decisions should include answers to at least the following questions.

- What are the desired program goals and philosophy?
- What is the program's description?
- What occupational tasks compose this health occupation (occupational analysis)?
- What student outcomes are essential?
- What program outcomes are desired?
- What constitutes an acceptable scope and sequence?

A summary flow chart for curriculum development is included as Figure 8-2. You will undoubtedly use or develop your own design. The above questions may seem complex at first. Obviously, each requires considerable thought. It is likely, however, that answers may be already available. It is strongly encouraged that you first review local, regional, and national

---

DEVELOPING A CURRICULUM (A PROPOSED MODEL)

Conduct a needs assessment
↓
Organize an occupational advisory committee
↓
Validate occupational analysis
↓
Develop program scope and sequence
↓
Identify core competencies
↓
Verify competencies
↓
Identify specifications for courses
↓
Develop course blueprints

FIGURE 8-2

resources. The following is a listing of suggested areas where curriculum-related information may be found.

- Educational Resources Information Center (ERIC)
  Contact: Local school media center specialist
  Products: Program abstracts, locations
- National Center for Vocational Technical Education Curriculum (NCVTEC)
  Contact: Local school media center specialist
  State department of public education
  Regional NCVTEC laboratories
  Products: Curriculum guides and materials from states
- Vocational-Technical Education Consortium of States (V-TECS)
  Contact: Local school media center specialist
  State department of public education (members only)
  Products: Objectives, test item banks, occupational task listings
- State departments of education
  Contact: Health occupations education state supervisor or education consultant
  Products: Curriculum guides, test item banks, instructional materials, program planning guides
- Commercial publishers
  Contact: Local school media center specialist
  Products: Procedure manuals, instructional materials, textbooks, teacher guides, student workbooks
- Professional organizations
  Contact: Local/regional/district/national presidents
  Products: Credential requirements, testing information, career descriptions

Although the previous listing is not all-inclusive, it can readily offer you a helpful beginning. Being able to adapt or adopt such materials can indeed reduce time consumption and costs. A word of caution, however. Be sure your group of experts verifies that the materials already developed are appropriate to the design and needs of the identified health occupations education curriculum desired.

For our purposes and in its broadest sense, curriculum is defined as a body of knowledge or a group of learning experiences necessary to a student's preparation for a given health occupation. More narrowly defined, it may be a written plan that identifies a scope and sequence of courses. Curriculum may also be synonymous with the term program, namely, a health occupations education program such as respiratory therapy.

Identifying an appropriate health occupations education curriculum is not difficult, but it does involve at least three initial steps: (1) Conducting a needs assessment, (2) organizing an advisory committee, and (3) creating a curriculum design or model. Such a process takes qualified people, money, and time.

References

Bloom, B. (1984). *Taxonomy of Educational Objectives.* New York: McCay.

Hass, G., J. Bondi, & J. Wiles (eds.) (1974). *Curriculum Planning: A New Approach.* Boston: Allyn and Bacon.

Houston, W. R. (ed.) (1974). *Exploring Competency-Based Education.* New York: McCutchan.

Maley, D. (1975). *Cluster Concept in Vocational Education.* Chicago: American Technical Society.

Raynor, N. (1990). *Secondary Health Occupations Education: Vocational Competency Achievement Tracking System.* Raleigh, NC: North Carolina Department of Public Instruction.

Rubin, L. (1977). *Curriculum Handbook.* Boston: Allyn and Bacon.

Winters, M. (1980). *Preparing Your Curriculum Guide.* Alexandria, VA: Association for Supervision and Development (Stock Number 611-80208).

Performance Objectives: What the Students Must Learn

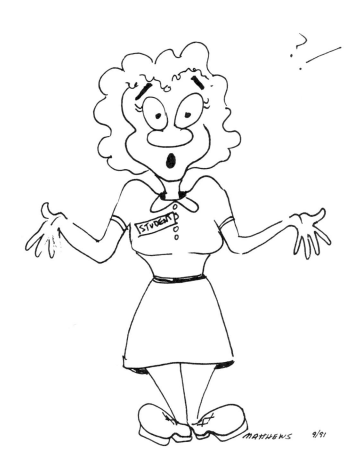

Evaluation of student performance is a topic of major concern to students, to parents, and to teachers. During the past ten years, a number of national reports have focused on the mediocrity of the curriculum and teaching in our schools. As teachers, we are interested in how well our students perform. Our interest is not only in how well students perform in relation to each other (a norm-referenced issue) but, even more important, in determining the extent to which they are able to meet externally imposed performance standards (a criterion-referenced issue). Some students may perform acceptably relative to other students in a group, but the entire group of students may not be able to meet external performance standards. This issue becomes even more critical in fields in which competent performance is mandatory in order to avoid potentially serious consequences such as in the health occupations education field.

☞ PERFORMANCE OBJECTIVES

Competent performance is measured by performance testing, which, in turn, focuses on skill outcomes. Skill outcomes reflect program objectives, meaning those competencies expected of students upon completion of the program. Skill outcomes may be found in most educational programs. For example, problem-solving skills are important in mathematics programs, and communication skills are important in language programs. In addition, skill outcomes are important in career-preparatory or vocational education programs such as agriculture education, business education, distributive education, health occupations education, home economics education, and trade and industrial education. Therefore, performance tests that measure skill outcomes are an important component in the evaluation of students for most educational programs.

Criterion-referenced measurement was popularized originally by Robert Glaser (1963) and is designed to evaluate mastery of a given skill or knowledge of a given performance objective. For the purpose of this chapter, a criterion-referenced measurement is one that measures what students know or can do compared to what they must know or be able to do in order to perform a specific task or procedure successfully. The standard by which students will be measured is the performance objective. Comparison between students is irrelevant in criterion-referenced measurement. For a review of the developmental and academic literature in criterion-referenced measurement, consult Alkin (1974), Berk (1980), Glaser and Nitko (1989), Hambleton (1974), Livingston (1972), Mager (1984), Meskauskas (1976), Panell and Laabas (1979), Popham (1971, 1990), and Swezey (1981).

Because the standard for criterion-referenced measurement is the performance objective, a brief description of objectives follows. One potential confusion about writing objectives is that the term objective is used in many different contexts. In an educational program, objectives are written for the overall educational program, for a specific course, for units of instruction, and for individual lessons. In addition, the work objective is used in program evaluation and management contexts to describe what the teacher or manager should accomplish during a specific period of time in relation to a group of students or other people. Some individuals use the term inappropriately to describe broad program goals or general intents of the educational program. To a certain extent, this variety of usage is understandable in that by definition, objective means an end of action. The term student performance objective refers to a statement describing the kind of performance to be achieved by students in a program. Such statements usually include three components: performance, condition, and criterion (Mager, 1984).

Performance

The performance part of an objective describes what the student will be doing. It must contain an observable response that can be measured. The following statements demonstrate the performance component of an objective.

- Demonstrate knowledge of the rationale for developing student performance objectives and the characteristics of properly stated objectives.
- Analyze and rewrite given student performance objectives.
- Identify each of the objectives on a given list as being primarily cognitive, psychomotor, or affective.
- Develop student performance objectives in each of the learning domains that contain statements of performance, condition, and criterion.
- Sequence a given list of student performance objectives.

Condition

The condition part of the objective outlines the circumstances under which the student will be required to perform the activity. This portion of the objective describes:

1. What equipment, supplies, or materials will be given to the student
2. What materials the student will be denied access to
3. What setting the performance must be demonstrated in
4. What information the student may be provided that will direct the action in a certain way
5. What amount of time will be allowed for the performance to be accomplished

The criteria part of the performance objective describes the degree of proficiency that must be reached in carrying out the performance; in other words, this part describes how well the student must be able to do the job. The criteria tell the student and the teacher what level of performance is required in order for the performance objective to be achieved. This part of the objective probably is the most difficult to write, but once done, it also provides the information necessary for planning how to evaluate student performance. There are several ways in which the criteria may be established, including:

1. Accuracy within a tolerance limit
2. Speed
3. Percent or number to be achieved
4. Reference to other material that identifies specific criteria
5. Maximum number of permissible errors
6. Degree of excellence
7. Any combination of these criteria

Following is a sample of performance objectives demonstrating the three components.

1. Dispose of a contaminated needle, according to your facility's policy, with 100% accuracy.
    a. Performance — dispose
    b. Condition — according to facility policy
    c. Criterion — 100% accuracy

2. Given a diagram, locate all of the endocrine glands found in the human body.
    a. Performance — locate
    b. Condition — given a diagram
    c. Criterion — all of the endocrine glands

3. Given a laboratory patient care unit, complete terminal cleaning of the unit correctly within one-half hour.
    a. Performance — complete terminal cleaning
    b. Condition — patient care unit
    c. Criterion — correctly within one-half hour

Objectives may dictate the type of performance testing to be used. Usually, performance testing includes the following types: (a) pencil and paper, (b) identification, (c) simulation, and (d) work sample. Pencil-and-paper tests are used to measure both knowledge and skill; that is, write a care plan, calculate a medication dosage, compute a patient's intake and output, or, from the previous objective, locate the endocrine glands on a diagram. Identification tests may be from simple to complex, from identifying the body organs to diagramming the flow of blood through the heart. Simulations emphasize proper procedure and may be used as a learning tool or as a final assessment of student performance, that is, role-playing a job interview or developing a sample diet for a resident. Work samples incorporate the highest degree of realism as students perform actual tasks under controlled conditions in either a laboratory or a job setting, for example, practicing bedside patient care skills in a laboratory, accompanying a home health nurse on patient assessment visits, or, from the previous objective, disposing of a contaminated needle according to facility policy. One or more test types can be used to measure a specific skill at various levels of instruction or upon completion of instruction.

☞ PERFORMANCE OBJECTIVES

Two types of performance testing—simulation and work sample—should include a checklist or some type of rating scale. Figures 9-1 and 9-2 demonstrate a common checklist approach to grading.

Student: _____

Date: _____

Directions: Place a check in front of each step as it is performed.

_____ 1. Review the physician's order.
_____ 2. Wash your hands.
_____ 3. Assemble equipment.
_____ 4. Identify the resident.
_____ 5. Provide privacy.
_____ 6. Explain what you are going to do.
_____ 7. Check to be sure the resident's hands are clean and dry.
_____ 8. Make handrolls from washcloths and give to resident to grasp.
_____ 9. Apply the mitt restraints.
_____ 10. Tie the straps to the bed frame using a square knot.
_____ 11. Check resident frequently, as restraint will prevent use of call signal.
_____ 12. Wash your hands.
_____ 13. Report the procedure, and record your action, following facility policy.
_____ 14. Remove restraints for ten minutes every two hours, and exercise the extremity prior to reapplication of the restraint.

FIGURE 9-1: *Checklist for Applying Mitt Restraints*

Student: _____

Date: _____

Directions: Place a check mark in the appropriate box.

	Additional Practice Needed	Satisfactory Performance	Comments
1. Explains procedure and elicits patient cooperation.	_____	_____	_____
2. Places patient's arm next to body with palm downward.	_____	_____	_____
3. Places first three fingers against radial artery.	_____	_____	_____
4. Feels for pulsation using gentle pressure.	_____	_____	_____
5. Counts for appropriate time period, using watch with sweep second hand.	_____	_____	_____
6. Records pulse and any unusual volume or quality.	_____	_____	_____

Comments:

Observed by: _____ Date: _____

FIGURE 9-2: *Sample Checklist for Radial Pulse*

Validity specifically refers to whether the instrument can measure what it was designed to measure. The rating scale can serve as a check to determine if the testing instrument uses the performance objective as the standard for criterion-referenced measurement.

Figures 9-3 and 9-4 use a type of rating scale. Performance tasks that use a rating scale are more difficult to construct and are more time-consuming than a checklist. These disadvantages along with the difficulty in assigning a letter grade to the rating scale have influenced many programs to adopt a pass/fail, satisfactory/unsatisfactory, or satisfactory/needs-improvement method of grading.

Mitstifer (1983) has developed a rating scale for performance testing instruments that describes specific criteria to be evaluated (Figure 9-5).

Achievement testing is important in all types and phases of instructional programs. Testing can tell teachers what skills and abilities students possess prior to the instructional program. During the instructional program, testing

Student: _____

Date: _____

Directions: Write in the appropriate number for level of performance of each activity.

PERFORMANCE LEVELS

Activity	4	3	2	1	0
1. Selection of Equipment	Selects proper equipment for each procedure	Usually selects best equipment for procedure	Needs some assistance to select best equipment	Usually needs assistance to select proper equipment	Never selects proper equipment for a procedure
2. Use of Equipment	Uses all equipment correctly	Uses most equipment correctly	Needs some assistance in using equipment	Usually needs assistance to use equipment	Always needs help to use equipment
3. Care of Equipment	Cleans equipment and returns to proper place	Usually cleans equipment and returns to proper place	Needs some reminding to clean equipment and return to proper place	Always needs reminding to clean and return equipment	Never cleans equipment or returns to proper place

Student Score

Activity 1: _____   Activity 2: _____   Activity 3: _____

Comments:

Observed by: _____   Date: _____

FIGURE 9-3: *Sample Rating Scale: To what extent does the student select, use, and care for equipment?*

Student: _____

Date: _____

Directions: Place a check mark in the appropriate box.

1 — rarely
2 — occasionally
3 — frequently
4 — consistently

	1	2	3	4	Comments
1. Has appropriate equipment.	___	___	___	___	_____
2. Explains procedure.	___	___	___	___	_____
3. Places patient's arm next to body with palm downward.	___	___	___	___	_____
4. Places first three fingers against radial artery and feels for pulsation.	___	___	___	___	_____
5. Counts for appropriate time period — 15, 30, or 60 seconds.	___	___	___	___	_____
6. Records pulse and any unusual volume or quality.	___	___	___	___	_____

Comments:

Observed by: _____ Date: _____

FIGURE 9-4: *Sample Rating Scale for Radial Pulse*

can tell which students are having difficulty with certain learning tasks. Upon completion of the instructional program, testing can tell how well each student has achieved the intended outcomes of instruction. Two types of testing are common to instruction: norm-referenced testing and criterion-referenced testing.

Norm-referenced testing emphasizes the measurement of individual differences in achievement and compares performance of the student to other students. It typically covers a broad area of achievement, and test items are selected that provide maximum discrimination among students. Easy items usually eliminated from the test. The level of performance is determined by

Student: _____

Date: _____

Directions: Rate the instrument according to the following criteria by placing an X in the appropriate blank.

Criterion	Description		Yes	No
Quality	Does it measure quality of the performance?			
		_____ Skill	_____	_____
		_____ Attitude	_____	_____
Efficiency	Does it measure efficiency of the operation?		_____	_____
Ease of use	Do the language, design, length, and degree of detail promote ease of use?		_____	_____
Achievement	Does it achieve the goals of monitoring of goals student progress, diagnosing, certifying, and evaluating instruction?		_____	_____
Adaptability	Does it serve, with little revision, for self-evaluation, peer evaluation, and instructor/supervisor evaluation?		_____	_____
Validity	Does it measure what it is designed to measure? ...		_____	_____
Reliability	Does it provide trustworthy or consistent measurement?		_____	_____

Recommendations for change:

Observed by: _____ Date: _____

FIGURE 9-5: *Rating Scale for Performance Testing Instruments (Mitstifer, 1983)*

relative position in some known group (e.g., ranks third in a group of 30 students).

The principal use of criterion-referenced testing is in mastery testing as its major emphasis describes tasks students can perform. Typically, it focuses on a limited set of learning tasks and includes all items needed to adequately describe student performance. No attempt is made to alter test item difficulty or to eliminate easy items to increase score variability. The level of performance is determined by absolute standards (e.g., demonstrate mastery by defining 90% of the medical terms).

Although both types of testing are important to instruction, this chapter addressed the use of criterion-referenced testing. Criterion-referenced performance testing provides the student with an individual assessment of one's endeavor against an externally imposed performance standard, the performance objective. The performance objective identifies what the student must do, in what circumstances, and how well. It reflects the skill outcomes or competencies required by graduates upon completion of a particular program. The criterion-referenced performance test is one path to be taken on the road to improved evaluation of student performance.

References

Alkin, M. C. (Ed.) (1974). *Problems in Criterion-referenced Measurement.* Los Angeles: Center for the Study of Evaluation, University of California.

Berk, F. A. (Ed.) (1980). *Criterion-referenced measurement: The state of the art.* Baltimore: John Hopkins University Press.

Glaser, R. (1963). "Instructional Technology and the Measurement of Learning Outcomes: Some Questions." *American Psychologist, 18,* 519–21.

Glaser, R., and A. J. Nitko (1989). "Measurement in learning and instruction." In R. L. Thorndike (ed.), *Educational Measurement* (3rd ed.). Washington: American Council on Education.

Hambleton, R. K. (1974). "Testing and Decision-making Procedures for Selected Individualized Instructional Programs." *Review of Educational Research, 44,* 371–400.

Livingston, S. A. (1972). A Classical Test-Theory Approach to Criterion-referenced Tests. Paper presented at the annual meeting of the American Educational Research Association, Chicago.

Mager, R. F. (1984). *Preparing Instructional Objective* (2nd ed.). Belmont, CA: Pitman Learning.

Meskauskas, T. A. (1976). "Evaluation Models for Criterion-referenced Testing: Views Regarding Mastery and Standard-Setting." *Review of Educational Research, 46,* 133–358.

Mitstifer, D. I. (November 1983). Educational Leadership Skills for Nurse Educators. Paper presented at an inservice staff development workshop for nursing faculty, Chambersburg, PA.

Panell, R. C., and G. T. Laabs (1979). "Construction of a Criterion-referenced Diagnostic Test for an Individualized Instruction program." *Journal of Applied Psychology, 3,* 255–61.

Popham, W. J. (ed.) (1971). *Criterion-referenced Measurement: An Introduction.* Englewood Cliffs, NJ: Educational Technology Publication.

Popham, W. J. (1990). *Modern Educational Measurement* (2nd ed.). Englewood Cliffs, NJ: Prentice Hall.

Swezey, W. R. (1981). *Individual Performance Assessment: An Approach to Criterion-referenced Test Development.* Reston, VA: Reston Publishing.

10

Competency-Based Education: Did They Get It?

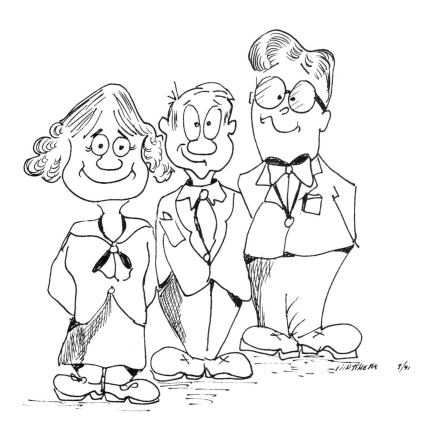

👉 DESIGN

Education in the United States is considered big business. It is funded with billions of dollars that pay for items such as salaries, buildings, supplies, instructional materials, staff development, and teacher education. Accountability for these funds is a given, not a choice. You, as one of many educators, are expected to provide documentation that justifies the expenditures necessary to initiate or maintain your health occupations education program. You must provide proof that the program in which you teach fulfills the purposes it was designed to achieve. A competency-based curriculum is one way this accountability may be measured.

Competency-based Education

Several definitions of competency-based education (CBE) have been written. A widely accepted definition, suggested by Stanley Alam, can be paraphrased as follows:

> Competency-based education is an instructional system designed to teach students to learn explicit knowledge, skills, and attitudes necessary for proficiency in the performance of a task or a group of tasks using individualized/personalized teaching/learning strategies and criterion-referenced evaluation methods.

What CBE Can Do

To explore more specifically what the previous statement means, let's analyze some essential elements of what CBE can do.

1. CBE is an instructional system that:
   - Affords both teacher and student accountability for learning and/or performance.
   - Facilitates the development and evaluation of a student's achievement of specified competencies.
   - Is composed of integrated parts, including competencies, objectives, supportive learning activities, resources, and testing.
   - Provides an instructional road map or blueprint for an identified body of knowledge, a group of learning experiences, or a curriculum's scope and sequence.
   - Is student oriented, not teacher focused, and based on outcome behaviors.

- Determines a student's rate of progress based on demonstrated proficiency and not time or course completion.
- Affords an accountable means to articulation/matriculation.

2. Competencies are broad, measurable statements that:
   - Reflect knowledge, skills, and attitudes to be demonstrated by a student.
   - Are stated in measurable terms making possible the evaluation of a student's performance or behavior.
   - Are made public, especially to students, in advance of their learning.
   - Identify the body of knowledge necessary to the preparation for a given occupation.

3. Criteria to be used in assessing competencies are:
   - Founded upon and compatible with preidentified curriculum competencies.
   - Explicit in reflecting expected levels of performance and mastery, given specified conditions.
   - Made public, especially to students, in advance.
   - Objectively focused.
   - Considerate of the student's knowledge relevant to basic and critical thinking skills.

Implied in this definition are other characteristics often found in CBE.

1. Instruction is personalized and individualized.
2. The learning experiences of each student are guided by feedback.
3. The emphasis is on exit, not entrance, requirements.
4. Instruction may be modularized.
5. The student is held accountable for performance, completing a curriculum when, and only when, he or she demonstrates the preidentified competencies.

For students, there is evidence that when they know in advance what is expected of them, their learning increases. Competencies provide important information about what is expected of them in the program. There is no guessing game between the student and teacher about what a program involves. Integrated within each competency statement are implied learning activities, which must be accomplished in order to successfully complete a program. The competencies also outline the criteria upon which a student is evaluated.

Consequently, students can determine at any point within a given program what they have accomplished and how much remains to be completed.

If students miss a portion of the curriculum for some reason, they can identify what must be done to complete the missed work. Or, if students have had previous experiences with given competencies, they can determine which ones they have already achieved, request testing, and, if successful, proceed to the remaining competencies.

For the teacher, a competency listing affords a valuable blueprint for planning and implementing the instructional process. It surely answers the questions: "What do I teach?" and "At what depth do I teach?" A comprehensive competency listing that covers all courses or individual ones identifies the knowledge, skills, and attitudes in which students must be proficient in order to perform those tasks that industry has verified are essential to a given occupation.

Having such information is especially helpful to the teacher who sometimes tends to stress certain curriculum content or skill development because of personal preference and not because a specific occupation requires that much emphasis. For example, a health clinician who has had extended practice in coronary care might spend extra time and energy teaching the circulatory system and less time on the nervous system. Both systems deserve at least equal time and energy. CBE offers a rational and systematic approach to delivering instruction and assessing student achievement founded upon what the health industry deems necessary.

For the potential employer, competency statements document those skills that graduates of a program can be expected to have. With access to computer capabilities, competencies and task listings can be entered, updated, revised, or deleted so as to match technological changes. In addition, a record of these competencies and the student's mastery level for each should be made available to graduates to share with potential employers, parents, guardians, or spouses.

For the program evaluator, a teacher's use of validated competency statements establishes a base for program evaluation. Questions about whether a program is fulfilling its goals, philosophy, and purposes or whether graduates are able to perform essential tasks may be reviewed through careful examination of how well students are achieving the competencies. Analysis of such information also can begin to identify program strengths and weaknesses in resources, methodology, learning experiences, student gains, and other essential components.

What CBE Cannot Do

Though CBE has many merits, it is only fair to discuss also what this instructional system is unable to do. Competencies are written in broad terms and reflect validated knowledge, skills, and attitudes. They do not define the teaching or learning activities that should be used to achieve them. Moreover, they do not specifically identify each occupation's tasks. The following example provides a case in point.

Competency Statement: Upon completion of the _____ program, the student will be able to apply medical asepsis with 100% accuracy in a health care setting.

Analyze the above statement. Do you see the following?

1. It is outcome based ("upon completion of the program").
2. It is student focused ("the student will be able to").
3. It relates needed knowledge ("apply medical asepsis") skills, and attitudes.
4. It affords conditions for ("with 100% accuracy in a health care setting").

You do not see a listing of teaching or learning activities. And you do not see medical asepsis broken down into specific occupational tasks such as handwashing, handling equipment, and handling supplies. Consequently, competency statements define what the outcome must be, but not how you will teach the material or how the student will learn it. As a classroom instructor, you will need to reduce each competency into smaller pieces of information and develop measurable lesson plan objectives.

CBE does not provide administrators with an easy approach for the elimination of teaching personnel in the event students fail to achieve expected levels of proficiency for all program competencies. It will, however, afford administrators and teachers alike a means to:

1. Assess exactly what the status is in terms of student achievement.
2. Identify the probable cause of such failures.
3. Provide a means for redirecting efforts or resources to improve given circumstances.

Among some educators there is disagreement regarding the strict use of measurable student outcomes as a sole means of evaluation and accountability. Arguments are that CBE limits students' applying or strengthening creative and critical thinking skills; that the development of values is given less instructional emphasis since many cannot be objectively evaluated; and that many teachers will "teach to a test" to ensure successful student competition. Such issues admittedly are debatable. It is wise for a new teacher to resolve such concerns on an individual basis with the help of experienced educators. One must always keep in mind that no one system serves every cause. Perhaps you will find to your satisfaction the best of both worlds for your students.

Responsibility for Implementing CBE

It is your responsibility as a teacher to plan for and manage a learning environment within which each of your students can achieve the competencies identified for your program. You are also responsible for testing or evaluating student performance and documenting the degree to which each student has developed proficiency or accomplished mastery.

As mentioned earlier in this chapter, you do not have this responsibility alone. The advisory committee you organized to assist in identifying an appropriate curriculum is invaluable to CBE implementation. In addition, your local administrators are equally accountable. This is especially applicable to providing planning time, a budget, staff, materials, facilities, supplies, and equipment. They are also responsible for ensuring each program is relevant both to student and community needs and to the occupational purposes the program was designed to meet.

The state education agency has a role in implementing CBE. You will recall earlier mention of access to program area specialists as consultants. Most likely the state education agency has prepared materials for you or can assist you in finding them. It is also the agency's role to offer you staff development or to recommend those individuals who can.

Developing a CBE Curriculum

In the event a competency-based curriculum is unavailable for the identified health occupations education program you desire to implement, one will need to be developed. You are reminded that CBE is an instructional system. As with any system, CBE involves several components or developmental steps. Do not assume that such a delivery system is developed single-handedly. Advisory committee members, state program consultants/supervisors, teacher educators, teachers, and local administrators are available and should be involved. From these groups, you may desire to select representatives to serve on a curriculum team. A word to the wise: Be sure to ascertain in advance your time frame for development, access to computer information entry, the budget, and other helpful resources. Maintaining a computerized progress/historical report of the developmental process will enhance your accountability.

STEP 1 • *Conduct an Occupational Analysis*

Logically, this step should have been completed when you identified an appropriate curriculum. It involves a comprehensive listing of every cognitive, affective, and psychomotor task in which a potential health clinician needs to be proficient in order to prepare for the identified health occupation.

Developing an occupations task list involves primarily those health clinicians who are actively employed in a health occupation. Selection of individuals from different health agencies in which this occupation is practiced is also recommended. This adds to the discussion of tasks and their applications. There is a process called simply developing a curriculum (DACUM), which may be used while conducting an occupational analysis and developing a CBE curriculum. There are available DACUM specialists who can be very helpful to you. Your local institution, university, or state education agency may be able to recommend someone.

STEP 2 • *Develop and Sequence Core Competencies*

A rough draft of possible competencies is prepared from a review of an occupational analysis, interviews with health clinicians in the identified health occupation, and available curriculum resources. The draft is submitted to teachers, teacher educators, curriculum specialists, program area administrators, and other appropriate practitioners for their verification, editing, additions, and/or deletions. (Remember—CBE statements should be written to reflect student outcome behaviors. Refer to the previous competency on medical asepsis.) Competencies from this revised and/or edited listing are once again submitted to practicing health clinicians in the health occupation for validation. Finally, a curriculum team reviews the verification and validation steps and makes the final decisions as to which competencies are core or supplemental and their sequencing within the identified health occupations program.

Decisions regarding which competencies are core or supplemental and their sequencing may represent a laborious, time-consuming activity. Core competencies are those most commonly practiced by all respective health clinicians in any appropriate health care environment. Supplemental competencies generally are those that are practiced by the health clinician but that may be unique to special health care environments or even reflect projected and/or futuristic health care delivery.

Sequencing of competencies may be influenced by several variables: from simple to complex behaviors, scheduling of courses within which competencies may be taught, weight or importance, and/or time needed to teach. It is important that the curriculum development team reach consensus on the criteria to be applied. Such information is valuable to a later staff development component.

STEP 3 • *Develop Course Sequences and Outlines*

Upon completion of step 1, a lengthy list of sequenced competencies should result, representing the entire identified body of knowledge or learning experiences necessary for the preparation of the identified health occupation practitioner. In most school settings, these competencies will need to be organized into a sequence of courses with identified course numbers and/or codes for whatever time frame is deemed necessary to complete them, namely, 12 weeks, 6 months, 1 year, 2 years, 4 years, etc. If the health occupation requires a college parallel curriculum to meet degree-granting requirements, consideration must be given to integrating appropriate academic or general education courses in the areas of, say, mathematics, science, and social studies into the total preparation time frame.

While the curriculum team is identifying courses, it is logical that it identify course titles and develop course outlines for the health occupation. This will facilitate and expedite the ongoing process. Because curriculum team members are also program specialists, their knowledge of content is reliable. Additional training with regard to curriculum writing may be needed, however.

STEP 4 • *Develop a Competency-based Test Item Bank*

For purposes of preassessment, interim assessment, or post assessment, a competency-based test item bank is recommended. Each competency should have at least one or a series of appropriate criterion-referenced test items.

Before initiating this step, be sure to research available test items. Upon receipt of any items, have the curriculum team or a selected test bank team screen these test items carefully for technical accuracy and content validity, and ascertain their reliability. Test items should measure the competencies identified.

A bank means that items may be deposited as well as withdrawn. Consistent updating is necessary to provide the most effective assessment process available. A system for reporting student performance is also necessary for communicating student progress, evaluating program strengths and weaknesses, and improving test items. Users of the test items must be afforded input into this assessment system. It should be noted that the sequence of this step in the curriculum development process is debatable. It is believed by some curriculum developers that it should be the final step since access to units of instruction (unit outlines, content, learning activities, resources) enhance the effectiveness of test item development. In contrast, others perceive development of units of instruction as a teacher's responsibility. You are advised either to use your own judgment in making this decision or to abide by your institution's policy.

STEP 5 • *Develop Program and Course Specifications*

If you consider the sequenced program and course competencies as a blueprint for instruction, then previous references to a comprehensive curriculum plan become clearer. An architect must develop a blueprint before construction can begin. Along with the architect's blueprint are construction specifications. This is also true of curriculum development. Program specifications include broader descriptions, and course specifications identify those specific to each course. Having such information at hand assists a teacher in effectively and efficiently planning instruction. Criteria for such specifications should include program title, code numbers, competencies to be taught, time length, teacher credentials, and resources. Review these carefully and differentiate the content.

STEP 6 • *Develop Program/Course Blueprints*

Reference has been made to a health occupations education blueprint. Blueprint information may be collectively applied to a format that identifies at a glance major program/course requirements. In addition, it is a very valuable planning tool from which a teacher can schedule, for example, an entire quarter-long, semester-long, or yearlong instructional plan. Moreover, it is an excellent marketing and accountability tool. Practically every major curriculum decision has been plotted on this blueprint, including time frames for teaching each competency or objective and the weight each carries per unit and for the course. Why is such weight important? Although there are several obvious reasons, a major one is that it more adequately conveys the number of test items to be incorporated into a given test for any given competency or objective.

STEP 7 • *Develop Units of Instruction per Course*

Some curriculum developers believe this is a teacher function, but development of units of instruction from previous program and/or course outlines can provide much assistance in conveying the thinking of a curriculum team and can standardize an instructional plan among the health occupations education programs of the same title. Units of instruction are the meat of a curriculum guide. It should be understood that this step is not intended to eliminate a teacher's creativity or teaching style. The format, which can vary, seeks to afford yet another piece of a curriculum blueprint, but with greater detail. Unit specifications may also be included.

Again, before embarking on the development of units of instruction, seek curriculum guides through the previously identified resources. They are likely available, but review them carefully to ascertain their compatibility with your identified curriculum.

STEP 8 • *Develop Supplemental Curriculum Resources*

There are many other instructional materials that a curriculum team might desire to develop or access through other resources. Such committed and creative individuals' ideas frequently outlast financial budgets. Examples of such resources are as follows.

- Course Calendar Instructional Plan

Helping a teacher to become an effective and efficient time manager is commendable. One approach to this achievement is through developing a course calendar instructional plan. Plotting a given course length on a calendar projects the number of days each unit of instruction should be taught and affords the teacher at a glance a mental clock for accessing student materials, inviting guest speakers, and ordering audiovisual aids.

- Class Progress Chart

Informing students in advance of expectations can assist them in achieving them. A class progress chart is simply a visual aid to assist students in accomplishing required competencies.

All competencies may be listed in a matrix format, and a bar graph can result that plots each student's progress. This matrix identifies specific competencies to be performed. Each student has an identification number that gives confidentiality but does not eliminate healthy competition. In addition, each student can plot progress as can the teacher.

- Individualized Learning Activity Packages

Integrating competencies, specific objectives, learning activities, and self-check quizzes into learning activity packages offers a self-pacing approach to individualizing and personalizing the instruction. Each student is given a package and primarily assumes responsibility for his or her own progress. The teacher's role is that of facilitator and evaluator. An advantage to this teaching/learning approach is that the teacher is more available to those students needing additional assistance. Activities should include both independent and cooperative learning opportunities.

Developing such packages is time-consuming and expensive, but they are considered an effective instructional tool. Investigate the availability of such resources before initiating development, and review them carefully to ascertain their compatibility with your identified curriculum competencies.

- Student Competency Record

Students receive report cards indicating their achievement or lack of it but the frequently used letter grades or Arabic numerals do not specifically convey the competencies in which a student may be proficient.

Developing a student competency record that identifies program competencies and a mastery level for each can be especially effective in communicating with parents and potential employers.

Curriculum Maintenance

Now that you have identified, developed, or accessed an appropriate health occupations education curriculum, you probably feel that your job is completed. Not so. Because your curriculum is based upon industry (technology) needs, community needs, and student interests and needs, these elements continue to change. Consequently, maintaining your curriculum becomes a cyclical process. Frequent assessment of the process and its products is essential to adequately prepare students for potential employment in the identified health occupation.

Advisory committee members can be a major resource in updating and upgrading competencies and content, but consulting them does not eliminate the need for continued surveys of a larger number of appropriate health clinicians and educators. In addition, follow-up on graduates can provide invaluable assis- tance for determining revisions. It is equally important to the developmental process to reassess at least annually the need to improve a competency-based curriculum.

Summary

Accountability in education is a given, not a choice. CBE affords an effective approach for educators, students, and the health industry to justify the preparation of potential health clinicians, given current and projected technological needs, community needs, and student interests. CBE represents an instructional delivery system that explicitly identifies the knowledge, skills, and attitudes necessary for proficiency in a task or a group of tasks. It supports individualized methodologies and criterion-referenced evaluation methods.

Developing a CBE curriculum may be considered a complex but not impossible task. Familiarity with its elements helps to accomplish the task in a rational, logical, and methodical manner. Most important are the involvement of advisory committee members, educators, and students and the use of available materials and resources.

Once CBE is implemented, critical to its success is reassessment of the process and products, at least on an annual basis. Change too, is a given and not a choice both in education and in the health industry. Preparation of potential health clinicians can be no more effective than the instruction they receive.

IMPLEMENTATION IN A VHO PROGRAM

There are many ways of implementing a competency-based, self-paced health occupations program in a postsecondary vocational center. Traditionally, health occupations training programs have been conducted using established beginning and ending dates, a lecture format, organized class activities and tests, class clinical experiences, and class graduations. The student who falters, is absent, or has a different learning style from the instructor's teaching style may be lost. Thus, a potentially successful student becomes a dropout.

Reenrollment must wait until the next class, maybe a year away. Because of some correctable setbacks, the individual who is otherwise "ready" has to be put "on" hold.

A successful option would be to consider converting your formal, traditionally taught program to a self-paced, modified, open-entry/open-exit program. Non-health-related vocational programs have utilized such a system for years.

This section describes two types of programs — one using a totally self-paced, open-entry/open-exit approach, and the other, a modified or "wheel," self-paced, modified open-entry approach. Both methods require extensive planning and organization in their administration and implementation.

Planning and Preparation

There are many models and resource materials published that go into detail on each aspect of implementing a self-paced, competency-based training program. This section introduces the reader to some practical basics that work. Further review and on-site visitation to operating programs are highly recommended.

First things first: Arrange a time allocation before starting this project. Total concentration and freedom from distractions are musts. The author completed the following activities in a three-week full-day time frame. But before starting, do the following.

Update the competency list: A thorough examination of the current content of the program must be made — reidentification of the specific competencies required for the occupation, steps needed for the student to achieve mastery of a competency, and willingness of the instructor to attempt a "change" in their instructional delivery system. The current state requirements must be reviewed to make sure that all "minimum" requirements are included in the program content.

Involve the program advisory committee: This is where the advisory committee comes in. The committee's job is to review the program competency list and content to ensure that what is taught is relevant to the local occupational job requirements. If the committee finds that certain content is not relevant to local needs or that other content should be added, the minutes of its deliberations and recommendations should be used in adjusting the competencies for the program. The recommendations should also be shared with the district and the state departments of education, so that when the time comes for official revision to program requirements, there are documentation and rationale to support the changes or updating needed.

Once the advisory committee evaluation has been completed, the competency list should be honed and trimmed. Each competency should be able to be taught within 3–30 hours of instruction. Competencies should be organized from the simple to the complex in groupings of related duty areas.

> Examples: All competencies relating to administration of medications should be grouped.
>
> All competencies relating to medical office insurance claim filing should be grouped.

Analyze the competencies: In order to be valid, a competency should be able to be measured objectively. How many of us judge a student's performance by our own value judgment or past experience? ("The only way is my way!") Have we established (and shared with the student) written criteria with which to measure a student's venipuncture technique — except that the student obtained a blue top vial of blood — without bruising the patient! This is where the instructor should examine the steps involved in evaluating a student's performance. What is the final outcome? Vital signs readings matched with what the instructor found? Ace bandage applied so gangrene wouldn't set in? Account ledger totals that add up to those on the teacher's answer key? Are we measuring a product (bandage and dressing) or a process (setting up a sterile field)? In addition, are we measuring the extent of theory or the knowledge of the student?

In a task analysis, the final method of evaluation of the specific competency is stated in the objective. Enablers or steps needed to meet the final competency level are determined. (How many of your old lessons did it take to complete instruction?) What do the students have to know (theory) about the competency? What do the students have to do to perform the competency?

Getting It All Together

This is a project that is best tackled during student holidays, spring break, or summer vacation. Curriculum development funds may be available — check with your supervisor. You will need work space to spread out and no distractions.

Now that the competency list and the task analysis have been accomplished, it's time to take stock of what you already have and what you will need to convert your program to self-paced learning.

If you've been teaching for any length of time, you have probably accumulated several file drawers full of handouts, article reprints, notes, folders on obscure but interesting subjects, samples, models, transparencies, and so on. All these things you use in your everyday traditional instruction. You may also have acquired a big notebook with your outlines and lecture notes.

Organization of all this material is the key!

- The first task is to label a bunch of file folders, each with the name of a competency identified for the program.
- The second step is to arrange the competency folders according to related groupings or duty areas: anatomy and physiology, legal aspects, vital signs, written communications, human behavior, front office duties, infection control. Arrange the grouping of folders on tables so you can read the labels.
- The next step is opening up all those file cabinets! Start sorting all the materials into the competency folders.
- This is where you start making a pile of those handouts, articles, and pearls of wisdom that don't fall into any specific category and that you can't part with. So set up a miscellaneous folder. If you find material that isn't current or appropriate, toss it. It will only hurt for a little while.

When you have created mountains of file folders, each stuffed with lots of materials, sort through your audiovisuals (tapes, filmstrips, videos), models, charts, operator's manuals, and adjunctive materials. Pile them on top of your folders or make a list of them as they relate to a specific competency folder and insert the list or paste it on the outside cover.

Take a look at your textbook. Are you using more than one? Is there another text that matches the content of your program better? Now is the time to think about changing texts. Hint: Have your reading specialist show you how to do a reading level on your text(s). An eleventh- or twelfth-grade reading level text is not appropriate for a seventh- or eighth-grade reading level student. (Editor's note: RightWriter Version 4.0 by MacMillian is a software package that quickly and simply evaluates the grammatical style and grade level of any material. Not only can you evaluate the grammatical and writing levels of personally designed material, but you may also key in text from books or articles for an evaluation.)

At this point, if you find that certain competency folders aren't very full, you may want to analyze the importance of these competencies. Are they actually an integral part of another competency, or have the competencies been overlooked and undertaught? On the other hand, you may find that some folders (competencies) need to be broken down into smaller competency statements. So, make some more folders. This is okay. These things happen. You are doing this for yourself and your students. Wait until you start writing!

Getting It in Writing

There are several ways to write self-paced instructional materials for your students. The learning guide or assignment sheet is the easiest and quickest way to accomplish it. Your purpose is to develop guides, not self-contained modules. These guides will tell the student to do certain activities, where to locate materials, what to do with them, and when to test.

Your students are going to be responsible for their own progress! You are going to become their learning manager and resource person. More on that later.

Take a competency folder—any one of them. Spread out the materials inside. Arrange them in order of sequence. Example: reading and studying concepts, audiovisuals, demonstration and practice, testing. Think about how you have presented these materials in the past. What were some of the activities you used to help your students learn the competency? Taking a blank sheet of paper, title it with the name and number of the competency. Start listing the activities in a logical sequence that will lead the student through to **mastery of the competency**. At this point, you may find that the content is too extensive for one series of instruction. Consider breaking this competency down into smaller more concise ones. Remember your 3- to 30-hour time span. (You'll find such adjustments will occur throughout this process.) Provide for self-checks of knowledge and practice time.

Note: Figure 10-1 includes a variety of learning activities to accommodate different learning styles of students. As you review these activities with the student, you may want to omit or add some for particular students.

Student: _____

Beginning Date: _____

Completion Date: _____

Competency 01.01 — Handwashing

1. In your text, read and study about bacteria and how they cause infection — *Bugs,* chapter 2, pages 12–13.
2. View the video, "Handwashing, the Video."
3. Arrange with your instructor to go to the computer lab to use the software "Handwashing, the Software." Bring the printout to your instructor.
4. Go to the resource file and obtain the folder "Handwashing, My Life." Read and study the article. Make notes for your notebook and return the folder to the file.
5. Check your understanding by completing the Student Activities at the end of the chapter in your text. Compare your answers with the contents of the chapter. If you didn't get 100%, review the chapter or see your instructor.
6. Have your instructor demonstrate handwashing techniques.
7. Practice handwashing.
8. Have a senior student evaluate your handwashing procedure.
9. Take Knowledge Test.
10. Take Performance Test.

FIGURE 10-1: *Sample Assignment Sheet*

Your school or district may require that all student learning materials be written in a special format. Student learning guides are different from one district to another. See the example at the end of the chapter for a complete guide. Your curriculum resource teacher can help you with development of your guides/assignment sheets.

Testing and Evaluation

Evaluate the written tests you have used in the past. The knowledge test should be revised to test the theory or concepts of the competency in question. You may elect to group several "level" or related competencies for a comprehensive written test.

A study guide listing major points may be developed for each written test. This guide should be shared with the student after the student has completed the learning activities. It could also be used for transfer students who are challenging competencies in order to receive credit for previous learning and or work experience. The author's feeling is that adult students need to know what is expected of them and need to be able to sort out the extraneous from the specific. You will find that distributing a study guide that lists topics/concepts to be included on written tests will be of great benefit to your students.

The performance test should be the most frequently used because the skill is the thing! A copy of the performance test should be given to students when they are given the competency assignment sheet or learning guide. That way, students know exactly the procedure (process) or product to be evaluated. It can be used by the peer evaluator during practice and by the instructor for the final performance. There is no room for guessing or judgment calls. Even substitute teacher has a guide to follow. With a checklist, a second teacher won't impose a new set of values if the performance test has all the criteria included in which to judge the performance.

Effects On The Instructor

Converting to a self-paced, individualized instructional program may give an instructor the initial feeling of giving up control over students. The students won't have the benefit of fascinating lectures well laced with war stories. In this new format, students need the instructor as much, if not more than in the traditional method. They become responsible for their own progress. New students need a time for adjustment and learning organizational skills. Advanced students need encouragement and support. The instructor becomes the resource manager, guiding and directing each student. The most frequently used method of instruction becomes one-on-one or small group. Much of the instructor's time is spent building a well-organized, professional learning environment.

Classroom arrangement: A typical classroom organized for self-paced instruction would include the following areas: quiet study, testing, demonstration and lab practice, small-group discussion, and audiovisual. In contrast to the traditional classroom, where enough pieces of equipment were needed for the anticipated enrollment, the self-paced classroom needs only enough equipment duplication to accommodate 4 or 5 students at a time (maybe fewer). The author's school originally purchased 15 microscopes and all the attachments for an enrollment of 15 students, and when self-pacing was implemented, 12 of the microscopes were put in storage. As students progress through the learning guides, some will work more quickly than others, and, eventually, a group who start together will soon diverge so that each works on a different competency! The room should be arranged so there are enough workstations containing equipment and supplies for each competency or competencies cluster. A quiet study area located away from the noisier end of the room is necessary for those students who need it. Study carrels, equipped with audiovisual equipment (slide/tape players, video projector, and head sets) should be arranged in a small grouping near audiovisual storage cabinets. A separate study carrel can be designated for written testing and should be located within easy view of the instructor's desk. Numbered files hold resource materials and assignment sheets/learning guides. Bookcases hold references texts, dictionaries, and models. Related charts, equipment, and samples should be labeled and displayed for easy location by the student. Collections of supplies (example: physical exam equipment) should be placed in labeled containers (plastic or heavy-duty cardboard boxes) and located in easily accessible areas. In general, all supplies and equipment (with the exception of hazardous or extremely delicate materials) should be out and available for student access. This will save time for the student and frustration (at the interruptions) for the instructor.

The student folders, testing material, and attendance records should be kept in a locked cabinet. Instructors should keep learning guides/assignment sheets locked also, so as to prevent students from helping themselves to more than one guide at a time. The instructor should be the one to dispense new assignment sheets in order to review them with the student and discuss the best approach to learning the new competency. Students should be working on one guide at a time during each class session. Testing (performance or written) should be accomplished as soon as possible after the student has completed the competency learning activities.

Classroom Management

Student orientation: New students will need a thorough orientation to the classroom and the concept of competency-based, self-paced learning. A tour of the classroom should be included for each new student. If these two things are not done, adult students may drop out quickly.

New students need a "home" seat and a place to put their books, notebooks, supplies. When students enter the classroom, seats should be designated. As students begin the day's activities, they will move about from one area of the room to another completing assignments but should have a place to come "home" to. Student lockers are recommended if more than one class is using the room at other times of the day or night.

Attendance: Attendance and promptness should be emphasized and checked at the beginning of each class period. Students should be encouraged to contact the school if they are going to be late or absent. This discipline is essential to success on the job in the future. The instructor is the role model.

Evaluating Student Progress

Another very important function for the instructor is to talk with each student at the beginning of each class day to identify goals for the day. The instructor can use the talks to plan for demonstrations, performance testing, and speakers; to schedule clinical experiences and assignment of rotations to other subject areas; and to verify the progress of the student. Such daily interviews help the instructor to encourage a student's progress and identify problem areas needing attention. A little notepad in the pocket of the instructor's uniform comes in handy for follow-up notes.

In addition to the daily interview, the instructor should set aside time at least every four weeks to meet privately with each student to evaluate the student's progress. Since most individualized learning materials will take from 3 to 30 hours to complete, a plan of completion can be established with each student. Students should be allowed to retake an unsatisfactory written or performance test 48 hours after the first attempt.

Scheduling

Variations in scheduling students should be available. Full-time students, half-time students, and part-time students can be accommodated in the same classroom. From the author's experience, enrollment will increase when choices for class times are given. When enrollment picks up, limitations on the variations in scheduling can be imposed. New students should be able to start at any time. An option would be to allow new students to start on a certain day during the week or a certain week during the month, especially if enrollment is high for the program. But in order to maintain the open-entry/open-exit concept, some flexibility on entrance dates is a necessity.

Benefits

Students complete the program individually throughout the school year instead of all of them at once. Employers have a constant selection to choose from due to this arrangement. Students can also enter throughout the school year—when they are ready and not when the school is ready. Students can enroll for portions of the program that may be needed for updating or for specific skill training while employed. Those who have to drop out for a period of time can reenroll and pick up where they left off. (Some discretion must be used in evaluating elapsed time.)

Conversion

Converting a traditional program to self-paced instruction is not easy, but it can make the difference between a failing program and a healthy one that meets students' needs for flexible scheduling. The following is a list of steps to follow in making the change.

- Organize materials according to the competencies included in the program.
- Prepare performance and knowledge tests for each competency (or group of related competencies).
- Make assignment sheets or learning guides that list directions and assignments for students to follow in achieving mastery of each competency.
- Rearrange files, bookcases, cabinets, and shelves to accommodate learning resources and equipment so they can be found easily.
- Visit a successful health occupations program that uses the open-entry/self-paced format.
- Prepare a new student-orientation plan.
- Evaluate, evaluate, evaluate—rewrite, rewrite, rewrite!

The Wheel

The following description is a natural evolution to the total open-entry/open-exit, self-paced, individualized classroom. It is called the Wheel, Figure 10-2. Please read on.

As a result of evaluation of the management of the original self-paced program, the concept of rotating small groups of students through different subject areas was developed.

Even though the program is competency based and self-paced (all students working on individual tracks, testing, and moving on at their own rate of learning), the concept institutes small groups (of no more than 6) that enter at the same monthly date, stay together, help each other, and feel a part of a family. We have seen the positive proof of peer-help keeping the group together. From it, the weaker student gains support and strength.

Each group starts on the third Monday of every month, except for the months of June and December. Each group starts at a certain position on the wheel

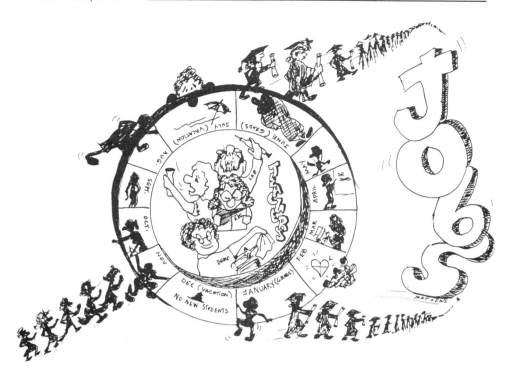

FIGURE 10-2: *The One-Year Wheel*

and progresses with the help of a flow chart and a calendar, knowing exactly where it should be at any given week in the 45 weeks of the program. Because of the need for more room, this center is limited to 51 students monthly, but a typical program has 56 students: 6 on externship for two months and 6 completing each month, thus allowing 6 new students to enter the program monthly. All students will complete the program in a year's time. No student will be slowed down. If a student is very fast, that student may jump into the group ahead; if students are slow, they fall back to the group that entered after they did. All students who have had this happen are happily accepted by the adoptive group. Thus, fast-track students feel able to complete the program in about ten months, and slower students extend their program if necessary. Students who are unable to handle the program are at all usually counseled out and encouraged to transfer to a more appropriate program. The attrition rate with wheel programs is low due to the customized self-paced approach.

The wheel concept requires more than one instructor. For example, in a medical assisting program, students rotate through ten different courses: Anatomy and Physiology and Medical Terminology, Human Relations, Administrative I, Administrative II, Clinical I, Clinical II, Laboratory Test Procedures, Basic X Ray, Employability Skills, and Externship. Due to the specialty of some competencies (lab and X ray), part-time instructors with appropriate credentials teach these areas. Students also attend portions of their program in other classrooms such as X ray room, computer lab, and employability skills lab and in off-site clinical experiences. One instructor is designated the clinical supervisor and visits the off-campus site to supervise the externs on a regular basis.

The authors' observations of this method of competency-based instruction have taken notice of the happiness of students. They feel responsible but not alone in their educational endeavor. They enjoy helping one another to truly understand, not just memorize. They have empathy for each other and feel team spirit. You can pick your friends, but not your family. These groups become family. There is no one-upmanship in terms of another group's place on the wheel. Students have become so busy keeping up with their own group that they don't have time to muse over what others are doing. This is a tough and demanding program and is not for the undedicated.

Author's note: The wheel concept was fully implemented during the fall of 1991. Complete evaluation of the results should be available next fall (the proposed publication date of this manuscript) when all students enrolled will have completed a full program using the modified open-entry/self-paced learning concept.

It has been the purpose of this chapter to discuss and to provide examples of a curriculum development process for any health occupations education program. Different from developing a pure science curriculum, a health occupations education curriculum is an applied science and founded on community needs, industry needs, and student needs and interests. Consequently, no single textbook, methodology, or resource material can effectively meet curriculum requirements.

Curricula, using CBE components are widely accepted. They offer an accountable approach to instruction and student achievement. Elements that compose the development of a CBE curriculum are discussed in detail with advice to the user. In addition, the user is encouraged to seek available resources and to carefully evaluate them for compatibility with the identified health occupations education curriculum before initiating the developmental process.

11

Legal Issues: What You Don't Know Can Hurt You

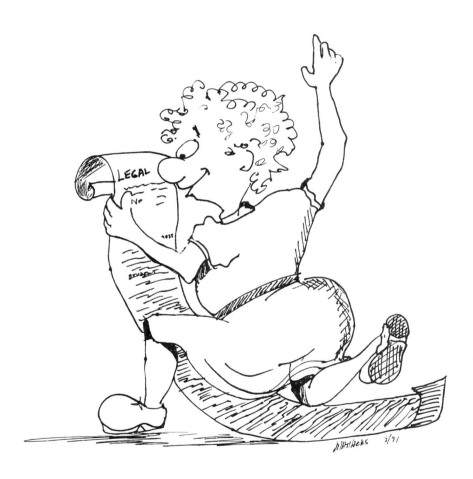

Over the past twenty-five years, vocational health occupations (VHO) teachers have encountered with increasing frequency certain legal challenges by students who are dismissed from their program. Because such dismissals threaten not only students' personal career goals but also their future employability, students are more likely to seek court action for resolution. Moreover, teachers face a dual dilemma. If they fail a student or place one on probationary status, they could be involved in litigation. On the other hand, if academic dismissal is not instituted, patient safety could be jeopardized.

As a teacher new to the world of education, you may hear from other staff some horror stories about students' threatening to sue your institution. Rather than approach your class and clinical experiences with fear and anxiety regarding possible lawsuits, you need to feel confident in your ability to determine basic competency in future health care workers. The following information will assist you to understand due process, tort liability, techniques for failing an unsatisfactory student, and the grievance process.

☞ DUE PROCESS AND ITS APPLICATION TO VHO

When students pursue legal action, they usually base their claim on violation of the Fourteenth Amendment's due process and equal protection clause. Dismissal cases involve either procedural or substantive due process rights. Procedural rights consist of the steps used to protect and guarantee the rights of citizens (Spink, 1983). These rights can be violated when an institution fails to provide a hearing prior to dismissal for disciplinary reasons. Often disciplinary action is taken when a student violates the institution's code of conduct. The landmark decision in *Dixon v. Alabama State Board of Education* (1961) afforded procedural due process in disciplinary cases for postsecondary students. In contrast, substantive due process focuses on academic deficiency in which the student fails to attain the required level of competency. To claim substantive due process, the intent of the law requires proving unfairness and unreasonableness in a teacher's or institution's decision regarding the dismissal.

Health occupations students may incur either disciplinary or academic dismissal. To determine whether disciplinary proceedings are appropriate, evidence must support that the student broke a school regulation or rule. In this type of dismissal, the student must be notified of the charges against him or her as well as given an opportunity for a hearing (*Goss v. Lopez*, 1975).

Because students direct their claim toward violation of substantive due process, we will concentrate on this area by discussing several cases and their implications for health occupations teachers. As stated earlier, under academic dismissal, the student fails to attain a specific level of competence. Limandri

(1981) believes *Connelly v. University of Vermont and State Agricultural College* established the basis for the courts to avoid judicial interference in the educational process unless the decision ". . . was motivated by arbitrariness, capriciousness, or bad faith." In *Greenhill v. Bailey* (1975), Bailey not only failed to hold a hearing but also in a memo had stated Greenhill "lacked intellectual ability." Whereas the court would not interfere in judging the student's academic performance, it did chastise Bailey for not providing notice of the charges. In addition, the court said an opportunity must exist for the student to clear his or her name and refute the allegations of academic deficiency before the academic body who is responsible for the dismissal (Niedringhaus and O'Driscoll, 1983).

The landmark case of the *Board of Curators of the University of Missouri v. Horowitz* (1978) addressed Horowitz's claim of deprivation of liberty and procedural due process rights. Horowitz, a medical student, claimed that she had not been permitted to see her clinical evaluations and was not notified of a dismissal hearing. The facts of the case include that she was given a warning, was placed on probation, and was told that she might be dismissed. Even though the school furnished her with additional clinical time, she still failed her final examinations. Subsequently she was asked to leave the school. The Supreme Court left the evaluation of her academic abilities up to her professors and stated that she had been given more due process than was required.

Nursing students' dismissal for clinical incompetence was challenged in *Gaspar v. Bruton* (1975), *Lyons v. Salve Regina College* (1975), and *Hubbard v. John Tyler Community College* (1978). While each case has its own unique circumstances, only Lyons won her case because the college breached the language in the student manual. Therefore, to avoid breaching students' due process rights, teachers and schools must inform students orally or in writing of their performance inadequacies and the subsequent effect on their academic standing. Moreover, ". . . the school's decision-making process must be careful and deliberate" (Niedringhaus and O'Driscoll, 1983, p. 158).

The courts have established that teachers are uniquely qualified to evaluate a student's performance in the classroom and clinical settings, and governing boards of schools have delegated this authority to teachers. Your health occupations department must develop course requirements and expectations for personal and professional behaviors before student performance can be deemed insufficient and warrant dismissal. More specifically, your department should complete the following steps:

1. Have all staff jointly develop theory and clinical student behavioral objectives.
2. Print the objectives in the course syllabus and student handbook as appropriate.

3. Review the objectives with students on entry into the program and during each subsequent school term.
4. Once the term has begun, do not alter these objectives.

In the clinical setting, you must establish criteria for such cognitive, affective, and psychomotor behaviors as fundamental knowledge, interpersonal relations, technical skills, integrity, and professionalism. You can probably think of many more measurements that are appropriate for evaluating a student's progress. Besides determining broad clinical requirements, carefully identify the criteria for satisfactory course completion as well as the consequences for unsatisfactory performance. You must decide your sources for evaluation input, for example, direct observations and clinical preceptors. In team-taught courses everyone must agree to use the same criteria. Reaching agreement is time-consuming, but once in place, your course will be solid and consistent. The author finds that by having detailed standards, students cannot easily claim they did not know what is expected of them.

After the criteria are set, determine the frequency for conducting formal evaluation conferences. The law requires that students be apprised periodically of their performance. With satisfactory performance, the minimum requirement consists of a mid-term conference and a final conference.

For written work, develop grading criteria, and publish them in the course syllabus before distributing the assignment to your students. Also, you should include your penalty for students who submit late written work. Be certain to use the criteria for grading your students' papers. If your department uses team-teaching and others in addition to you will be grading the written work, it becomes even more important for everyone not only to agree with the criteria but also to apply them. Students tend to compare the evaluative comments on their papers. When grading inconsistency becomes apparent, grievances are likely to follow. Some departments promote the concept of a second grader for failing papers. If a mechanism is not in place for the student to redo the paper in order to achieve mastery of such concepts as the nursing process, this practice can save you from defending your grade to your school administrators. It is wise to make a copy of the failing paper and place it in the student's file until the student fails or graduates. Although the student may pass your term, he or she may be on academic probation the next. Having examples of prior unsatisfactory work not only assists the next instructor in thoroughly evaluating the student but also may provide the foundation for winning a grievance.

Procedural due process rights must be published in your school's catalog and student handbook. All new faculty and students should receive a copy of the handbook on beginning employment or a program of study.

Now, take a moment to look at your institution's catalog and your department's student handbook, and try to answer the following questions. Are graduation requirements clearly specified? Do the publications contain the student grievance process? Within your department, is the process reviewed with the students? Does each student have a copy of the student handbook?

With legal precedence being set by such landmark cases as Horowitz and Connelly, institutions must continue to deal fairly with students and accept internal accountability for their decisions and their decision-making process. Once you have identified, written, published, and reviewed your evaluation criteria with the faculty and students, no one should be misled as to a program's requirements for satisfactory performance.

☞ REDUCING TORT LIABILITY

Lessner (1990) defines tort law as someone being at fault for an act. Negligence or malpractice is the one category of tort law that commonly involves health occupation professionals as well as VHO teachers. Health professionals are held to a higher standard of care than the ordinary citizen. If injury occurs to a patient, one is judged by the "reasonable man" test, which defines ". . . the standard of care that a reasonable person would give in a particular set of circumstances" (Lessner, 1990, p. 30).

Generally, VHO teachers are not liable for the acts of students in the clinical setting. However, you and your institution will be held liable if either (1) you assign a student a specific task that the student did not know how to perform or (2) you were not aware of the student's inability to perform the skill. If your school requires that students demonstrate minimal skill competency in your skills laboratory before they can practice the skill on their own, then you are not liable.

Once the initial skill-check is passed, the student accepts the responsibility for demonstrating the skill correctly in clinical practice. If students are unable to perform skills correctly, they should be sent back to the lab for additional practice and a second skill check. The author's school has instituted a formal skills remastery plan for this purpose. Students cannot perform the skill in clinical until they demonstrate mastery. They are given one week in which to master the skill. If again they cannot demonstrate the skill correctly, they could be dismissed for the term. However, such drastic measures are reserved for students who cannot demonstrate several skills as well as practice at the current level of expectation.

Students should receive an appropriate assignment and adequate supervision from their clinical instructor. Many times you cannot observe everything the student does. Often other health care professionals in the facilities informally evaluate your students, not as an affront to you but because they are liable and concerned for patient safety. To facilitate their assistance, share your clinical objectives and expectations with them. Typically these professionals and their feedback cannot be part of the formal evaluation process. Therefore, be careful of the type of feedback you seek from them. You could be breaching the student's due process rights. In addition, if students deem an institution is not offering reasonable, good-quality health care, it is your responsibility to investigate and perhaps change health care facilities placements.

When students are working in the health care system, they are employees of the facility. To ensure this fact, you must have contracts between your institution and each health care facility in which you place students. In essence, the contract requires the health occupations teacher to supervise students in such a manner that guarantees patient safety. By allowing a student to practice in an unsafe manner, you and your institution are in a legally vulnerable position.

Generally, contracts contain broad statements regarding each party's responsibility toward students and are renewed every year. At the beginning of an academic year or before using a new clinical site, review the facility's contract. You will find these contracts in your director's office. Clarify any questions you have concerning the language or implied level of supervision. You are held accountable for each facility's contract.

An additional concern is that all equipment within both facilities be safe for student use. The contract should contain a clause regarding the level of responsibility of each party in the event of injury. With the increasing incidence of patients with hepatitis and AIDS, both institutions need policies addressing the student's, teacher's, and facility's responsibility in case either the student or instructor the develops a health problem.

If your institution promotes students' practicing skills on each other, another problem may arise. When this is a standard policy, you need to state it in your syllabus or student handbook. Students have the right to refuse such invasive procedures as blood drawing, subcutaneous or intramuscular injections, nasogastric tube insertion and intravenous needle insertion. Dismissing a student for refusing to participate in these practices, could engender a student grievance, which the student would probably win. Moreover, if a student suffers injury during a practice session, you will be liable. Check your state laws regarding whether an informed consent form is necessary from each student who volunteers to be a "patient."

Malpractice is the most common tort law affecting health occupations teachers. Whether working in clinical as a health care practitioner or as a clinical teacher, your practice will be judged according to the "reasonable man" test. If your health profession requires state licensure, students do not work under your license. However, you are liable for the students' actions when you fail to provide adequate supervision or to assign appropriate tasks based on students' current level of ability.

☞ FAILING AN UNSATISFACTORY STUDENT

Teachers are hesitant to recommend remedial work or to fail the student who is performing below minimal standards in the clinical component of a course. Reluctance arises in a teacher because clinical evaluation is subjective and often is based on limited observations, and fear exists in being accused of having a personality conflict with the student. Hesitancy is compounded further when clinical objectives are broadly stated in the syllabus, leaving room for open interpretation.

Failing students who are performing poorly is mentally and physically draining. You need to spend more time planning clinical experiences and closely supervising them. Extra conferences must be held with the student either in the clinical setting or in your office. Even more time is spent in the ritual of psyching yourself up for these confrontations (Symanski, 1991). An added burden is realizing that you must leave competent students to fend for themselves while you concentrate on the poorer student and you may resent spending all the effort on a student who in all likelihood will not graduate.

As a new teacher or even a seasoned veteran, you may want to blame yourself for the student's inadequacies. You may find fault with the curriculum, say the workload does not allow you to spend time with your students, or say your personal or home situation distracts you from high-quality teaching. Always remember that you are the professional and you know what constitutes competent practice. Just as you have a sixth sense in your practice, your intuition about student performance is usually correct, too.

Be careful of becoming immersed in a doom-and-gloom attitude over failing a student. Yes, students can face financial and personal hardship because they must wait a year before returning to the health occupations program. However, keep asking yourself: Is this student safe in the health care setting? Does allowing him or her to continue for financial reasons justify not only the burden you place on the next instructor, who will be the clinical supervisor, but also the ethics of permitting an incompetent student to work with patients?

Sometimes following a student failure, the student will heave a big sigh of relief and state that health occupations was not his or her choice, but parental pressure forced a health career decision. You may find a returning student, who has failed previously, still has unresolved anger and bitterness. You will have difficulty convincing such students how much improvement there has been in their clinical performance. A positive response comes when dismissed students are able to work in a related health career field for at least a year or so. On returning to their original health care field of study, these students show increased self-confidence in their abilities and themselves. Such students become better health care providers than had they been allowed to struggle on toward trying to complete the program originally.

You may find other teachers in your program who have never failed a student. They may become hostile and angry toward you, and you may hear such remarks as: "You are just too critical" or "That student did very well in *my* clinical rotation!" They believe you are taking unnecessary and drastic action. After all, they will tell you, not every student is perfect. You must keep in mind, though, that perfection is not what you are seeking but rather minimal safe competency.

You may even be in conflict with yourself over this issue. By being a health care professional, you see yourself as caring and nurturing. You'll ask: How can I fail a student and still remain caring and nurturing? Your approach to students, while you are guiding them through remediation and possible failure, always remains humane. However, caring for and nurturing of patients must be taken into account, too. It is not humane, let alone ethical, to allow an incompetent student to practice on patients.

Although you will encounter teachers who are opposed to failing students, seek the opinions of those who do support your cause. During the process of handling an unsatisfactory student is not the time to engage in philosophical battles over viewpoints about failing students (Symanski, 1991). Seek your administrative director for advice and guidance. The director should be knowledgeable and supportive about your decision as long as you have adequate documentation and have preserved the student's due process rights.

It is hoped that you will not be pressured to pass a student just to maintain program enrollment numbers. Occasionally such a request is made because the dismissal occurs early in the quarter or semester. Most postsecondary institutions receive federal finances based on their FTE (full-time equivalent) by the fourth or sixth week of the quarter. One director, half-seriously, told the teachers not to dismiss anyone until after the fourth week of the quarter.

Now that you are more familiar with the emotional issues surrounding student dismissal, let's turn to the actual process. To determine student competency or deficiency, a well-developed, concise evaluation instrument and anecdotal notes are absolutely essential. Anecdotal notes contain factual observations, not interpretations of student behavior that you do not like. Even though notes are time-consuming, they provide you and the student with actual documentation of the events. Because clinical supervision is hectic, keeping notes seems overwhelming. The following guidelines are suggested to ease the process.

1. Keep a notebook with each student's name listed on a separate page.
2. Following direct observation or quizzing of a student, stop for a few minutes and jot down your observations of the student's behavior. If

you wait till the end of the day or rotation, key observations will be forgotten, and on trying to decide whether the student has consistently demonstrated a pattern of poor performance, you will have to spend endless time trying to recall significant data.

3. Note positive and negative behaviors. When evaluation instruments contain only negative behavior, you can be accused of having a personality conflict with the student.
4. Transfer your anecdotal notes to the formal evaluation form. Some instructors can write directly on the evaluation form. You will find that when you sit down to write an evaluation, in the quiet of an office, you can remember additional information about the student's performance that you would not have recalled in the busy clinical setting.
5. Be sure each anecdotal note is dated on the evaluation instrument. When a student displays below-average competency, you have accurate details to develop a progressive plan.
6. Keep a record of each student's clinical assignment and additional learning activities.
7. Keep all anecdotal notes and evaluation instruments until each student graduates.

Some departments use rating scales on their evaluation instruments. While they provide numerical data to make decisions unless there are complete descriptions of each numerical value, the evaluation is still subjective. In one nursing program, we changed from numbers to a detailed description of each clinical objective that outlines minimal competency. This is a tedious process, but the efforts have rewarded us when making a remedial plan or failing a student.

Besides written documentation, the importance of effective communication, not only when performance is satisfactory but especially when unsatisfactory cannot be overstated. Whether communication consists of informal feedback in clinical or formal written evaluations and conferences, the student must be given ample time to respond. To verify the student's understanding, Majorowicz (1986) recommends that the student reflect on the student-teacher conversation overnight, summarize the major points, and meet with the teacher the next day to clarify any misunderstandings.

Unfortunately, communication with a student can be turned against you. For instance, when a student is informed at mid-term that his or her performance is unsatisfactory, common student reactions include "You don't like me;" "You always watched me so you could fail me;" "You make me so nervous—how could I function?" Frequently students will scapegoat their incompetencies at a grievance hearing by using these same reasons. Do not react. Keep your conversation focused on the facts.

When a student performs below the minimal standard, you must have a process in place for handling this. First and foremost, be sure you conduct a well-thought-out assessment of the student's deficiencies. If you doubt your conclusions, you may want another clinical instructor to evaluate the student. Even when you choose not to seek a second evaluator, it may be helpful to discuss your concerns with a colleague or director. Some schools and teachers believe this practice violates the student's rights. However, many grievance committees look more favorably on the teacher who willingly sought assistance for helping the student. Our program discusses student concerns in our team meetings for the purpose of helping the teacher brainstorm a more comprehensive plan of action.

Once you have a plan in mind, your next step is to arrange a meeting with the student. Each department determines whether the student and teacher meet alone and/or with the department director. If you had assistance in developing your plan, you may not need to include the director at the initial meeting. However, if your plan is to permanently dismiss the student from clinical and the program, the director must be present. Depending on your school's policies, the student is placed on academic warning, which may be less severe than probation, or probationary status. To ensure that the student's rights are not violated, use a stepped approach in addressing academic or clinical deficiencies. This process allows the student ample opportunity to improve the deficiencies. However, even with the stepped approach, you can bypass the lesser step when the student makes a major error or causes harm to a patient.

Regardless of whether you use a stepped approach or move directly to probation, when you meet with the student, each deficiency is described and an appropriate improvement plan is discussed. Figure 11-1 is an example of the student progression plan that we use in our nursing program.

Including instructor actions illustrates that the plan is a collaborative effort. Administrators and school boards prefer to see that you are making a conscious effort to help the student improve. In addition, note the time frames and consequences that are listed. This gives the student a definite period of time in which remediation must occur and describes the outcome if improvement does not occur. Remember to document referrals to counseling or other appropriate institutional resources such as tutoring. Although this does not stop a student from filing a grievance, it does show that you did not act in bad faith or in a capricious or arbitrary manner.

One suggestion is to develop a generic plan with lines for the student and instructor name(s); course title; date; and student, teacher, and director signatures. These plans can be printed on NCR (no-carbon-required) paper so

EXAMPLE

Problem

Violation of Chemical Safety

1. 4/10/91 8:00 a.m. John entered H.R.'s room to administer an IM medication. He failed to check the patient's armband or double check the medication record before giving the med. I reminded him to follow the "Five Rights of Administering Medications."

2. 4/10/91 10:30 a.m. John was giving his 10 a.m. medications when he discovered that he had omitted H.R.'s 9:00 a.m. Digoxin. MD was notified. Digoxin was given at 10:45 a.m. and an incident report was filed.

3. 4/17/91 John was unable to state the side effects and rationale for his patient receiving Procardia, Apresoline and Aldomet. He stated he did not have time to research his medications even though he received his assignment on 4/16/91.

Plan of Action

1. John will administer all medications following the "Five Rights of Administering Medications."

2. John will develop and implement a plan to avoid omitting medications in the future.

3. At the beginning of each clinical shift, John must be prepared to state each drug's action and side effects as well as correlate all medications and IV solutions to the patient's diagnosis.

4. The instructor will observe John administer medications to all of his patients for one week (4/24 & 4/25/91).

5. If no further violations of chemical safety occur by the end of the quarter (June 7, 1991), this plan will be discontinued.

6. If further violations of chemical safety occur, John's progression in the second-year will be reviewed by the second-year team and the director of nursing.

FIGURE 11-1

that a copy can be given to the student and another placed in the student's file. Having a generic form increases consistency among your fellow teachers. To decrease the time spent in hand-writing a plan, develop the plan on computer, and print it directly onto the generic form.

All parties involved in teacher-student conferences should sign and date the written document. Signatures do not make the document a binding contract but serve to verify that the conference actually occurred.

Once a plan is instituted, you must follow it to the letter. Remember, the student's outcome will be either meeting the improvement plan, progression to probation, or failure. When failure results, assist the student through the grieving process. Until the student can reach the acceptance phase, he or she will feel a tremendous loss of self-worth. To assist the individual in reaching acceptance, emphasize his or her positive attributes. Even with your positive approach, do not expect the student to feel positive toward you as you end your student-teacher relationship. Most students will not view their failure as a learning and growth experience.

Although failing an unsatisfactory student is difficult, you do not fail students; they fail themselves. When evaluations are based on sound professional standards and judgment and are conducted without malice, the courts uphold your decisions. The key intervention strategies are to establish concise course requirements; use complete documentation and communication techniques; and provide feedback as well as the opportunity to correct the deficiency in a timely manner.

HANDLING STUDENT GRIEVANCES

When a grievance occurs, your institution's and department's policies regarding grading, expectations, and dismissal are reviewed for appropriateness and fairness. Grant (1989) recommends the following steps before a grievance is filed:

1. Review your grading criteria for how clear they would be to a lay audience.
2. Use standard forms and language across all clinical courses.
3. Be sure your institutional policies for student grievances are not ambiguous.
4. Ensure that dismissal criteria within the department are clearly stated and presented to students in a handbook on entry into the program.

Students who file a grievance must follow your school's policies. Usually this means providing a written statement that describes the problem, the reasons why the grade is unfair, and a proposed solution. Incomplete statements should be returned to the student for revision. Do not try to interpret what the student is saying. It is not your duty to rewrite the student's grievance for clarity.

The next step is to submit the statement to your department's director, director of students, instructional director, and/or student/faculty grievance committee. Of course the exact process will depend on your school's administrative structure. Regardless of the specific policy in your school, however, always keep the higher levels of administration informed of progress as the grievance proceeds through channels.

In most instances, grievances are resolved at the director's level. When they progress upward into your school's administrative ranks, do not assume your administrators are knowledgeable regarding the function of health occupations students in the clinical setting. Furthermore, they may not be familiar with the legal precedence regarding the grading of students (Grant, 1989). Even though your records are clear and concise, you will still need to explain why the student failed your program.

Be prepared to explain your anecdotal notes on the evaluation instrument. You will need to correlate the clinical evaluation to your course and clinical objectives. If the student is appealing a theory grade based on tests and/or written papers, again, your course objectives and grading criteria must be explicit. Otherwise, the administration will have difficulty upholding your decision.

If your school uses a student-teacher grievance committee, you may have to appear to explain your actions. Generally, academic hearings that are not of a disciplinary nature are informal and not viewed as courts of law. When your presence is required, the committee's chairperson should meet with you beforehand to explain what you should prepare and what is expected of you at the hearing.

During the hearing, only those directly involved with the process should be present. Whether or not your institution will allow a parent, spouse, or lawyer present at the appeals process is an individual decision. From my own personal experience, having support for the student may appear more humane but is more nerve-racking for you.

If you must participate in a formal hearing, you should first meet with your school's legal counsel. If you believe the attorney may not be your ally, you can hire your own lawyer. But this can be expensive. The author recommends developing a working relationship with your school and its legal assistance. They carry more weight than you do alone in academic hearings. Also, this is your golden opportunity to educate them on the inner workings of health occupations and its students so that the next teacher will have less difficulty with a grievance.

The atmosphere of the hearing be made friendlier by using a round table rather than a formal courtroom setup. Either a secretary or a tape recorder is used to record the proceedings. At the beginning, the chair summarizes the appeal, which is followed by separate statements from you and the student. Separate testimony facilitates a freer exchange between the committee members and the person presenting the evidence.

Don't forget — the burden of proving arbitrariness and capriciousness is on the student. However, you must be able to answer the committee's questions concerning the student's claims. Even though an impartial decision should be made based on the facts, your behavior (verbal and nonverbal) during the hearing can add or subtract from the student's claims. After all the testimony has been heard, the committee will make its decision. Sometimes more information is requested from you after the hearing. This may be frustrating, but you need to comply to ensure a fair decision for you and the student.

Appeals and hearings should be resolved as expeditiously as possible, preferably before the next school term begins. If you think reaching a resolution will be lengthy, you might want to consider temporarily reinstating the student. Such consideration may be appropriate when appeals are based on theory examinations. If the student won and subsequently missed several weeks of the next term, which would hinder his or her satisfactory completion of the program, the school can be sued for further damages. However, when dismissal is based on unsatisfactory clinical performance, re-placing the student in clinical would be a negligent act on the part of the teacher.

During the middle of the grievance process, you start to feel overwhelmed and possibly ambivalent. You may feel personal and professional pressure to turn back your attention to your other students and duties. The longer the appeals or hearing process takes, the more eager you become for a resolution. During this period, don't jump to alternative solutions merely as a means to end the grievance. For an alternative to acceptable, ". . . it cannot violate the student's rights by requiring something that is not required of other students," and it ". . . should not set an unacceptable precedent" (Majorowicz, 1986, p. 36).

In summary, students are more knowledgeable about their rights nowadays, and the frequency of grievances is increasing. When a grievance is filed against you, be prepared to assist your school administrators in understanding how health occupations students differ from those in nonvocational programs. Be articulate about your course and clinical objectives; know how your decision relates to the objectives and grading criteria.

Don't be afraid to seek assistance from either your school's legal counsel or your colleagues who have been through a grievance hearing. Don't choose alternative solutions just because you are afraid of the grievance process. Remember — the student cannot simply claim but must prove that you acted in bad faith or in a capricious or arbitrary manner.

Student dismissals based on academic deficiencies are upheld by the courts, provided that you do not violate the student's due process rights. Teachers, especially in the health occupations field, are viewed as being qualified to decide whether the student has met the program's academic requirements. To ensure their rights, develop, publish, and review your course requirements and behavioral objectives with them after they begin each new course. When unsatisfactory performance occurs, develop a plan and furnish an opportunity for the student to improve. You should include specific guidelines, time frames, and consequences on which to judge whether satisfactory improvement has occurred. If dismissal results, students have the right to express their disagreement through the grievance process, which must be fair and impartial to you and the student. After resolution, determine whether any of the program's requirements are vague or unrealistic. Also, the department should review its student progression process and whether the grievance might have been avoided. Adhering to legal precedence may seem overwhelming at first, but once you are familiar with it, you will feel more comfortable with your teaching career.

References

Board of Curators of the University of Missouri v. Horowitz, 435 U.S. 78 (1978).

Dixon v. Alabama State Board of Education, 294 F 2d 150 (5th Cir. 1961).

Gaspar v. Bruton, 519 F. 2d 843 (10th Cir. 1975).

Goss v. Lopez, 419 U.S. 565 (1975).

Grant, A. B. (1989). "Dealing with a Student Grievance." *Nurse Educator, 14*(6), 13–17.

Greenhill v. Bailey, 519 F. 2d 5 (8th Cir. 1975).

Hubbard v. John Tyler Community College, 455 F. Supp. 753 (1978).

Lessner, M. W. (1990). "Avoiding Student-Faculty Litigation." *Nurse Educator, 15*(5), 29–32.

Limandri, B. J. (1981). "Academic Procedural Due Process for Students in the Health Professions." *Journal of Nursing Education, 20*(2), 9–18.

Lyons v. Salve Regina College, 422 F. Supp. 843 (1975).

Majorowicz, K. (1986). "Clinical Grades and the Grievance Process." *Nurse Educator, 11*(2), 36–40.

Niedringhaus, L., and D. L. O'Driscoll (1983). "Staying within the Law: Academic Probation and Dismissal. *Nursing Outlook, 31*(3), 156–159.

Spink, L. M. (1983). "Due Process in Academic Dismissals." *Journal of Nursing Education, 22*(7), 305–306.

Symanski, M. E. (1991). "Reducing the Effect of Faculty Demoralization When Failing Students. *Nurse Educator, 16*(3), 18–22.

12

The VHO Teacher's Role in HOSA: Advising in a Hands-Off Format

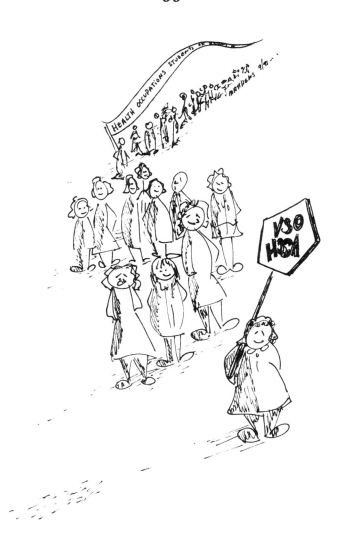

Health Occupations Students of America (HOSA) plays an essential part in a successful health occupations program, and every vocational health occupations teacher should be a HOSA adviser. Consider HOSA an *integral* part of the curriculum. HOSA is organized on the local, state, and national levels: the local chapter is part of the state organization, which in turn is affiliated with National HOSA.

BECOMING A CHAPTER ADVISER

Occupational theory and tasks necessary for health care practitioners' programs are dictated by the health care professions. HOSA chapters provide opportunities to harness student power, promote leadership, and share authority. In pursuit of activities encouraged by HOSA, students leave the classroom situation and practice skills in leadership and interpersonal relations as well as occupational topics. Watching the development of these skills among individual students represents one of the many benefits for advisers.

Utilization of the full potential of HOSA requires study and planning. Use the HOSA handbook for orientation to the organization, its philosophy and goals, and its components. The handbook sets forth the value of the organization in providing realizable standards and directions for teacher and student as well as the information for getting organized. Select a realistic number of HOSA's components to include in plans for the school year. The other necessity is the state HOSA handbook. Request this with recent addendums or publications and schedules before the school year begins. These selections and schedules will fill in the program of work for the year.

Involvement in HOSA can be hard work, but it is also exciting and well worth the effort. Volunteer for the annual state conference. This affords a means of understanding how HOSA operates through the contributions of its various advisers. Judging or cochairing a competitive event on the regional or state level can be a future endeavor.

Other sections in this chapter address specific topics that experienced HOSA advisers have identified as central to the success of a local chapter. Adopt and adapt the suggestions as they seem pertinent to your program, chapter, and school district goals.

USING THE HANDBOOK

The Health Occupations Students of America National Handbook functions as the major resource for the establishment and success of a chapter and for its relationship to the state and national levels. It is easy to use, uncomplicated to read, and routinely updated. Make it a priority purchase for the chapter. It is divided into three sections, each published as a separate document, which facilitates its use and revision as needed. Sections can be purchased (from HOSA Related Materials Service) as a whole or separately when latest editions are required. The three sections embody all that is needed to understand the organization and to make it an integral part of your instructional program.

Section A

National HOSA — the Organization is the shortest of the sections and has three parts. Review General Information for the basics of the work; the purposes; the organizational chart; the emblem, motto, and creed; the official uniform policy; the membership categories; the state affiliations; and the geographic areas. Explanations about HOSA, INC., as a legal corporate body, its national officers, and the national headquarters are also included. The next part contains a history of HOSA and the constitution and bylaws. In the Appendices of this section are found practical aids for installation ceremonies, duties of the officers, and report forms for chapter activities.

Section B

National Competitive Events is the largest and most frequently updated and expanded section of the handbook. Guard these pages religiously, because they contain vital information for advisers and students in preparing for participation in competitive events. Note the categories of related events, occupations skill events, individual leadership events, and team leadership events. The rules, procedures, equipment, and materials are periodically revised to incorporate the latest changes in practice, thus ensuring that students are competing by current standards. Using the event guidelines that are appropriate for the health occupations program in classroom situations for all or selected members will enrich the program and promote participation by students. The judges' rating sheets are excellent step-by-step procedure evaluations that are functional for innumerable situations.

Section C

Guide to Organizing and Managing a HOSA Chapter is invaluable for the vocational health occupations teacher who is to be a HOSA adviser. It is practical, technical, instructional, and the final piece to bring about full integration of HOSA with the occupational program.

The national handbook is not the only guide for advisers to use. Textbooks and state publications have suggestions, lesson plans, and activities that are serviceable and effective for developing the participation and leadership that result in successful ventures for advisers and students. Use these as appropriate and time-saving measures. However, remember that the HOSA national handbook in its latest edition is the final authority used by HOSA leaders and supporters.

☞ ORGANIZING A CHAPTER

Establishing a Chapter

Organizing a chapter has two interpretations: a function to establish a chapter and a process that is repeated annually. Organizing a chapter can be compared to a roller coaster ride, with the excitement of the climb to the peaks, the fearfulness of the descent to the valleys, the necessity to hold on tight, and, when the ride is over (the year has ended), the exhilarating feeling of accomplishment. The high spirits that come with the end of the year constitutes the impetus to take on the process for the next year.

No year is the same as any other. Membership changes, there are different ideas to try, and the HOSA organization itself grows and expands its activities and aims. The decision to join opens up a world that is fascinating, frustrating, and fulfilling. It requires decision making, delegating, and delineating. It necessitates clarifying, cajoling, and congratulating. Becoming an adviser for any of the vocational student organizations can provide these thrills, but the affinity of working with leaders in the same industry is found only within HOSA. The insight gained from association with members of many health occupations from other geographic areas is phenomenal.

If no chapter exists, then the school principal or student activities administrator is the one to see. Knowledge of local administrative policies is crucial to a good beginning. Compare these with the goals of HOSA to rule out any conflicts. The purposes, structure, constitution, and bylaws are in the aforementioned national handbook, which it is assumed you have purchased or to which you have access. HOSA requires that all members be affiliated with the national organization in order to receive the rights and privileges that affiliation confers. Therefore, a commitment to full membership puts the chapter in good standing. Following administrative approval, the next step requires the state adviser or administrator to request a charter. Request also the state handbook, publications, and/or program of work. Within these references are found many recommendations, lists of responsibilities, and suggested activities for new advisers.

The state adviser or administrator is a resource person who can answer specific questions or put you in touch with experienced advisers. Many chapters welcome the opportunity to assist in the formation of new chapters, so be sure to ask if this service is available. Assistance with leadership activities, competition preparation, community projects, and classroom integration may be nearby.

Organizing Students

Organizing the students is a step-by-step procedure. The task is easiest when the adviser is also a teacher in a VHO program. In that case, the membership can be 100% of the class members, the time for meeting and activities becomes part of class time, and the curriculum reflects the HOSA component. When members must be recruited from the general school population, the participants and the meeting times will be unique to the situation. In either case, information-giving sessions must be planned, student committees must be formed, and the process of developing leaders must begin. The national handbook is a succinct source of ideas. Use HOSA publications and materials, visual aids, guest speakers, question-and-answer sessions, discussions, and, of course, enthusiasm to capture student interest and shift responsibility to student leaders. Use the constitution and bylaws of the state until there is opportunity to develop them for the new chapter.

Organizing the Chapter

With a few variations, organizing the chapter annually parallels establishing a chapter. When there are returning members, they become the most likely committee members for reorganization. Some functions remain identical annually. Meetings should be held weekly at first to facilitate dispensing of needed information. Open each meeting formally with the HOSA creed, and close with the motto. Be on time, be prepared with an agenda, and accomplish some piece of work. Keep notes or rotate the assignment of taking minutes. These are the hallmarks of a successful chapter.

Meetings can be held for many reasons other than a regular business meeting in the beginning. Use game formats to increase participation and camaraderie among members. Workshops for officer candidates are productive. Include campaign materials and campaign speeches to build momentum and make HOSA goals relevant to members. Plan lessons in parliamentary procedure because this usually needs to be taught and is well worth the effort early in the year. Form committees in small groups to accomplish work that will be brought to the full membership for approval. Involve the members, perhaps the executive committee, in planning the program of work on a calendar that includes state meetings and conferences. In this way, responsibility and direction for the year are shared.

Chapter activities are learning activities for members. The ceremonies, the committee reports, the parliamentary procedures are all ways to develop student confidence and expand horizons. Connect chapter endeavors to classroom activities, to the future, to occupational performance, to understanding varying roles in the health occupations, and to community needs. These are the purposes for which the HOSA organization exists.

☞ INTEGRATING HOSA INTO THE CLASSROOM

Early in every health occupation instructional program the course of study dictates that lesson plans be presented to define the occupation and explain its contribution to health care and its place on the health care team. The credentials of the occupation (e.g., registration, licensure, certification) and professional organizations are often discussed. This is the time to present HOSA as the vocational student organization for health occupations students. If the textbook being used does not have a section describing HOSA, then use state publications, flyers, or parts of the HOSA handbook to present the purposes and goals.

Information Session

Plan an information session and point out that the professional standards and ethics of HOSA are similar to those of the professional organizations. Explain that a HOSA chapter will constitute that part of the curriculum that offers students opportunities for interesting activities and direct input. Select from Section C in the HOSA handbook the content to cover in introducing HOSA. Discuss as thoroughly as possible the benefits of HOSA membership.

Following this correlation of HOSA with professional occupational organizations in what is perhaps the introductory unit of the instructional program, set aside a time each week for continuing organizing activities. These hours should now be designated as HOSA.

Integrating HOSA

If the existing curriculum does not have a unit, topic, or module for HOSA, one should be written. The objectives of the unit are active participation in leadership activities, competitive events, and educational and community services. Evaluation of student progress or performance will depend upon specific objectives chosen from the guidelines of the state and/or national organization. Leadership activities are the business meeting, officer duties, committee membership, and volunteering — there is something for everyone! Competitive events include the general rules and regulations, categories, and guidelines found in Section B of the national handbook. However, much of the instruction, practice, and simulation is included as part of the strategies and task competencies of the curriculum.

The preferred method is for the HOSA program of work to be a part of the instructional program — an intracurricular component. In actuality, some meetings, practice sessions, activities, and conferences take place outside regular class hours and are not strictly counted as curriculum hours.

The planned organizing activities must be upbeat and capture the interest of the new members. One suggestion is a participatory session using role-playing. Prepare an agenda and scripts for officers, for committee chairpersons (program, fund-raising, social, etc.), and for members. Incorporate parliamentary procedures into the script, such as make a motion, second the motion, table the motion, call for a vote, appoint a committee, and the like. Either choose students or solicit volunteers to play the roles and read the script. The topics of the script should spark interest and encourage involvement. This activity can be a lively demonstration of the components of HOSA and how the work of HOSA is accomplished.

Independent study or review of resource activities can be used for individual or small groups of students to find more information on the components of HOSA. This assignment provides an early opportunity for the instructor to observe students' preferred methods of learning. In addition, it may represent a more efficient dissemination of the information in the national and state handbooks, the filmstrips on HOSA and parliamentary procedures, and publications sent out spring and fall by HOSA. Plan that reports of the findings be given at the next scheduled meeting time.

When this strategy is successful, it is time to begin the flow of communication from students and the shift of responsibility to student leaders. Ask leading questions or ask for motions to decide what the group sees as important to do next. The democratic process is at work. Should the whole group view certain filmstrips? Is an officer workshop needed? Are students ready to form an organizing committee? Is it time to distribute applications for office? Which lessons in parliamentary procedure are needed?

The foregoing takes preparation by the instructor/adviser, but remember that much of this information is available in the national handbook. Student power has been tapped, potential leaders have been uncovered, and a model for the regular meeting has been demonstrated.

Officers

Campaigning for office can be fun for many members. Officer candidates need campaign managers and workers. Allot the time for campaign planning, posters, literature, and speeches at the end of school day, with most of the work to be done after school. Look to other faculty members for help for the candidates: media specialists, graphic or commercial artists, data or business department faculty, guidance personnel, and English and related subject instructors.

Guidelines about enlisting assistance for conducting the actual election are included in Section C of the national HOSA handbook. The student activities director or the principal will probably be willing to take part in installation ceremonies. (See Section A the handbook.) After installation, the new officers will assume the duties to give the chapter structure, and the membership will make decisions, develop a program of work, raise funds for dues and other needs, give the chapter direction, and form committees to assist all of the above.

Time is an important consideration. Using class time ensures consistency. However, administrative policy or the curriculum itself may dictate constraints. One time slot a week should be reasonable. In the beginning of the year, informational and organizing activities will be needed each week. Thereafter, if only one time slot is available, use the time for committee meetings one week, with the business meeting scheduled for the next week.

The outline for regular business meetings should follow the agenda as explained in Section C, Part 3, of the national HOSA handbook. Forms for the secretary's minutes, treasurer's report, and committee reports are in the Section C Appendices. In these regular and special meetings, many activities are happening, including practicing parliamentary procedures, choosing service projects in the school or community, setting up committees, and starting fundraising. The adviser will want to encourage volunteerism and identify educational programs such as blood pressure screening, health lessons in an elementary school, and cardiopulmonary resuscitation demonstrations. Note also the list of suggestions for local activities in the Section C Appendices. Discussing a list similar to this can be a stimulus when members are hesitant to contribute ideas or, on the opposite side, when ideas have strayed from the chapter goals.

Plan to attend the student and adviser fall leadership training conference held in the district or at the regional level of the state. Meeting health occupations teachers and students from other schools builds a sense of belonging. The expenditure for this should be in the budget or in the student activities fund. In advance of the conference, prepare the leaders — usually the officers — for the conference agenda and the activities. Assign them to the sessions they are to attend. The shy ones may not follow directions because they do not want to be in a session alone. Accept this, if it happens. There will be other gains in experience that will surface as the year continues. After the conference, plan how to share the information with the general membership.

Competitive Events

Meanwhile, curriculum topics in the health occupations instructional program have continued to be introduced. It is time to introduce another HOSA component: competition. The national HOSA handbook Section B focuses on the National HOSA Competitive Events Program and the four categories offered. The state holds competition in the spring to determine who is eligible to go to the national competition, but the preparation for students begins much earlier.

Competition is a normal part of the workplace. Competition in HOSA is a way for members to prepare for the workplace. It is also a means of gaining recognition for competency in occupational tasks and related topics. Competition requires a quest for excellence, and it rewards competitors with increased confidence and a sense of accomplishment. The opportunity to compete should be offered to all members. Preparation can be fit into class time, and the appropriate guidelines can be used in several parts of the VHO curriculum.

Become familiar with the occupational skill events as they are presented in the national handbook. Be sure those used are the latest revisions. Select those that are relevant to the program. In other words, identify those events with the skills that are being taught in the VHO program. As these skills are taught and evaluated in the program, introduce the HOSA rating sheets also.

Another means of promoting competitive events is to use one or more of the event skills as quarter or mid-term practical examinations. In this manner, all class members are being prepared for competition. If craft advisory members can be scheduled to be the judges, this sets up a local competition within the chapter and provides excellent experience for the next levels of competition.

The benefits of encouraging competitive events are many: adherence to an accepted step-by-step procedure, use of scored rating sheets, penalties and disqualifications, repetition for a reason, confidence in performance, cooperation among classmates, reinforcement of appropriate occupational attire, and encouragement of maturing attitudes. Review with students the introductory information of Section B as well as all parts of the event guidelines.

Students may enter one event in each category of competitive events. Look for occasions to use the leadership events also. Introduce and use the speaking rating sheet when students are giving oral reports. Use the job-seeking event rating sheet in the curriculum or for a grade. Encourage students to enter related or team events.

It is not possible for one adviser to be everywhere, so this is where delegation is necessary. Assign students to help one another practice by being in turn the patient, the judge, or the interviewer. Use other faculty members for the same purposes. From these experiences, students will learn responsibility and independence. Both students and adviser will gain insight from the discussions that take place before and especially after the competitions. Success is achieved even when awards are not won. However, winning at one level qualifies the participant for the next level. These are exhilarating experiences that you should not miss.

Resources

Computer Disk

Notgrass, Troy: Parliamentary Procedure, Extension Instruction and Materials Center, University of Texas at Austin, 1986.

2 Apple disks, instructor's guide, pad of score sheets. To provide practice in applying parliamentary procedure knowledge and skills in simulated situations.

Filmstrips

HOSA Filmstrips: National HOSA, 1983.
   3 color filmstrips, 2 cassettes.

1. National HOSA Competitive Events
2. HOSA Serves the Community
3. Promoting Your HOSA Chapter Activities

Meetings: Parliamentary Procedures in Action, Eye Gate Media, 1978. 4 color filmstrips, 2 cassettes, lesson plan.

A. How to Run an Orderly Meeting
B. What Officers Do and Why
C. How to Use Robert's Rules of Order
D. Your Meeting Organized or Disorganized

Zeiss, Cathy. *An Introduction to Robert's Rules of Order.* Arthur Merriweather, 1980. Color filmstrip (82 frames), cassette, script.

Video

HOSA: Helping Members Become the Best They Can Be!, Hosa People Development Video Series, 1990.

☞ LOCAL OFFICERS' PERSPECTIVES

"As local president, I learned the importance of having leadership qualities. The responsibilities I was given were sometimes overwhelming, but always fun. I am glad I took the job because, in a small way, I believe I made a big difference."

— Vikki Dishman

"Being a secretary in HOSA helped me become more comfortable talking in front of a group of people. It helped me become aware of the process and responsibilities of a secretary. It also gave me the opportunity to become a better person and speak out, instead of keeping things to myself."

— Kathy McConnell

"HOSA has brightened my future by making me an outstanding person and by making me feel good about myself. I have had a great time making friends and making somebody out of myself."

— Danny Qualls

"The experience found in HOSA has been overwhelming. I was able to meet new people, learn new things, compete, and win. There is nothing that compares to the fun involved in HOSA. I highly recommend it to others!"

— Suzanne Decker

"HOSA has helped me open up more. It also helped me with talking to other people I did not know. Attending regional and state conferences helped me get along with other people. It also taught me that everyone is equal."

— Crystal Pippin

"HOSA gives you a chance to meet people, go to leadership workshops, attend regional, state, and national conferences, and participate in various community projects."

— Vickie Bilbrey

"HOSA has changed my life. It has shown me leadership and teamwork. It showed me that teamwork is needed to have a successful club. I am proud to be a member of HOSA."

— Gina Campbell

SECONDARY SCHOOL STUDENTS' PERSPECTIVES

"The health occupations education class I took my senior year really influenced me. We had in-class training along with training at a local nursing home. The class prepared me by letting me know what to expect in the nursing profession."

— Carol Burgess

"I learned a lot from health occupations education. I got hands-on experience, which is far better for anyone than just sitting in a classroom with our nose in books."

— Candy Baker

"The things I gained from my experience in health occupations education were learning the risks and challenges that health career workers face. I also learned of the patience and care they have to have in order to work in this career."

— Yvonne Hickman

"Health occupations is fun and educational. You make several new friends. I got a head start on my career by learning skills and then getting firsthand experience. Because of this class, I have a job."

— Christie Kirby

"This class taught me how to become a more responsible person. It taught me the importance of people and how to take care of them and their feelings."

— Nickie Gunter

"Health occupations education has helped me learn what the health field can offer. It helped me learn patience and responsibility."

— Callie Watts

"I use every day what I learned in health occupations education. I think I've gone far since I've taken this class."

— Melissa Williams

Terms of Importance to HOSA

Conferences — Local, regional, state, and national conferences are held to conduct competitive events, to elect officers, and to carry on other HOE/HOSA business. Local events are usually conducted in a school setting. Each state then conducts regional and state events. The national event is held in June in different states on a rotational basis.

Leadership workshop — A workshop conducted to train officers, to inform students about competitive events, and to relate other information to HOE/HOSA members.

President — An elected officer who presides over the meetings and represents HOE/HOSA at various events.

Reporter — An elected officer who prepares written information about HOE/HOSA for publication.

Secretary — An elected officer who keeps the minutes of all meetings.

References

Birchenall, J. M., and M. E. Streight (1989). *Health Occupations — Exploration and Career Planning*, Chapter 1: Health Career in Review; Gaining Your First Experience. C. B. Mosby.

Gerdin, J. (1991). *Health Careers Today*, Chapter 2: Developing Workers for Change. Organizational Behaviour. C. B. Mosby.

Health Occupations Students of America: National Handbook. Section A: National HOSA — The Organization. Section B: The HOSA National Competitive Events Program. Section C: Guides to Organizing and Managing a HOSA Chapter.

    Health Occupations Students of America
    6309 North O'Connor Road, Suite 215, LB #117
    Irving, TX 75039-3510
    800-321-HOSA

New Jersey HOSA Handbook: New Jersey Association Health Occupations Students of America.

Robert, H. M. (1981). *The Scott, Foresman Robert's Rules of Order*, Newly Revised. Scott, Foresman.

Simmers, L. (1988). *Diversified Health Occupations* (2nd ed.). Appendix A: Vocational Student Organizations. Teacher's Resource Kit. Leadership, Entrepreneurship and Parliamentary Procedure. Albany, NY: Delmar.

Sloan, J. R. (1981). Medical Assistant. Section A: Orientation, Unit II: HOSA, Division of Health Occupations Education. Oklahoma State Board of Vocational Education.

13

Health Occupations Students of America: Our Vocational Student Organization

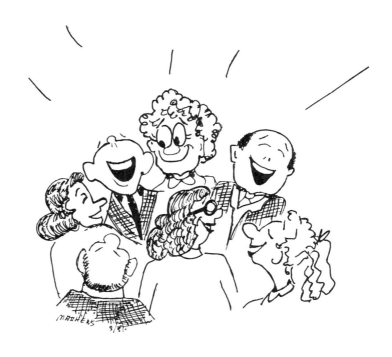

☞ UNDERSTANDING VSOs IN GENERAL

Vocational student organizations (VSOs) are the vehicles by which students expand their experience in vocational education. A list of VSOs is provided in Figure 13-1. Under the guidance of advisers and administrative policy, students may become members of the school club or chapter, participate in state-sponsored activities, and qualify to attend the national conference. Students gain experience in the democratic process as they elect officers, work in committees, develop projects, perform civic services, and participate at the local, state and national levels. In addition, they receive recognition for achievements through the organizational structure of the VSO. This background should encourage future participation in the professional and community organizations of their chosen career area.

VSOs are recognized by the U.S. Department of Education. Some are specific to occupational areas and others are for students enrolled in any trade, industrial, or technical courses. Both secondary and postsecondary students are included in the membership. Educational, professional, and industrial organizations support VSOs in many ways and provide a link to the world of work. Local community leaders volunteer time, talent, and materials for VSO activities, thus promoting liaisons between school and industry.

VSOs have many similarities, though their statements of goals or purposes may differ slightly. VSO activities promote the development of employability and occupational and communication skills. They enhance instructional programs with career information and job-seeking preparation as

---

BPA — Business Professionals of America — (1988) (formerly VOECA — Vocational Office Education Clubs of America, 1966)

DECA — Distributive Education Clubs of America (1947)

FBLA-PBL — Future Business Leaders of America, Phi Beta Lambda (1937)

FFA (formerly the Future Farmers of America) (1928)

FHA-HERO — Future Homemakers of America (1945)

HOSA — Health Occupations Students of America (1976)

NYFEA — National Young Farmer Educational Association (1982)

OEA — Office Education Association

PAS — Postsecondary Agriculture Student Organization (1978)

TSA — Technology Student Association (1988) (formerly AIASA — American Industrial Arts Student Association, 1965)

VICA — Vocational Industrial Clubs of America (1965)

FIGURE 13-1: *Vocational Student Organizations Recognized by the U.S. Department of Education*

well as occupational skill development. Competitive events in leadership, related areas, and occupational categories add another dimension and opportunity for growth.

In some schools, more than one VSO is approved and active. This can generate a healthy competitive spirit for the benefit of the school as a whole. Advisers can share techniques, successes, and problems. Administration can set parameters, assign resources, and encourage participation. Recognition programs that combine the VSOs not only bring community members, parents,

---

I Believe in Vocational Education. I teach it by choice and not by chance. I believe in the ability of vocational education to develop better, more useful citizens; and I am convinced of its necessity in a democratic society.

I Believe That Vocational Student Organizations Are an Integral Part of Vocational Education; that they are essential to a vocational student's education. As such, I will do everything within my power to ensure that my students' leadership and personal skills are developed to the same degree as their technical skills.

I Believe That Vocational Student Organization Activities Should Be Designed by the Students for the Students, and that my major function as advisor is to assist and guide students in developing and conducting such activities. It is my duty to structure the activities so that they build the characteristics of cooperation, leadership, citizenship, and patriotism.

I Believe That My Leadership Role Is of Utmost Importance in demonstrating to students the skills that they will need to become effective members of today's American society. Therefore, I will strive to set the highest personal moral and professional standards possible.

I Believe in the Worth of the Individual; that every student is important. I shall not neglect the student who falls behind or the one that speeds ahead. I shall never knowingly hinder the education of any student, and I shall strive to provide the opportunity for every student to gain recognition through participation in my vocational student organization.

I Believe in Vocational Student Organizations and in their ability to improve the individual. I shall continually endeavor to improve my skills as an advisor and shall never, despite temptations to the contrary, deny my students access to this essential educational ingredient. I proudly accept my responsibilities as vocational teacher and advisor — I shall not fail in either responsibility.

FIGURE 13-2: *Vocational Student Organization Advisor's Creed proposed by Paul R. Vaughn, Rosco C. Vaughn, and D. Lanette Vaughn, 1990, in* Handbook for Advisors of Vocational Student Organizations, *2nd edition, published by the American Association for Vocational Instructional Materials (AAVIM)*

and friends to the school but also bring together diverse students to appreciate the accomplishments of one another.

VSOs provide many opportunities to develop the skills desired by employers. Those traits that are sought after, such as cooperation, self-confidence, initiative, flexibility, dependability, commitment, and conflict resolution ability, are the outcomes of successful participation in the activities of a VSO. Students attend meetings, participate with their peers, exchange information, attempt confidence-building tasks, put forth and evaluate ideas, adjust to changes, prepare for competitions, and handle disappointments in the course of active membership. Advisers build networking contacts, hone managements skills, become change agents, and assist others to share visions of new horizons.

Entrepreneurship is a recent undertaking for the VSO viewed as essential for future employees to experience and understand. Training in this area prepares students to think and adapt in settings requiring a slightly different set of leadership skills. References are available that detail learning activities in entrepreneurship as well as leadership for inclusion in VSO programs.

Parliamentary procedure is a traditional endeavor in VSOs. All state and national conferences follow protocol using Robert's Rules of Order as reference. Local chapters do a service to their members when they follow parallel procedures. VSO handbooks, teacher's resource kits or manuals, simplified references, and visual aids assist local advisers in selecting informative and learning activities to include early in the school year and to foster throughout the programs of work.

REVISITING THE DEVELOPMENT OF HOSA

Health Occupations Students of America (HOSA) has become a strong, healthy, ever-growing, 44,000-member organization in 33 states and the District of Columbia. It is goal-oriented, with sights on the future, and serves secondary, postsecondary, and collegiate students and alumni in widely diversified health care delivery fields.

It is difficult to realize that the initial idea for this national group began only as "a gleam in the eye" of a few caring and farsighted health occupations education leaders back in the sixties and early seventies. HOSA:

- was first formed by the original six charter states at the Organizing Meeting in Cherry Hill, New Jersey, in November 1975;
- was officially formed by Constitutional Convention held in Texas in November 1976;
- included official participants who were state supervisors/advisers, teachers, and over 300 student leaders;

- comprised only six states, with nearly 600 student members; and
- focused on limited supportive nursing, dental, medical, and related occupations programs, as well as organized prevocational programs in health careers approved by the state department of education.

Pre-HOSA History

Let us examine the record. In 1957, the then U.S. Office of Education realized that educational programs in health fields were growing throughout the nation at a pace that warranted the appointment of the first health occupations specialist, Helen K. Powers, to supervise this field. As programs expanded, organizational needs, among others, began to emerge for students enrolled in these programs.

Early needs were met through Future Nurses Clubs and VICA Vocational-Industrial Clubs of America, organized in the sixties in some states. The demand grew for a group giving attention to the specialized needs of health occupations students as such programs diversified. An organization called Health Careers Clubs gained national strength, especially in Alabama, New Jersey, New Mexico, New York, North Carolina, and Texas. These focused specifically on health-career-oriented programs operating in academic high schools.

Programs continued to grow and diversify, with many offerings established in vocational and technical schools/centers across the land. Health occupations educators also began to see the need for a united organized effort to consider common and unique concerns. Thus the American Vocational Association (AVA) emerged as a logical locus for such a group. Beginning as a subgroup of the AVA's New and Related Services Division, Health Occupations Educators (HOE) soon reached the 1,000-member level to qualify as a separate division. The HOE Division was born in 1971, with Dale J. Petersen (of Iowa), as its first president; Petersen also served as vice president of HOE on the AVA board.

One of the new division's first concerns was consideration of the potential "club" needs of its youth (students). A task force was appointed by President Petersen to:

"1. Study student clubs.

2. Determine how they might better serve HOE students.

3. Examine whether a new organization is needed."

Joan B. Stoddard (Oregon) chaired the task force, with Catherine Junge (Texas) and Jack Hatfield (Kentucky) as members.

A study was commissioned by the task force and coordinated by James L. Navera of the Oregon Board of Education, entitled "A Tensibility Study for a Vocational Youth Organization for Health Occupational Education." Its report, submitted to the HOE Division and entitled "Position Paper on Student Organization in the Field of Health Occupations Education," stated:

> ... the nature and relationships of student organizations should be determined at the state and/or local level. The HOE Division of AVA should serve a facilitating role in assisting the various state and/or local groups to develop the type of organization each deems most appropriate to their setting. In addition, this Division should achieve a liaison role among the states and facilitate any desired affiliations with national organizations.

During the December 1973 AVA meeting, one program feature was entitled HOE Student Organization, Health Careers Clubs of New Jersey, and a Special Interest Group Session was scheduled on Student Organizations. This division endorsed the creation of a youth leadership organization for health occupations. The second HOE vice president, Wilma B. Gillespie, appointed a Core Planning Group, whose membership represented those states with established student organizations (New Jersey and Texas) and those in the process of organizing (Alabama, Indiana, and New York).

The Core Planning Group, later termed a task force, met in July 1974 at the Brown County State Park in Nashville. The following December, one HOE Division AVA Special Interest Group Session centered on further discussion of the outcomes of the July meeting and on the Texas Association of Health Occupations Students. Cochairmen for this event were V. Devine Bauer (Alabama) and Mary Holstein (Indiana).

With momentum on the rise, the division's Policy Committee in March 1975 accepted a "Task Force Report on a Health Occupations Student Organization." At the same time, the Policy Committee endorsed the recommendation "to encourage those states with viable statewide student organizations to cooperate in forming a charter organization" and "gave teeth" to this recommendation by establishing a Student Organization Planning Committee, charged as follows:

> To facilitate the efforts by states who now have viable HOE student organizations to 1) expedite seeking a national charter, and 2) devise ways to assist other states in their organizing efforts.

Joan M. Birchenall, director of HOE in the New Jersey State Department of Education served as chairman of this committee, whose members were the HOE state supervisors in Alabama, New Jersey, New Mexico, North Carolina, Oklahoma, and Texas, or their designees.

This committee lost no time in arranging a November 1975 meeting in Cherry Hill, New Jersey, composed of eighteen representatives from the six states with HOE student organizations. Participants included the HOE state supervisor or state adviser and the student president from each state (Alabama, New Jersey, New Mexico, North Carolina, Oklahoma, and Texas). The student presidents exercised their voting power and carried a motion to form the American Health Occupations Education Student Organization (AHOESO, later to be changed to HOSA). They further discussed goals, objectives, and membership, formed committees to draft a proposed constitution and bylaws, and established a plan to hold a Constitutional Convention in Texas in November 1976.

In December 1975, the report of committee actions at the Cherry Hill meeting was accepted by the HOE Division Policy Committee and by the HOE Division during its Annual Membership Meeting. Further, during this AVA Convention an ad hoc seminar gave division members and others the opportunity for a lively discussion of decisions, ways other interested states might organize, and plans for the Constitutional Convention.

HOSA—The Beginning

The Inn of the Six Flags in Arlington, Texas, was the site of the exciting Constitutional Convention held November 10–31, 1976, which gave formal structure to the new student organization. Joan M. Birchenall (New Jersey) presided, as the crucial elements of the organization were formalized. The name was shortened to the one the organization bears today, Health Occupations Students of America — HOSA, as the bylaws were adopted. In addition, delegates elected the first set of national officers, with Lynne McGee of North Carolina as the first national HOSA president. They also chose, maroon, medical white, and navy blue, as national HOSA colors, which prevail today. Further, they designed a contest to identify a national HOSA motto and a HOSA emblem. Finally, Oklahoma was selected as the site and spring 1978 as the date for the first national HOSA conference. The spring date during the 1977–78 year was designated to provide time for dissemination of information, for state and local organizing efforts, and as a culmination of the first full year of HOSA.

The initial, sponsoring national Board of Directors consisted of the HOE state supervisor or state adviser from the six organizing states, the AVA HOE Division vice president, and the president of NASAHOE (National Association of State Administrators of Health Occupations Education), also a HOSA sponsor. The last organization now includes both state and local HOE supervisors and is known as the National Association of Supervisors and Administrators of Health Occupations Educations.

During the first three years, HOSA board chairmen were elected from among the six organizing states. North Carolina's state adviser, Linda Watson, was the first board chairman, from November 1976 through 1978;

Lois Graham, New Jersey's state adviser, served during 1978–79, and Oklahoma provided its state advisor, Mary Randall, for the academic year 1979–80.

With HOSA now duly constituted, it remained for its structural aspects and programming to be more fully identified, defined, and expanded. We will now examine the development of selected aspects of the expansion.

National HOSA Management/Headquarters

In the early years, the state education department of the board chairman for that year provided the national headquarters for HOSA. Thus, the first National HOSA Headquarters was located in Raleigh, North Carolina (November 1976–Spring 1978); the second, in Trenton, New Jersey (1978–79); and the third, in Oklahoma City, Oklahoma (1979–80).

It soon became evident that the management of this rapidly growing organization required more attention than could be provided through any one state's already busy education department. The HOSA Board of Directors advertised for bid proposals for an organization to serve HOSA in a managerial capacity. Four proposals were submitted and their representatives invited to make a presentation during the board's meeting at the New Jersey conference (June 1979). Following considered discussion, the board selected Kenora Enterprises, with Ken and Nora Smith as owner/managers.

After legal aspects of contract development were resolved, and records transferred, the first national HOSA office was established in Wilmington, Delaware, in October 1979, under the direction of HOSA's first national management team, Ken and Nora Smith. In summer 1982, Kenora Enterprises moved its location and national HOSA headquarters to Washington, D.C., giving HOSA a presence in the nation's capital.

Over the years, the HOSA board has asked Kenora to assume increasing responsibilities. Under Kenora's inspired guidance, the organization thrived, growing from a membership of 19,013 and 18 states at the close of the academic year in 1979, to 29,058 members in 27 states in 1982, when Ken and Nora Smith found it necessary to resign as HOSA's managers.

A Search Committee, appointed in 1982 by then board Chairman Barbara James of South Carolina, worked with Kenora to refine the description and functions of a management firm for national HOSA, with Ruth-Ellen Ostler (New York) as chairman. Bid proposals were solicited, and 12 received from individuals and firms all over the country. Their representatives were invited to present their proposals during the board's meeting at the Sixth National HOSA Leadership Conference in San Antonio, Texas.

It was at that time that National HOSA's second national management firm was selected: Leadership Development Institute, Inc. (LDI, Inc.), of Oklahoma City, Oklahoma, with Dr. Jim Koeninger, president, and Karen Elias, vice president, effective summer 1983. Creative and experienced in leadership development activities, in public relations approaches, and in use of diversified media, this management team built on the firm foundation that had been established by Kenora Enterprises. It assisted HOSA both in reaching its now well-recognized and respected status and in giving service to HOE students.

Since 1985—when the HOSA board decided to continue management firm coordination in preference to establishing a separate headquarters—Dr. Koeninger and Ms. Elias have been officially designated as HOSA's executive director and associate director, respectively.

In August 1986, the location of LDI, Inc., and HOSA headquarters was changed to Fort Worth, Texas, and in 1989, to its current site in Irving, Texas. HOSA offers a toll-free number to maintain contact and deliver a variety of services to its members, advisers, and state organizations: 800-321-HOSA.

National HOSA Motto/Emblem/Creed/Uniform Policy

The April 1978, the First Annual Leadership Conference produced numerous decisions basic to the operation of a student organization. The first policy regarding uniforms, consisting of navy slacks/skirt, vest, and jacket; white blouse/shirt; and maroon scarf/tie, was established. Minus the vest, and with scarf optional, this policy remains today.

The Delegate Assembly in Oklahoma adopted the original motto, which was submitted by the Florida State Association of HOSA and read: "The hands of youth mold the health of tomorrow." Even before the 1979 Annual Conference in Cherry Hill, New Jersey, it was recognized that HOSA serves adults as well as youth, and the 1979 Delegate Assembly carried a motion to substitute "HOSA" for "youth," so the current national HOSA motto now reads, "The hands of HOSA mold the health of tomorrow."

In 1978, the official emblem also was adopted by Delegate Assembly action. The design is still used today and is described as follows:

> "The circle represents the continuity of health care; the triangle represents the three aspects of humankind well-being—social, physical, and mental; and the hands signify the caring of each HOSA member."

Colors, of course, are maroon, medical white, and navy blue. This design was submitted by the Tennessee Association of HOSA. The HOSA emblem/logo was registered with the U.S. Copyright Office in 1980.

It was not until the Third National HOSA Leadership Conference, held in Asheville, North Carolina, in 1980, that HOSA's official creed was adopted, as submitted by South Carolina's state HOSA. The HOSA creed can be found in Figure 13-3.

I believe in the health care profession.

I believe in the profession for which I am being trained and in the opportunities which my training offers.

I believe in education.

I believe that through education I will be able to make the greatest use of my skills, knowledge, and experience in order to become a contributing member of the health care team and of my community.

I believe in myself.

I believe that by using the knowledge and skills of my profession I will become more aware of myself. Through fulfilling these goals I will become a more responsible citizen.

I believe that each individual is important in his or her own right: therefore, I will treat each person with respect and love. To this end, I dedicate my training, my skills, and myself to serve others through Health Occupations Students of America.

13-3: *HOSA Creed*

Recognition by U.S. Department Of Education

HOSA was one of two new student organizations (the other was, the American Industrial Arts Student Association — AIASA) recognized by the then U.S. Office of Education in September 1977 as it issued its new policy statement, designed to endorse all vocational student organizations. Ernest L. Boyer was commissioner at that time. Such endorsement has been reaffirmed periodically, as in 1988, under Secretary William J. Bennett, and again in 1990, under Secretary Laura F. Cavazos.

National HOSA Board of Directors

From the time of its first set of bylaws, HOSA has provided for an adult sponsoring group. As specified in the present board bylaws, the object of this group ". . . shall be to sponsor the student organization Health Occupations Students of America (HOSA) and to promote and sponsor the HOE — HOSA partnership."

In 1980, incorporation of HOSA was transferred from New Jersey to Delaware, and the Board of Directors was reorganized as HOSA, Inc. This body and its Board of Directors was formed to be the legally responsible agent for the student organization of HOSA. At the third conference, in North Carolina (1980), the HOSA bylaws and the HOSA, Inc., bylaws were revised from those of the original board. Exempt status for the organization also was achieved.

Initially consisting of a relatively limited membership of HOE state supervisors, advisers, and student officers, with selected affiliate nonvoting representatives, the HOSA, Inc., Board of Directors now includes broad membership composed of state and local advisers, student officers, health care industry representatives, and HOE students.

Regarding national HOSA competitive events, the founders of HOSA believed initially that HOSA should feature leadership development programs and activities, not contests. Thus, no competitive events were included in the bylaws and meeting plans established at the 1976 organizing meeting.

However, as additional states became interested and were chartered, numerous requests for some competitive events were received, and the first Competitive Events Committee was appointed prior to the 1978 meeting. This resulted in four events being scheduled for the First Annual Leadership Conference in Oklahoma (1978). All focused on general health issues and across-the-board leadership development aspects of HOE programming: a HOSA poster (health issue), extemporaneous speaking, informative speaking (now called prepared speaking), and job interview (now, called job-seeking skills).

Responses were so favorable that during the Second Annual Conference in New Jersey, demonstrations and exhibits of three more events were presented: HOSA Bowl, Best HOSA Chapter, and Outstanding Chapter — the latter two evidenced by scrapbooks. None of these was adopted until HOSA Bowl finally progressed through another demonstration (1983, Sixth Conference, Texas), piloting (1984, Seventh Conference, Florida), and, as a regular event in 1985 at the Eighth Conference in Tennessee. The Outstanding HOSA Chapter event also followed the now-in-place plan for new events, and was a regular event in 1987 in Texas at the Tenth Conference.

It was not until the Fourth Annual Leadership Conference in New Mexico in 1981 and in Illinois in 1982 that Competitive Events Demonstrations and Pilots began in earnest in more specialized health-related areas and in very specific health skills areas. They resulted from much greater HOE program diversification represented by increasing numbers of members throughout the nation.

Therefore, by the Sixth Conference in Texas in 1983, four categories of events, each with several subcategories, were well established and had become an expected part of the national leadership conference each year:

I   Health Occupations–Related Skills: five regular events and one pilot
II Health Occupations Skills: Six regular events
III Individual Leadership Skills: three regular events
IV Team Leadership Skills: two regular events and two demos

New events continue to be suggested by states that assume responsibility for the demonstration and piloting stages of a proposal event. The total number of events has increased.

All events are coordinated by the Competitive Events Committee and the headquarters staff, with a lieutenant in charge of each category. The first Competitive Events Handbook Section was published in 1983 and has been revised several times, the latest in 1990. A complete list of currently offered events is given in Figure 13-4.

Category I — Health Occupations Related Events
    Dental Spelling
    Dental Terminology
    Extemporaneous Health Display
    Medical Spelling
    Medical Terminology
    Standard First Aid/CPR
    First Aid/Rescue Breathing

Category II — Health Occupations Skill Events
    Dental Assisting
    Medical Assisting — Clerical
    Medical Assisting — Clinical
    Medical Laboratory Assisting
    Nursing Assisting
    Practical Nursing
    Surgical Technology
    Advanced Nursing
    Dental Laboratory Technology
    Respiratory Care
    Veterinary Assisting
    Opticianry

Category III — Individual Leadership Events
    Extemporaneous Speaking
    Job-Seeking Skills
    Prepared Speaking
    Extemporaneous Writing

Category IV — Team Leadership Events
    Community Awareness Project
    HOSA Bowl
    Parliamentary Procedure
    Outstanding HOSA Chapter

FIGURE 13-4: *National Hosa Competitive Events*

References

Minutes of HOE Division, AVA, from its inception in 1970.

Birchenall, Joan M. "History of Health Occupations Students of America." Paper delivered at AVA HOE Division Luncheon, December 1, 1977.

"Ad Hoc Seminar on AHOESO." Transcript of Presentations and Discussion, AVA Convention, Anaheim, California; Joan M. Birchenall, Chairman; December 9, 1975.

"Introducing AHOESO," Paper summarizing action taken at Planning Committee meeting in Cherry Hill, New Jersey. Presented at Ad Hoc Seminar on AHOESO, December 9, 1975.

"1980 Special Awards to Recognize Past/Current Leadership, HOSA." Script for presentation of awards to honor all individuals and state associations instrumental in the planning and founding of national HOSA and in its first three years. Third Annual National HOSA Leadership Conferences, Asheville, North Carolina, June 8–12, 1980.

"Development of HOSA," National HOSA Handbook, Section A (1st ed.). Irving, TX: Health Occupations Students of America, (1st ed.). 1982 (rev. 1985).

"1900–2000: A Century of Progress for Health Care Personnel." National Health Occupations Education Curriculum Conference, Sacramento, California, 1990.

"Historical Development; National HOSA Competitive Events Program," *HOSA Management Resource Guide* pp. 2–22. Ft. Worth, TX: National HOSA, 1987.

National HOSA Handbook, Section A — National HOSA — The Organization," pp. 3–78. Fort Worth, TX: National HOSA, 1985; 1988. Section A — "National HOSA — The Organization; Section B — "The HOSA National Competitive Events Program" (1st ed. 1982, rev. 1990); and Section C — Guide.

HOSA Magazine. Selected issues. National HOSA: Irving, TX.

VISION. Selected issues. National HOSA: Irving, TX.

NLC Guide, 1992. National HOSA: Irving, TX. *HOSA Directory, 1991–92.* National HOSA: Irving, TX.

"HOSA Board and Committee Minutes." Selected years. Irving, TX: National HOSA, 1976–Present.

HOSA Leaders Update, 1979–1983 (Delaware and North Carolina). Irving, TX: National HOSA.

Vaughn, P. R., R. C. Vaughn, and D. L. Vaughn. *Handbook for Advisors of Vocational Student Organizations* (2nd ed.). Athens, GA: AAVIM, 1990.

14

Vocational Education: Our Umbrella

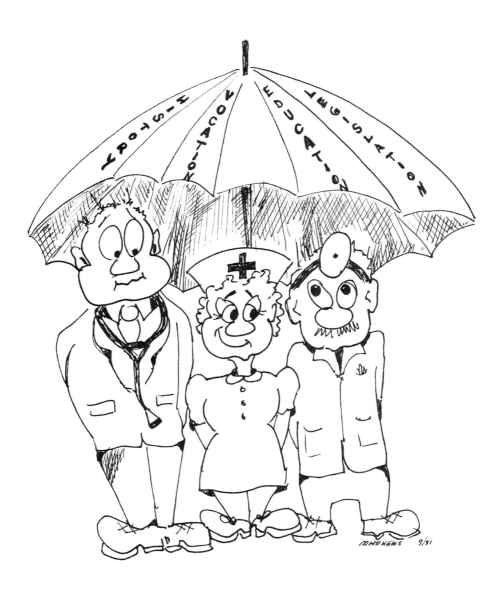

HISTORY OF VOCATIONAL EDUCATION

There are some people who consider that any education that prepares one for work is vocational education. However, vocational education as defined by federal legislation is education at a level less than the baccalaureate degree level, which prepares one with initial job-entry skills. So, where did vocational education come from? How did training for work end up in our schools? How did it become separate from traditional academic education?

The movement for federally funded public vocational education gained its momentum in America somewhere between 1876 and 1917. During that time, social, political, economic, and philosophical factors all conjugated in a unique chain of events that led to the passage of the 1917 Smith-Hughes Act, the "Magna Carta" of present-day vocational education. But vocational education has been around much longer than that.

Apprenticeship

Since early civilization, training for work has been a doctrine handed down to each successive generation. In earlier times, such training was conducted by families, from father to son, and from mother to daughter (Evans, 1971; McClure, Chrisman, and Mock, 1985). As vocations became more complex, families could no longer handle this preparation alone. New systems had to be developed for training the young for work.

One answer came in the form of apprenticeship training. Those who wished to enter a certain vocation had to first join the appropriate guild and become an apprentice to a master in that guild (Chambers et al., 1987). An agreement usually lasted seven years, with the apprentice normally living with the master. The master would provide food, lodging, and vocational and moral training. Upon completion of the apprenticeship period, and with satisfactory progress, the apprentice became a journeyman. After completing a "masterpiece," the student could either become his own master or continue working as a journeyman (McClure et al., 1985).

Colonial America

As the concept of universal education gained momentum in England and as the presence of merchant and crafts guilds waned, settlers arrived in Colonial America. The settlers brought with them many educational theories and practices reflective of their English ancestors; however, the systems they set up in Colonial America were not exact duplicates of those of the world they left behind (Pulliam, 1991).

Vocational education was more prevalent in the middle colonies than in others. Local private schools often taught such practical skills as merchandising, bookkeeping, navigation, trade, mechanics, and geography (Pulliam, 1991).

In the period following the American Revolution, two types of secondary educational institutions became prominent: the Latin gammar schools and the academies. Latin schools were attended by boys who planned on going to college. Their classic curriculum consisted mainly of Latin.

Benjamin Franklin opposed the classical, liberal education offered in the Latin schools, preferring instead education related to the professional affairs of life. In this interest, he founded an academy in 1751. Designed for those not going on to college, the academy offered practical subjects in English rather than Latin and offered training in manual skills such as bookkeeping, carpentry, farming, and printing (Ornstein and Hunkins, 1988). Such academies were eventually replaced by public high schools.

Early American Vocational Education

During the 1800s, a great many European educator reformists helped set the stage for the vocational educational movement by introducing progressive ideas and influencing American educational philosophy. One of the more prominent reformers was the Swiss educator Johann Heinrich Pestalozzi. Influenced by Rousseau, Pestalozzi believed that schools should emphasize the natural development of youth (Ornstein and Hunkins, 1988). In 1774, Pestalozzi developed the Neuhof Industrial School, a farm school for poor children. The children were trained in farming, handicrafts, and general education based on Pestalozzi's pedagogical belief that children learn through sensory stimuli rather than through words (McClure et al., 1985; Ornstein and Hunkins, 1988). Because of his beliefs, Pestalozzi is often called the father of manual training (Feirer and Lindbeck, 1964).

At the 1876 Philadelphia Centennial Exposition and World's Fair, countries from around the world came to exhibit their newest innovations and advances, but the Russian exhibit stole the show. Featured were tools that had been made by students using a new system developed by Victor Della Vos, director of the Moscow Imperial Technical School. Della Vos had been searching for a more efficient method for teaching his students the trades. It was common to have students learn trades in a workshop setting where they would construct items as apprentices. But Della Vos felt that the apprentice workshop method was overly expensive and inefficient (Cremin, 1964). Della Vos founded a new form of shop in which students were taught each skill needed to complete the whole. The skills were arranged in a logical manner, and a series of graded exercises was developed that, upon mastery of each, students could progress to the next level. Della Vos was teaching the use of the tools and principles of a trade without actually having students work as apprentices in the trade itself (Cremin, 1964).

One of the visitors at the 1876 Exposition was John D. Runkle, president of Massachusetts Institute of Technology. After seeing the Russian display cases and learning the new system, Runkle immediately took the idea back home. At MIT he recommended the construction of similar shops. Shortly thereafter, MIT's School of Mechanical Arts was formed based on the Russian system (Cremin, 1964). This new method of teaching the mechanical arts proved to be extremely successful, and Runkle was an enthusiastic supporter of the system (Feirer and Lindbeck, 1964).

Runkle was not alone in his excitement over the new system. Calvin M. Woodward was a Harvard-educated faculty member at Washington University in St. Louis, who was finding ineffective the system he used to train apprentices for engineering trades. On June 6, 1879, Woodward opened the St. Louis Manual Training School for Boys, an affiliate of Washington University, based on Della Vos's theories of teaching (Feirer and Lindbeck, 1964). In this school, boys learned the proper use of tools without an immediate vocational goal. The students were offered a mixture of liberal and manual training, but the emphasis was on expanding the students' experiences in using their hands rather than on specific vocational training (Feirer and Lindbeck, 1964). Hence the movement became known as the manual arts movement, the "art" representing the nature of the manual training. Woodward quickly became a proponent of this new system of training.

Together, Woodward and Runkle pushed to have the manual arts introduced into the public school system. In 1877, Runkle spoke before the National Education Association (NEA) to explain the new system (Cremin, 1964). Gradually, the word spread, and manual arts training became buzz words. With the progressive ideas of Pestalozzi and Froebel fresh in their minds, educational reform leaders began to see hope for the manual arts training system. By the turn of the century, manual arts training in the public schools had become a hotly debated issue.

On one side were those who felt that the manual arts movement held the key for making education more relevant and individually oriented. On the other side were those still holding to the thought that an academic, liberal education was the only form of education that should be offered in the public schools. And a new dimension had been added. There was a new group that now wanted to go one step beyond manual arts training. This group wanted to see specific job skill training offered, and it wanted public funding for this vocational training. The adherents felt that the United States needed to provide for those students who were not being served by public education (the ones who dropped out or did not go on to college). It was clear that the United States now believed education was the natural right of all, and funding for public education had indeed been incorporated into law in every states. The question was what type should this education be?

☞ FEDERAL VOCATIONAL EDUCATION LEGISLATION

In the late 1800s, some sought federally supported vocational and trade education. And they wanted to see separate vocational schools established. The slogan for their movement became "equality of educational opportunity" in place of "equal education for all" (Barlow, 1965). The proponents of vocational education felt that equality of educational opportunity meant providing training and skills that would be appropriate for each and every student, not just those going on to college (Barlow, 1965). Earlier, in 1862, Congress passed the Morrill Land-Grant Act, which established the agricultural and mechanical colleges, but there had been no changes in the curricula of lower levels of education (Schaefer and Kaufman, 1971). Now the movement for reformation of the public school system had begun.

Precursor Events

In 1896, the National Association of Manufacturers (NAM) formed and quickly joined into support trade education in the schools. By the 1900s, NAM was the nation's most outspoken advocate of trade education (Cremin, 1964). In 1905, NAM appointed the Committee on Industrial Education to study and promote the issue. It supported practical education but was not sure of the ability of professional educators to run such a program (McClure et al., 1985). NAM wanted to see vocational education under a separate system run by representatives of workers, farmers, and employers.

The American Federation of Labor (AFL) was the largest labor organization at the turn of the century (McClure et al., 1985). It advocated educational reform but had mixed feelings about vocational education. The AFL supported the concept of vocational education in the schools but did not want a separate system that was controlled by managers and employers. In fact, the AFL did not like the concept of a dual educational system of academic and trade schools because it felt that trade schools provided an avenue for management to sidestep organized labor and provide low-wage workers (McClure et al., 1985). At the time, the United States was in the midst of its industrial revolution, and the factories were in dire need of skilled workers. The AFL wanted vocational training, but it wanted publicly controlled vocational education to be included together and as part of public education.

In 1906, the National Society for the Promotion of Industrial Education (NSPIE) was formed. The society's membership quickly grew, and the NSPIE did much to increase U.S. attention to industrial and trade education. Moreover, the NSPIE served to unite various groups to lobby for a federal vocational education bill.

The AFL and NAM joined forces in 1910 to lobby for trade instruction in the schools. The AFL issued a report that year entitled *Industrial Education* in support of publicly funded and controlled vocational education (Gompers, 1910). And in 1910, the NEA publicly joined the others with its, *Report of the Committee on the Place of Industries in Public Education* (1910), which referred to the importance of vocational education for those students going into industry after school. Support came from everywhere — from citizens, educators, politicians, social workers, businesspeople, and laborers (Greenwood, 1978).

Charles A. Prosser became secretary of the NSPIE in 1912 and together with other educational leaders and various organizations began the push for the appointment of a national commission to study the issue of federal aid for vocational education. Prosser had admired Pestalozzi and based his own philosophy of education on Pestalozzian principles (Greenwood, 1978). Prosser advocated a curriculum based on individual needs, interests, and abilities and had long been a staunch proponent of vocational education. Together, Prosser and his associate Snedden had developed a strong vocational education system in Massachusetts and now sought to bring this system to all youth via the federal government.

In 1914, President Wilson finally appointed the Commission on National Aid to Vocational Education. The commission consisted of four congressmen (Senators Carroll S. Page and Hoke Smith and House Representative S. D. Fess and D. M. Hughes) and five vocational education leaders, one of whom was Charles Prosser (Schaefer and Kaufman, 1971). The commission found that vocational education was imperative for students not going on to college and that the only way to stimulate the growth of vocational education was to provide federal funds to support it (McClure et al., 1985).

Smith-Hughes Act

The commission's recommendations were incorporated into the Smith-Hughes Act of 1917, which authorized funds for states for vocational education in agriculture, home economics, and trade and industry. States did not have to accept the funds, but if they did, they had to match them. In addition, all funds had to be publicly controlled. The act also established a federal board to oversee the provisions of the act. The Smith-Hughes Act marked the beginning of a federally supported system of vocational education that still serves students today at the secondary and postsecondary education levels. Whereas it may have been the manual arts movement that began the push, and whereas Prosser, Snedden, and organizations like the NEA and the NSPIE might have helped drive the push, and whereas labor, the AFL, the NAM, and the industrial revolution might have added fuel, and whereas Pestalozzi's and Froebel's philosophies might have fanned the fire, it was not any one of these factors alone but the conglomeration of all these factors that form the history behind the passage of the Smith-Hughes Act of 1917. The founding of vocational education in the U.S. can't be attributed to just one group or person.

The following year, the NEA's Commission on the Reorganization of Secondary Education issued its famous *Cardinal Principles of Secondary Education* (1918). Influenced by the federal concern for vocational education, the commission included vocations as one of the seven major objectives of secondary education. The nation had finally begun to change its educational philosophy.

Further Acts and Amendments

In the years since the passage of Smith-Hughes, Congress has continued to refine vocational education. The George-Reed Act of 1929 and the George-Ellzey Act of 1934 adjusted the distribution of funds. The 1937 George-Deen Act increased expenditures and added distributive education to the list of vocational subjects. And in 1940, under the threat of war, the National Defense Training Act (also known as the Wartime Production Act) provided wartime vocational training for thousands of workers in defense industries (McClure et al., 1985).

By the end of World War II, tremendous numbers of wartime workers were no longer needed, and the United States was faced with the prospect of high unemployment unless something was done. Congress responded by passing the Servicemen's Readjustment Act (also known as the G.I. bill) to retrain World War II veterans. This training also included vocational training.

The 1946 George-Barden Act (also known as the Vocational Education Act of 1946) amended the George-Deen Act. It increased federal aid and gave states more flexibility for the development of vocational programs and activities.

The Health Amendments Act (1956) signed by President Eisenhower amended the George-Barden Act to include practical nursing and other health occupations programs. This legislation is the basis for including health occupations as one of the vocational education areas; practical nursing was the first health field identified in federal vocational education legislation.

During the 1950s, Russia's launching of Sputnik raised fears that America was losing the technical race. This was perceived as a national security threat, so Congress passed the National Defense Education Act in 1958 to address the need for more technical education.

The 1960s saw a major shift in social and educational philosophy, which influenced the direction of vocational education legislation. All legislation affecting vocational education between 1940 and 1960 had meeting the nation's manpower needs and society needs as its principal objectives (preparing for war, combating unemployment, keeping technologically advanced).

But in the 1960s, Congress passed several laws to better the condition of citizens who were suffering because of the economy. The United States became humanity oriented. The Area Redevelopment Act (1961) was passed to help areas that had experienced long-term unemployment. It stressed the need for the Department of Labor and vocational education agencies to cooperate in helping those in depressed areas.

In 1962, the Manpower Development Training Act was the Congressional response to President Kennedy's call to help those who had lost their job to machines and economic problems. It provided for the training and retraining of individuals to work within the community. The 1962 Public Welfare Act provided training for welfare recipients so that they might obtain gainful employment. The Trade Extension Act of the same year provided for training of displaced workers. The 1963 Higher Educational Facilities Act earmarked funds for technical institutions as well as community colleges to update vocational facilities.

During the Kennedy era, Congress passed the Vocational Education Act of 1963. In addition to adding business education to the list of vocational subjects, the act required states to submit state plans and specified some of the areas that money was to be spent in.

In 1968, the Vocational Education Act Amendments repealed all previous vocational education acts except for Smith-Hughes. This act made funds available to states on a matching basis to meet the needs of:

1. High school students needing postsecondary vocational/technical education.

2. Individuals needing training or retraining to keep or advance in their positions.

3. Nonhigh school students needing training to enter the job market.

4. Disadvantaged individuals.

Funds were made available for teacher training, supervision, guidance, evaluation, demonstration products, and development of instructional materials. The act also created the National Advisory Council on Vocational Education and procedures for evaluating state plans.

The Vocational Education Act Amendments of 1974 and 1976 provided support for nurse training, part-time employment of trainees, training of the handicapped, and training of the disadvantaged. It was also the first time that sex discrimination was forbidden in programs receiving federal funds.

By the late 1970s, several reports were critical of vocational education. Programs were seen as expensive. Many students did not get jobs in the area that they had trained for, and no data surfaced to suggest that students who attended a vocational program were any better off than their high school dropout counterparts.

Federal cutbacks in the early 1980s were matched by cutbacks in state funding for vocational education. And a new rash of education reform reports had surfaced suggesting that the philosophy of education should be a back-to-basics approach and a return to traditional academic curricula. In response, Congress revamped vocational education with the Carl D. Perkins Act of 1984 as follows.

1. To assist states to expand, improve, modernize, and develop high-quality vocational education programs.
2. To ensure that individuals who are inadequately served under vocational education programs are assured of access to high-quality vocational education programs.
3. To promote greater cooperation between public agencies and the private sector in preparing individuals for employment.
4. To improve the academic foundation of vocational students.
5. To provide vocational education services to train, retrain, and upgrade employed and unemployed workers in new skills.
6. To assist the most economically depressed areas of a state so as to raise the employment and occupational competencies of its citizens.
7. To assist states in utilizing a full range of supportive services, special programs, guidance counseling, and placement.
8. To improve the effectiveness of consumer and homemaking education.
9. To authorize national programs designed to meet designated vocational education needs.

The Perkins Act was reauthorized in 1989 and completely rewritten in 1990. One of the most noticeable changes was in the name of the act. In 1990, it was renamed the Carl D. Perkins Vocational and Applied Technology Education Act Amendments of 1990. Along with the name change came a change in the purpose. In place of the nine objectives stated in the 1984 act, the 1990 amendments contain a single statement of purpose:

> It is the purpose of this act to make the United States more competitive in the world economy by developing more fully the academic and occupational skills of all segments of the population. This purpose will principally be achieved through concentrating resources on improving educational programs leading to academic, occupational, training, and re-training skill competencies needed to work in a technologically advanced society (Section 2).

As we near the end of our century and enter the next, it appears that vocational education may have a new direction. The 1990s appear to be the decade when the duality of vocational education and academic education will merge to form one combined education for all students. We do not know what the twenty-first century will bring, but as vocational educators, we can look back on our rich history and realize that the introduction and development of vocational education forever changed the course of education in our country.

References

Area Redevelopment Act. Statutes at Large, Vol. 85 (1961).

Barlow, M. (1965). The Challenge to Vocational Education. *Vocational Education, the Sixty-fourth Yearbook of the National Society for the Study of Education, Part I.* Chicago: University of Chicago Press.

Barlow, M. (1967). *History of Industrial Education in the United States.* Peoria, IL: Charles A. Bennet.

Bennet, C. A. (1937). *History of Manual and Industrial Education 1870 to 1917.* Peoria, IL: Charles A. Bennet Co., Inc.

Brubacher, J. S., and W. Rudy (1976). *Higher Education in Transition* (3rd. ed.). New York: Harper and Row.

Carl D. Perkins Vocational and Applied Technology Education Act Amendments of 1990 (1990).

Carl D. Perkins Vocational Education Act of 1984., 20 U.S.C. SS 2301. (1984).

Chambers, M., R. Grew, D. Herlihy, T. Rabb, and I. Woloch, (1987). *The Western Experience.* New York: Alfred A. Knopf.

Commission on the Reorganization of Secondary Education (1918). *Cardinal Principles of Secondary Education.* Washington: U.S. Government Printing Office, Document #1004.

Cremin, L. A. (1964). *The Transformation of the School: Progressivism in American Education.* New York: Alfred A. Knopf.

Drost, W. H. (1967). *David Snedden and Education for Social Efficiency.* Madison, WI: University of Wisconsin Press.

Eaddy, K. M., D. B. Mock, and R. G. Stakenas (1985). *Educating Hand and Mind: A History of Vocational Education in Florida.* Lanham, MD: University Press of America.

Evans, R. N. (1971). *Foundations of Vocational Education* (1st ed.). Columbus, OH: Charles E. Merrill.

Feirer, J. L., and J. R. Lindbeck, (1964). *Industrial Arts Education.* Washington: Center for Applied Research in Education.

Finch, C., and J. Crunkilton (1984). *Curriculum Development in Vocational and Technical Education: Planning, Context, and Implementation (2nd. ed.).* Boston: Allyn and Bacon.

Gadell, J. (1972). *Charles Allen Prosser, His Work in Vocational and General Education.* Unpublished doctoral dissertation, Washington University.

George-Deen Act of 1936. Statutes at Large, Vol. 49 (1936).

George-Ellzey Act of 1934. Statutes at Large, Vol. 48 (1934).

George-Reed Act of 1929. Statutes at Large, Vol. 45 (1929).

Gompers, S. (1910). *Industrial Education.* Washington: American Federation of Labor.

Green, T. M. (1955). A Liberal Christian Idealist Philosophy of Education. *Modern Philosophies and Education.* Fifty-fourth Yearbook of the National Society for the Study of Education, University of Chicago. Chicago: University of Chicago Press.

Greenwood, K. L. B. (1978). *A Philosophical Rationale for Vocational Education: Contributions of Charles A. Prosser and His Contemporaries from 1900 to 1917.* Unpublished doctoral dissertation, University of Minnesota.

Hawkins, L. S., C.A. Prosser and I. C. Wright (1967). *Development of Vocational Education* (5th ed.) Chicago: American Technical Society.

Health Amendments Act of 1956. Statutes at Large, Vol. 70 (1956).

Higher Education Facilities Act of 1963. Statutes at Large, Vol. 77 (1963).

Krug, E. A. (1969). *The Shaping of the American High School, 1880–1920.* Madison, WI: University of Wisconsin Press.

Lazerson, M. (1971). *Origins of the Urban School: Public Education in Massachusetts.* Cambridge, MA: Harvard University Press.

Lazerson, M., and W. N. Grubb (1974). *Education and Vocationalism: A Documentary History, 1870–1970.* New York: Teachers College Press, Columbia University.

Manpower Development Training Act of 1962. Statutes at Large, Vol. 76 (1965).

McClure, A. F., J. R. Chrisman, and P. Mock (1985). *Education for Work.* Rutherford, NJ: Fairleigh Dickinson University Press.

Miller, M. D. (1985). *Principles and a Philosophy for Vocational Education.* Columbus, OH: National Center for Research in Vocational Education, Ohio State University.

National Defense Training Act of 1940. Statutes at Large, Vol. 54 (1954).

National Education Association (1910). *Report of the Committee of Ten on the Place of Industries in Public Education.* Washington: National Education Association.

Ornstein, A. C., and F. D. Hunkins (1988). *Curriculum: Foundations, Principles, and Issues.* Englewood Cliffs, NJ: Prentice Hall.

Public Welfare Act of 1962. Statutes at Large, Vol___ (1962).

Pulliam, J. D. (1991). *History of Education in America* (5th ed.). New York: Macmillan.

Schaefer, C. J., and J. J. Kaufman (1971). *Vocational Education; Social and Behavioral Perspectives.* A report prepared for the Massachusetts Advisory Council on Education. Lexington, MA: Heath Lexington.

Schubert, W. H. (1986). *Curriculum: Perspectives, Paradigm, and Possibility.* New York: Macmillan.

Servicemen's Readjustment Act of 1944. Statutes at Large, Vol. 58 (1944).

Smith-Hughes Act of 1917. Statutes at Large, Vol 39 (1917).

Snedden, D. S. (1921). *Sociological Determination of Objectives in Education.* Philadelphia: J. B. Lippincott.

Violas, P. C. (1978). *The Training of the Urban Working Class: A History of Twentieth Century American Education.* Chicago: Rand McNally College Publishing.

Vocational Education Act of 1946 (George-Barden Act). Statutes at Large, Vol. 60 (1946).

Vocational Education Act of 1963. Statutes at Large, Vol. 77 (1963).

Vocational Education Amendments of 1968. Statutes at Large, Vol. 82 (1968).

Vocational Education Amendments of 1974. Statutes at Large, Vol. 88 (1974).

Vocational Education Amendments of 1976. Statutes at Large, Vol. 90 (1976).

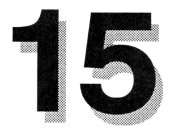

15

Health Occupations Education: Our Focal Area

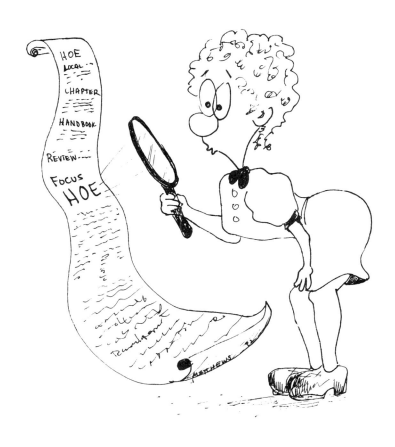

[*Editor's Note: This section is a series of excerpts taken from work by the late Elizabeth E. Kerr, Ph.D., in (Joseph Hamburg, ed).* Review of Allied Health Education: 2, *Permission for use was generously granted by the University Press of Kentucky.*]

☞ REVIEWING HOE IN GENERAL

Need for Health Care

At the turn of the century, health services in this nation were provided almost entirely in homes and doctors' offices and almost exclusively by only three categories of health workers: physicians, dentists, and nurses, who numbered about 350,000 in all. Commensurate with the tempo of social change and technological advance, health care settings have expanded progressively first to hospitals and nursing homes and more recently to extended care units, home care programs, and ambulatory care areas such as community or neighborhood clinics and rehabilitation centers.

Today the efficient and effective delivery of high-quality health care requires the competencies of a broad spectrum of workers: autonomous primary professionals, who carry the greatest burden of legal responsibility for the care provided, and a variety of allied health personnel—professionals, technicians, assistants, and aides—whose work supports that of the autonomous primary professionals. The level of educational preparation required of these workers varies according to the functions they are expected to perform. Therefore, programs preparing health care personnel range from doctoral-level preparation to short-term, on-the-job training.

The term "health occupations education," through popular usage in recent years and as treated in this chapter, means specifically the education of workers whose roles are supportive to health professionals and do not require a baccalaureate degree. Until recently, health workers generally have tended to fall into five distinct categories:

1. Autonomous primary professionals: physicians, dentists
2. Professionals: medical technologists, physical and occupational therapists, nurses, medical social workers
3. Technicians: dental laboratory technicians, dental hygienists, environmental technicians, respiratory therapy technicians, associate degree nurses (by definition of the nursing profession)
4. assistants: dental assistants, medical office assistants, practical nurses
5. aides: nurse aides, orderlies, physical therapy and occupational therapy aides, dietary aides

When considered by level of responsibility or autonomy, the five categories of health workers tend to regroup into three:

1. Autonomous primary professionals, generally prepared in medical and dental colleges of public and private universities
2. Professionals, increasingly being prepared at four-year colleges and universities in health specialty departments and in schools of allied health professionals
3. Supportive health workers (technicians, assistants, and aides), prepared in many different types of programs located in a variety of administrative settings

The ever-increasing utilization of workers in the latter group has contributed substantially to the numerical growth of identifiable occupations in the health field, a growth that has been dramatic over the past fifteen to twenty years.

Unquestionably, therefore, health occupations education (HOE) is vital to the preparation of an adequate force of workers to meet the health care needs of this country. Its continued viability and productivity must be ensured in light of the U. S. Department of Labor's 1970s prediction that by 1980, 80 percent or more of all service occupations would require less than four years of college. Indeed, this forecast has major implications for our predominantly service-oriented health field. (Editor's Note: More recently this figure was 84 percent for all workers—*Occupational Outlook Handbook*, 1990, p. 9).

Programs

HOE is the composite of less-than-baccalaureate-degree preparatory and supplemental (continuing education) programs that prepare and upgrade personnel in the provision of health care. These programs—ranging from short-term offerings to two-year associate degree programs—are administered predominantly by public community/junior colleges and vocational-technical institutes in cooperation with state departments of education, though some are administered by hospitals and private schools. And, increasingly, secondary schools (meaning middle schools and high schools) are offering programs to provide students with opportunities both to explore careers in the health field and, as appropriate, to prepare themselves for selected health occupations. The rapid expansion of vocational-technical education, especially in community college settings, has contributed immeasurably to the growth and quality of HOE, now an identifiable component of this branch of education.

Probably the greatest single stimulus to HOE, however, came with the passage of the Health Amendments Act of 1956, which, in essence, amended the 1946 George-Barden Act by including Title II, Vocational Education in

Practical Nurse Training. Its purpose was to improve the health of people by helping to increase the number of adequately prepared practical nurses. This act provided $5 million to be used as matching monies awarded by the federal government to cooperating states for the development of practical nursing and "other health occupations education" programs.

For the first two years, matching was based on a ratio of 3:1, and for the remaining three years, on a dollar-for-dollar basis. Whereas these monies could be used to support any HOE program "of less than baccalaureate level," by far the greatest portion was used for practical nurse education; consequently, the act often is referred to as the Practical Nursing Act. This act required that each state accepting these funds employ a professional nurse to serve as the state supervisor (consultant) for HOE.

The Vocational Education Act of 1963 (P.L. 88-210) authorized appropriations of up to $225 million annually for occupationally oriented programs of all types except for those "generally considered professional or as requiring a baccalaureate of higher degree." This act prompted a rapid expansion of HOE, and within the U. S. Office of Education, HOE was transferred from the trade and industrial branch and established as an independent arm of the Bureau of Adult, Vocational and Technical Education. A similar reorganization has been made in most state divisions of vocational-technical education.

Despite rapid growth in the number and types of HOE programs following passage of the Health Amendments Act of 1956, by 1965 the need for highly competent workers prepared in HOE had become even more urgent. A shortage of health care personnel already existed and was expected to become more acute in view of the 1965 amendments to the Social Security Act and the health legislation that funded a nationwide attack on heart disease, cancer, and stroke. In an effort to help ease the shortage, HOE was encouraged both to expand its existing programs and to create new types of programs to broaden the scope of occupational roles.

Teachers

Growing along with the number of HOE programs and students being served has been the need for teachers and administrators to staff these vastly expanding efforts. Vocational-technical education has played a prominent role in teacher education, particularly through the establishment of inservice education offerings to assist health professionals–many in transition from health practitioner roles to roles in education–in gaining the necessary competencies for effective teaching.

With the broadening of federal legislation to include HOE, vocational-technical funds, although not earmarked specifically for teacher education in this area, were used within the general intent of the legislation to prepare and upgrade HOE teachers. Such offerings were conducted by four-year colleges and universities both during the academic year and in summer sessions.

Within the past several years, many educational institutions formally engaged in vocational-technical teacher education, and many private colleges as well have modified these types of specific programs to offer credit for previous work experience. Completion of an HOE preparatory program is now applicable toward a baccalaureate degree. Such programs parallel traditional university offerings but recognize previous work and education experience as the major components of a traditional teacher education program. Universities assume responsibility for the liberal arts core requirements for a Bachelor of Arts or Bachelor of Science degree. Such programs are currently identified as inverted degree or two-plus-two programs and provide for a logical and systematic articulation of existing community college and hospital-based programs as the major components of a university degree. [*Editor's Note: Several of the authors completed their Bachelor's degree using this approach.*]

Efforts to provide teacher education for HOE educators have moved from haphazard endeavors to a highly developed and valuable delivery system. This system addresses the basic teaching needs of health workers entering the field of HOE either with or without a baccalaureate degree but also for articulation with the graduate level of preparation. Further, current efforts to introduce and develop competency-based teacher education programs are being pioneered in many instances by universities with active departments of vocational-technical education in which HOE instructional personnel are being prepared.

In the attempt to provide adequate health services to all at a reasonable cost, there have been, and will continue to be, changes in patterns and practices in our health care delivery system. These changes, in turn, are requiring corresponding adjustments in our education system, since it is expected to prepare the needed number of health workers at varying levels of competency.

From kindergarten through high school, more effort must be directed to the development of curricula providing orientation to all types of health careers and to the dissemination of information on roles of health workers and the preparation required for each role. For students who express interest in a health career, secondary schools should provide the opportunity for in-depth exploration of those careers most in keeping with those students' interest, motivation, and abilities. As appropriate, schools should provide high-quality preparatory programs for those not planning to continue their formal education after leaving high school but electing to work in an entry-level health occupation. Such programs necessarily will be limited in number and scope because of existing legal requirements and program approval standards. Another potentially limiting factor, and one deserving careful consideration, is the maturity level of students.

At all levels of post–high school education, opportunities for preparation for a health career should be available not only to recent high school graduates but also to mature men and women, including those seeking a second or third career: former military personnel, members of minority groups, handicapped persons who can complete a preparatory program satisfactorily, persons from central cities and rural areas, those from so-called fringe areas of society, and those who need remedial work to make them eligible for existing programs. Potential students should have the opportunity to make a wise choice from among the various health careers, whether the choice be one requiring initial preparation or one allowing advanced standing in a program by virtue of previously achieved education and/or experience. This calls for knowledgeable guidance personnel and for school admission officers who espouse the concept of career mobility and who, in cooperation with the faculty of the educational programs, will make appropriate and reasonable decisions when considering applicants in the admission process.

To ensure increased opportunities for career mobility, some traditional patterns and relationships must be changed. It is imperative that more progress be made nationwide in providing strong linkages to increase traffic between vocational- and technical-level preparation and between technical- and baccalaureate-level preparation.

Indeed, there are increasing demands nationally for inservice and continuing education programs to upgrade or retrain professionals, technicians, assistants, and aides for careers in the health field. Therefore, these types of educational programs must be offered at all education levels — vocational, technical, baccalaureate, and graduate. More and more, states are requiring that practitioners of health care achieve a prescribed number of continuing education units to qualify for relicensure. Educational institutions must ensure that continuing education is accessible to all health workers who need and want it.

Opportunities for career advancement, based on previous formal preparation and competencies gained in employment, are slowly becoming more available, but the development of curricula especially designed to facilitate progression in the health careers must be accelerated.

For too long there have been barriers limiting the accommodation of many who desire initial preparation for a health career and blocking opportunities for career mobility within the hierarchy of health workers. Too often, organized groups at each rung of the ladder have erected obstacles aimed at fending off encroachment by other workers. Certain barriers are maintained by tradition and by concepts more appropriate to a guild in the Middle Ages than to a modern profession; they have no justification other than to protect the positions of those already ensconced. Upward advancement is hampered when skills, knowledge, and attitudes acquired in pursuit of one occupational goal are not applicable toward a higher goal and when work experience is undervalued. This is extremely discouraging to aspirants, who should be challenged with promise at every entry level.

Curriculum developers must embrace two major concepts that are central to providing expanded career mobility opportunities: accommodation and articulation. Here, accommodation means providing what is needed or desired for an adjustment of differences, making goal-directed movement possible. Both an attitude and a process, it implies generosity and flexibility in the adaptive aspects of planning and implementing. Accommodation is educationally and administratively prerequisite to the development of new curricula for students with diverse backgrounds and indeed to total program development. Operating at various program entry points, it necessitates highly skilled counseling with astute assessment of educational records and career histories followed by a plan of study tailored for each student or group of students. Individualized plans should be developed jointly by student and faculty and should be compatible with the career goal of the student and with the admission and graduation requirements of the educational institution. Provision should be made for the use of evaluative procedures to determine existing competencies. Articulation is the system of links and connections that provides a network mechanism for vertical and horizontal movement in and through the various territories of the education system.

To further foster the ladder and lattice concepts, educators must promote and provide for increased traffic among the several educational systems: general, vocational-technical, and professional. When accommodation fosters articulation, it can be expected that such traffic will indeed increase and lead to true career education.

It is imperative that all health careers educators accept two basic principles: (1) the educational system that prepares health care personnel must respond to the real needs of our health care delivery system in terms of both the number of workers needed and the functions they are expected to perform, and (2) within this educational system, there must be appropriate and effective correlation among and between these various levels of preparation. Just as the health care system must provide comprehensive health care, the educational system must provide comprehensive programs in health career education. Following are five guiding statements toward this end.

1. Occupational choice and career development constitute a continuous activity; each person starts an individual pattern in the early years.

2. The public school has the major role in enhancing each individual's occupational opportunities as a part of one's development in becoming a productive and contributing member of society.

3. To maintain occupational options, each individual not only must be aware of vocational opportunities but also must be able to obtain preparation for entering the occupation.
4. Participation in educational activities has become a life-long activity; programs for preparation, upgrading, retraining, and maintenance of competencies are required at all performance levels.
5. Comprehensive programs in health occupations education require continuous interrelationships among all levels of education, health specialties and services, and health agencies and associations.

In the past decade there has been a substantial shift in administrative responsibility for health careers education — from health service agencies to public educational institutions. This shift embraces the philosophy that the cost of educating health workers should be charged to the public tax base rather than to patients. It requires new alliances between the agencies and institutions; their collaboration and collective resources are essential to the success of preparatory, continuing, and inservice education programs that are endeavoring to prepare the number and types of health workers needed.

Citizen-consumer participation is particularly appropriate to the concept of a public-professional partnership in matters related to health care. Increasingly, and rightfully, users of health services are seeking not only involvement in the formation of broad public policies pertaining to the quality and availability of health care but also more direct and active participation with providers in health care settings. The laity should be encouraged and given the opportunity to become involved in the planning and evaluation of health careers programs. Indeed, a program and its purpose and objectives should be developed and maintained within the context of the community and known by the public it serves.

Greater efforts must be expended to build an adequate corps of qualified and effective instructional personnel for health careers education. Too few universities have undertaken programs to enable health practitioners to become accomplished teachers in the health field. And supervisors, consultants, and administrators for health careers education are also in short supply. Educational opportunities and planned experiences to increase skills for these positions must receive greater attention.

In general, the current structure of accreditation of specialized fields of study is geared to an anachronistic perception of accreditation as a private activity, accountable only to the professional organizations by which it is sponsored, conducted, and controlled. Particularly in health careers programs, insufficient responsibility in the expansion of accreditation has resulted in the duplication of accrediting agencies in the same health field. Because of this duplication and the inherent fragmentation, both the efficiency and the efficacy of the accreditation process have been hampered. There is little evidence to suggest that positive steps are being taken to improve this situation. Where is the needed action?

Credentialing is one of the stickiest wickets in the health field. The present system of licensing health care personnel is being questioned, and some feel that it risks breakdown if faced with public confrontation. Effective changes in credentialing practices are slow in coming about, primarily because of vested interest resistance. Much discussion has been devoted to the certification, registration, and licensure of health care personnel. Can our current practices be validated, or even justified? Many believe they cannot. Is the licensure process truly protecting the consuming public by ensuring minimum safe-practice standards? Many doubt it. Too long we have assumed that safe practice and high-quality care result from completion of a program and passage of an examination that tests ability to memorize and recall information. Greater effort must be devoted to conducting research to determine the specific competencies needed for safe practice in a given health career.

Any and all efforts to meet the health care needs of our society today require creative and innovative leadership. The ideas and plans of those in the vanguard of new movements may be challenged by those more comfortable with the status quo. Leaders must be alert to, and knowledgeable about, the issues and be actively and forthrightly involved in the planning and execution of actions to resolve them. These actions must be devoid of two devastating maladies: the illogical love of the old and the illogical fear of the new. These diseases manifest themselves by procrastination — the art of keeping up with yesterday — and must be eradicated.

The challenges, while staggering, are surmountable with the concerted action of leaders representing all levels of health care providers and health care educators, along with the support of their respective associations, health facilities, educational institutions, and voluntary agencies, in addition to organized labor, government, and industry.

No longer can any single one of these groups plan unilaterally; all must work in concert lest separate courses of action build new rigidities into a system that is already in desperate need of more flexibility. It is imperative that there be open and continual communication within and between them, for only through their sustained cooperation and collaboration will it be possible for existing barriers to be lowered, conflicting opinions to be resolved, and plans for the future to be formulated and then carried out wisely.

☞ DESCRIBING HOE AS A DIVISION OF AVA

The American Vocational Association and Its Relation to a Teacher

"Are you a professional?" As a clinician making the transition to becoming a teacher, you are likely to reflect on your clinician's background first. Most likely your response is a resounding "Yes, of course I am!" As an educator now, you desire to be known as a professional in this environment as well.

When we ponder the notion of being a professional or professionalism, various philosophies surface. By and large your belief system and values emerge. Professionalism is demonstrated, however, through acts that endorse high standards and the application of moral and ethical behaviors.

As a clinician, you believe that patients have the right to high-quality care. As an educator, you believe that students have the right to the best education you and the system can provide. Being the best at anything requires dedication, determination, and daring. Of course, these traits result from hard work. Preparing and executing lessons that reflect the most current practices or state-of-the-art technology are no easy task. They especially demand of educators the need to stay abreast of the latest trends in both education and the health field. How does a professional do this? One of the most effective ways is being actively involved in a professional organization that best serves your interests and needs.

Searching for an Appropriate Professional Organization

A good deal of research is being conducted today to determine what it is that current members and potential members desire in a professional organization. Consumers are more careful in their selections and wish to invest their money in a single organization, if possible, to serve their specific needs and interests.

David R. Bywaters, author of *Total Marketing: An Approach for the Future*, discovered in his surveys that potential members are not initially concerned with a wide array of services unless those services focus on their specific needs. According to survey results, the following areas were of most importance.

1. Access to continuing education that includes supportive and useful materials.
2. Access to specific solutions to specific problems.
3. Legislative influences that affect change and improve individual environments (e.g., salary, resources to do a better job, career mobility).

4. Availability of literature that reflects the latest and projected trends as well as how-to information, such as books, journals, and periodicals.

The ASAE Foundation conducted a think tank conference and determined that if professional organizations were to continue as a strong force in the future, they would need the following characteristics.

1. Be proactive not reactive.
2. Be led by a vision and visionaries.
3. Reflect diversity of membership.
4. Demand a high level of accountability.
5. Have a board of directors concerned with future actions rather than evaluative of past actions.

What do you consider important when selecting a professional organization? Do you compare your specific needs and interests to the services that any organization can provide? Are you easily influenced to select an organization because your school, department, or supervisor tells you to?

These are serious questions that require your attention. Another, more obvious question is "What can any organization offer me personally and professionally now that I am a health occupations educator?"

Making the Right Choice

The above final question ultimately places you, like others who used to be practicing clinicians, now educators, in a quandary. As a dental hygienist, respiratory therapist, or nurse, you probably feel that membership in your career-related professional organization is a must. Even while you were experiencing postsecondary/collegiate preparation, no doubt you were a member of a student organization that reflected your career goal. It was the expected thing to do.

Now, however, being a health occupations educator removes you from being a practicing clinician. You are an educator of a vocational education program. You need to associate with educators or teachers with similar functions, learn as much as you can about the latest teaching methods, and become involved to effect change. What kind of professional organization best serves these needs and interests now? Do you give up your affiliation with your career-specific organization to join some educationally related one? Obviously the choice is yours to make. And perhaps, given your current responsibilities, you do need to affiliate with both kinds. But just as there are numerous health-related professional organizations from which to choose, there are also many educational ones. How do you make the right choice and spend your money wisely?

The American Vocational Association: Purpose and Structure

Important to making the right choice about a professional educational organization is the recognition of what kind of educator/teacher you are now. Regardless of the program in which you are currently teaching, you are considered a health occupations educator. This needs to be stressed.

Health occupations education (HOE) is funded primarily with vocational education monies, including your salary, equipment and supplies, and instructional materials. This places you in the generic category of vocational educator. Consequently, the search for and the selection of an appropriate organization should be based on its ability to serve your needs and interests as a vocational educator and more specifically as a health occupations educator.

The American Vocational Association (AVA) is a professional organization of and for vocational educators. It is a national organization with state-chartered associations, headquartered in Alexandria, Virginia, in its own building, and led by an executive director and staff. An elected AVA Board of Directors, composed of a president, president-elect, and vice presidents from all vocational programs (including HOE) govern the association.

The mission of AVA is to provide educational leadership in developing a competitive work force. Its purposes are to provide:

1. Professional development that encourages career development, professional involvement, and leadership among members
2. Program improvement that fosters excellence in vocational-technical education
3. Policy development that advocates national public policy to benefit vocational-technical education
4. Marketing that keeps both the public and private sectors informed about vocational-technical education.

The above mission and purposes are implemented through annual plans of work by the membership. You might still be asking at this point, "How does AVA relate to a health occupations teacher?" This is an excellent question! Of course you desire associating with others more allied to your responsibilities, and AVA recognizes this.

Although AVA collectively represents all vocational educators, its structure includes subdivisions. One of these is the AVA-HOE Division. This is the one for you.

The division has a governing body composed of elected leaders from three groups: teachers, administrators, and teacher educators. It is called the AVA-HOE Division Policy Board. Chaired by a division president/chairperson and other officers, it is their function to address the business issues that concern the organization and its membership. Operating policies founded upon the AVA's constitution and bylaws strictly identify the means by which member representation is elected and represented and business is conducted. These policies safeguard against special interest groups' controlling the division. The president serves as vice president on the AVA Board of Directors. This ensures communication linkages with divisions.

The AVA-HOE Division also has associated organizations. One is the National Association of Health Occupations Teachers (NAHOT). This is another way to strengthen communication and networking with individuals more allied to your area of responsibility.

The AVA-HOE Division is guided by an annual Management Action Plan (MAP). It is an extension of the annual AVA Program of Work but is designed to address those goals and objectives related to the special needs and interests of health occupations educators.

The AVA, its divisions, and its associated organizations are productive primarily through committees. Committee structure is duplicated at each level of the association, with chairpersons serving on division and AVA committees. Again, this ensures continuity of communication within the association and among its members.

Specific Benefits

Organizational structure is inherent in any professional association. It is its major source of communicating, especially with a diverse membership. It also serves to accomplish goals, resolve critical issues, and influence legislation in a collective, unified manner. Every member has the right to communicate concerns directly to AVA, to his or her respective division, to his or her affiliated organization's leadership, and through the state- or regional- level leadership.

So you have a professional association, but if you are not one of its leaders or committee members, are there any other benefits you can realize? Good question! The answer is yes. Included with your membership are such things as the monthly *Vocational Education Journal,* filled with articles that keep you abreast of the latest happenings in vocational education and exemplary programs. In addition, you receive four issues per year of the *AVA-HOE Division Newsletter.* At additional but reasonable costs are other benefits: group insurance plans, including malpractice insurance for you while supervising students in clinical areas; member loans; numerous books, research papers, newsletters, video and audio tapes, marketing supplies that assist in student recruitment, and association paraphernalia; attendance at conventions, conferences, and seminars; leadership development; and personal and professional development opportunities.

Major benefits to all vocational educators, however, rest primarily on the association's legislative impact. The AVA holds its own when lobbying for its members in Washington. It is the only professional organization that aggressively seeks to influence the creation of laws and policies that provide you with resources to do your job, a critical consideration when selecting a professional organization.

Make a Difference

Given the above information, it is hoped that you will strengthen your professionalism by affiliating with the organization that is committed to your needs and interests as a vocational educator and more specifically a health occupations educator. More important is your active involvement in AVA at the state, region, and national levels. This is one way you can make a difference! The first step is to contact your state's organizational leadership and especially your HOE Division president. Talk with this individual, gather information, and request a membership application form. If you are unable to do this, then write or make a toll-free call to AVA headquarters. You owe it to yourself and to your students to be the best professional you can be, which includes being an active member in your professional education organization: the American Vocational Association, Health Occupations Education Division.

Call or write to: Membership Department, American Vocational Association, 1410 King Street, Alexandria, VA 22314; 703-683-3111 or 800-826-9972 (outside the Alexandria area).

Professionalism is demonstrated through the practice of high standards and moral and ethical beliefs. Making and continuing a successful transition from clinician to teacher includes active involvement in a professional organization designed to meet your specific needs and interests.

Research indicates that consumers of professional organization memberships seek first the services and benefits most suited to their individual needs and second, those that benefit others. Surveys have shown that potential members and current members desire a professional organization that is proactive, not reactive; has visionary leadership; is involved in legislation and public policy; offers specific answers to specific problems; affords personal and professional development; and provides group rates for insurance programs.

Health occupations educators are inclined to exhibit strong allegiance to their career-specific professional organizations first. Many do not consider themselves vocational educators, but, for example, dental hygienist instructor, practical nursing instructor, or medical office assistant instructor.

It must be made clear that transition from clinician to health occupations teacher in a high school, community college, technical college, or university has created not only a career move but also a change in title. You have become a significant part of vocational education as a vocational educator. It behooves you to investigate carefully your relationship to and support of an appropriate professional association.

HOE programs are funded primarily through vocational education legislation. This legislation includes funding for health occupations instructor/teacher positions/salaries, facilities, instructional materials, and laboratory equipment. The AVA is one organization that places lobbying for such legislation as a priority on its agenda. Its past record is indicative of its success.

In this day of costly memberships in any professional organization and the limitations on anyone's investments, making the right choices is difficult and sometimes confusing. Your relationship to the AVA and especially the HOE Division constitutes an initial commitment to serve you. By affording you personal and professional opportunities and your active involvement, this organization can contribute to strengthening you as a professional. This strength should make a difference with your program, with your students, and with the quality of care that future health care workers will provide for consumers.

References

AVA. *American Vocational Association* (Constitution, Bylaws, Program of Work, Organization Chart). Alexandria, VA: author.

AVA (1991). AVA-HOE Division Management Action Plan. Alexandria, VA: author.

Bywaters, D. R. (November 1985). "Total Marketing: An Approach for the Future." *A&SM*.

Flanders, R. (August 1970). "Employment Patterns for the Seventies." *Compact*, p. 7.

Greenfield, H. I., and C. A. Brown (1969). *Allied Health Manpower: Trends and Prospects*. New York: Columbia University Press.

Myers, E. M. (March 1990). "Future Vision." *Association Management.*

U.S. Department of Health, Education and Welfare, Public Health Service (1970). *Health Manpower Source Book, Section 21, Allied Health Manpower, 1950–80*. PHS Publication No. 263. Washington: U. S. Government Printing Office.

U.S. Department of Labor (1990). *Occupational Outlook Handbook 1990–91*. Publication No. 2350. Washington: U. S. Government Printing Office.

Webster's New World Dictionary (2nd ed.) (1980) Cleveland, OH: William Collins and World.

16

Perspectives of VHO Professionals: From the School to the Federal Level

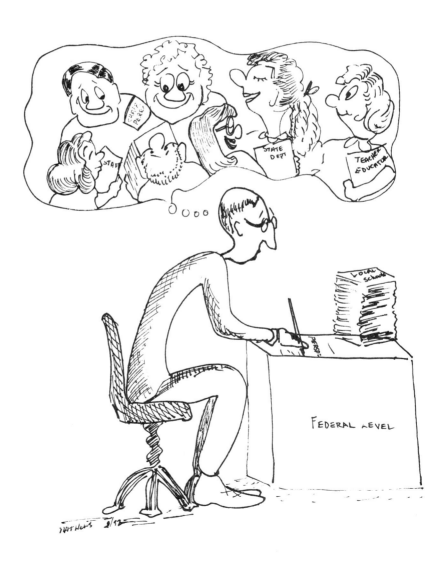

Each student chooses an individual path through the education maze (Figure 16-1). In order to properly prepare and inform your students about career choices you must be familiar with the educational model for VHOs at the community, state, and federal level (Figure 16-1). This chapter will assist you in understanding these organizational structures and how you "fit."

☞ MIDDLE SCHOOL TEACHER

How does one explain the nature of working with middle schoolers? The "M" word has been known to send shivers down the spines of the strongest educators! Puberty, hormones, experimentation, power struggles, challenging, crying, brooding, loving . . . The list could go on and on and on. The single descriptive word this author can use to explain the middle school animal is dynamic. Middle schoolers experience daily changes and mood swings that surprise and intrigue adults, many of whom no longer remember those experiences.

These students take "orientation" and "exploration" career classes in various vocational fields for varying time periods according to the educational model adopted by their school. The teacher of middle schoolers and the youngsters themselves have to be very flexible to fit into the constantly changing plans sweeping through the educational community. A school system may have only one educational concept for class divisions, and the next county or city over might have multiple concepts. Some schools (or districts) follow the K–5, 6–8, 9–12 model; others use K–6, 7–9, 10–12 (often referred

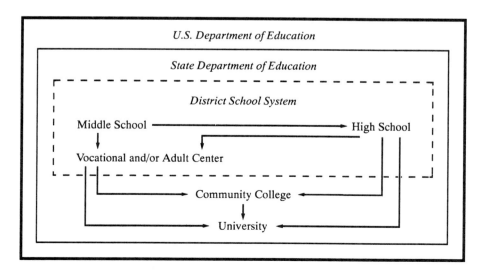

FIGURE 16-1

to as the junior high systems), or K–8, 9–12, or K–7, 8, 9–12, or K–12, or . . . The reason behind a community's selecting a particular program may be to alleviate overcrowding in a small community school, to cut back on instructional help, or to separate emotionally and physically diverse students: prepubertal students, pubescent students, and older teenagers.

Orientation

The orientation program you will teach may run from two weeks to nine weeks in length. Remember — orientation is meant to do just that, to orient students to the wonderful careers available to them in the world of health care. The old story about the snake oil salesman is pertinent to orientation classes: The traveling vendor made his first monthly stop at a small country store in the dead of winter. Only one elderly man was sitting in the rocking chairs on the front porch. To prove his worth, the salesman gave his very best spiel, extolling the virtues of the ointment and condemning the use of medical doctors. At the completion of the show, he shook the farmer's hand and asked, "Were you moved by the speech?" The farmer squinted his eyes and shrugged his shoulders saying, "When I go out to feed the cows and only a couple show up, I'll be darned if I'm gonna empty the whole truckload of hay for them two scrawny thangs."

New vocational instructors tend to want to share everything they know about their wonderful field with every child who enters their class. Don't overwhelm orientation students; just whet their appetite to enroll in your exploratory program (Figure 16-2). Use videos, computer programs, guest practitioners (preferably parents), career games, and other exciting, enticing ideas to tease students into investigating health fields further. Middle school students are curious and very interested in real-life applications for what they are learning. Use anecdotal stories from your life to intrigue them. Be real with them. They will question your ability to teach a subject if you don't have some real-life applications to tell them about.

One Middle School Vocational Model

Orientation class:	Grade 6 — three weeks in every vocational- and academic-based enrichment course, two at a time.
Exploration class:	Grade 7 — twelve-week classes in six of the previously studied orientation programs, usually not of the student's choice.
	Grade 8 — eighteen-week-long (one semester) courses in four subject areas consisting of two personally chosen electives and two forced electives (team electives).

FIGURE 16-2

Exploration

Exploratory programs are generally lengthier than orientation programs. An exploratory course may be from twelve to eighteen weeks in length. The purpose of the program is for students to explore or delve into the experiences of careers available to them. Remember that these student are in the building, concrete operations stage of their life (refer back to chapter 5 on adolescents and Piaget's work). Let them take temperatures, fill out charts, make hospital beds, take blood pressures, perform emergency room interviews, and triage a simulated bus, train, or plane wreck.

A middle school in Orange County, Florida, suffered the tragedy of a school bus that got pushed off an overpass above Interstate 4. Two marvelous things saved the lives of many of this author's former students. One, was that a group of medical professionals who had been meeting on International Drive, a block away, were just adjourning, and this myriad of doctors and other medical professionals spontaneously stopped and anonymously rescued the trapped and injured youngsters from the wreckage, immediately administering first aid. (If you were involved, thank you for helping "my children.") Second, a group of high school students had two weeks before besieged a local hospital after being "rescued" by paramedics from a simulated bus wreck. Thanks to the help of concerned teachers and interested students who had used this hands-on approach, local medical personnel had just recently trained in triage medicine.

Utilize the vocational student organization in your district or state to augment your instruction. Making the organization's chapter an integral unit of your instruction gives middle school students a goal to aim for in grade levels and makes learning a thrilling democratic experience. They can relate better to peers sometimes, instead of always having to listen to adults.

Resources

You have many human resources available to you in your teaching. Former colleagues in health care, students' parents in the field, advisory committee practitioners, other vocational instructors at your school, health teachers from other schools, students who have moved on to higher levels of health care instruction, and vocational student organization advisers and members represent some of the people you can call on to help you develop and maintain an effective and efficient program.

You don't have to buy all the tongue depressors, alcohol, ace bandages, or stethoscopes you need. Local practitioners, advisory committee members, and retail or wholesale dealers are usually more than thrilled to be asked to donate used or new equipment and supplies to teach prospective consumers and employees. Ask and ye shall be given, but be sure to applaud and thank your benefactors, publicly and privately.

The first couple of years of teaching in the system may be frustrating. You want to know every student and help them all. "But, I have them only two weeks," you say. If you do the best job you can in those two weeks, you will awaken their interest either in valuing health care workers in their world or in becoming a health occupations professional.

You may also be the only one in your field at your school. Other vocational teachers there have similar programs but with a different focus. The ten-year business education teacher can help you understand the chain of command at your school. The agriculture instructor can guide you through the purchase order process or explain the tenure process to you. Ask the technology teacher to show you how the "wheel" of orientation classes rotates, when your grades have to be ready for the next teacher, and what you are to do with hall passes and attendance records. You all have the same goal: to offer all of the students at your school a peek into the window of knowledge that each has available. You may guard the window well and keep them from gazing into it, or you may open the curtains and let them experience the warmth of the rays shining through it.

Wheels, quarters, semester finals, changing classes, lockers or no lockers, teachers as advisers, peer counselors, changing clothing for physical education, athletic competitions, and student organizations clutter the minds of teachers and students alike. Use your resources, human and material, accept the students for what they are at the moment, use your instincts to explore the vast realms of health occupations, and rely on your students to educate and inform you about the field you love!

☞ HIGH SCHOOL TEACHER

High school students are expected to make career decisions and take appropriate prerequisite courses. However, this is in contrast to the American tendency to prolong adolescence. As a result, it is not surprising that many are not sure about a specific career. A study by Ebrite (1986) of 6,640 tenth and eleventh graders in a Midwestern state revealed that 22 percent of the students were interested in a health career. Of the 5,204 students not interested in a health career, 39 percent (2,030) had not decided on a career, 1,509 said they did not know about health careers, and 623 responded that their family did not want them to have a health career. A family's desire for the student affected 46 percent of the students' decisions.

The VHO teacher can utilize the characteristics of this age group to develop effective classroom activities. The get-acquainted activities that get a class off to a good start include ones that help students get to know each other personally. Students create personal collages illustrating their life and then present the collages before the class or hang them up and let the others in the group match students with their collage. Personal bingo is another way to assist students in getting to know each other. The bingo spaces are filled with names of hobbies, and class members sign their name in the space of the hobby they participate in. Students may describe themselves in a speech as if they were describing what they look like to a stranger who will be meeting them at the airport. Pair students up and give them one minute to look at each other. Then have them turn back-to-back and describe each other. Two important get-to-know-you activities are having students search out and write down their long-term and short-term goals and assisting them in finding out who they are and their own attributes. The goals are periodically evaluated to assist students in staying on track.

Peer pressure and the need for group acceptance indicate a need for frequent small-group activities such as planning, minilectures within a small group or that are presented to the entire class, and designing bulletin boards. It may be productive to rotate group members during various group activities. This allows every member in the class to work directly with every student in the class, and the rotations assist them in getting ready for the real world of work in which they have to associate with a variety of people.

To help students formulate appropriate VHO values, frequent discussion is critical. They must hear themselves think aloud and respond to others in order to clearly define their own values. Scenarios where students are asked to make choices can be used. Examples are ethical and legal situations or decisions that may occur in a medical facility, including the situation of drug abuse by a coworker, inappropriate patient care, sexual harassment, emergency assistance, and euthanasia. The instructor must maintain neutral ground as the facilitator of such discussions. Students may see others' point of view, helping them realize that there are other ways of looking at the situation. They also take a look at their own feelings about issues they may not have thought about.

To assist students in developing abstract thinking, the classroom activities can include planning the care of a fictitious patient. Students are asked to plan the care from admission and physical examination to discharge, including surgery if they see fit. This activity allows them to see consequences to actions and assists in developing critical thinking skills.

Developing a HOSA chapter gives students the opportunity to compete in a positive manner that is reflected in defeat as well as in winning. Students must believe your expectations are high and that disappointment only comes with lack of trying, not with defeat. Assist them in realizing the positive aspects of the competition and cooperation, such as gaining new skills, meeting other students with similar goals, and, most of all, personal growth.

ADULT VOCATIONAL CENTER TEACHER

Teaching a VHO program is by all standards a very rewarding career. Teaching a VHO course in a vocational-technical (vo-tech) center is a multi faceted job. The vo-tech center provides an opportunity for all types and levels of education, and it offers almost anyone the means to acquire the knowledge and skills needed to obtain employment in a health career field. Teaching health occupations in a vo-tech center presents many challenging and unique situations (never any problems, just new and unique challenges).

VHO programs offered in vo-tech centers range from single- instructor to multiinstructor programs. And all of them require that instructors be organizers of time, people, equipment, supplies, and budgets.

Student Placement into a VHO Program

At the beginning of each new term, the first obligation of a VHO instructor is to assume the role of placement counselor. As professionals in a specific area, we are called upon to assist the official student counselor in the proper placement of applicants to our program and ensure that state and national requirements are met prior to students' enrollment in the program. The instructors also assist the counseling personnel in providing information about the VHO programs offered at the center. This assists the counselors in guiding students into programs in which they will be the most successful. Counselors do rely on instructors to help in the placement of prospective students into the VHO programs.

Program Preparation

OKAY! Now that we have our students identified and enrolled, it is now time to change roles again — now we are purchasing agents. The teacher in a vo-tech center is responsible for ordering the supplies and equipment that are needed to make the VHO program operate, in effect, assume the output and production standards of the specific occupation being taught. Vo-tech instructors have to request and receive bids on supplies and equipment, select the specific type and style of equipment that the health care industry is currently using, and attempt to duplicate or simulate industrial settings for students.

Public Relations

Here we go again. (And class hasn't even started yet!) Now we take on the role of the public relations officer. A very important aspect of the VHO program is its advisory committee. Without an active and functional advisory committee, it would be almost impossible to have an up-to-date, vital VHO program. The instructor has to visit professionals related to the program not only to seek advice and input but also to promote the VHO program. After many visits, phone calls, and letters, it becomes the responsibility of the VHO instructor(s) to select the advisory committee members who will benefit not only the program itself but also the students and instructors individually. The selection and composition of an advisory committee constitute an ongoing concern that the VHO instructor should never stop considering. The instructor should continue making contacts and promoting the benefits of vocational training long after the original committee is organized.

Student Diversity

Vocational teachers have a wide variety of students in terms of socioeconomic level, ethnicity, age, gender, and other characteristics. Some programs comprise only secondary students, and some only postsecondary students. Then there are the programs that combine both secondary and postsecondary students in one classroom. Secondary students may be in the classroom for only part of the day, and postsecondary students all day or all evening.

Curriculum Development

Let's not stop yet! Another role that many vo-tech health occupations educators assume is that of curriculum development specialist. The curriculum needs revision regularly to teach the required competencies. The educational level of the vo-tech student must also be taken into consideration for the type of curriculum selected. Areas of study may need to be simplified to be understood, using relevant terminology so that students reach the required level of competency. Remember this: we are educating students to work with and assist personnel in highly technical fields.

Job Placement

Now let's change roles again and become job placement specialists. One of the first areas a student needs to know about in order to be employable is proper work ethics. The VHO teacher will most often assume the role of the employer in order to establish characteristics that all health care employers expect to see in their workers. Vo-tech teachers should be willing to accept the job placement specialist role during visits to all places where potential positions for students exist, because this oftentimes results in trying to match a student with a particular job or a particular type of employer with a particular type of student. Above all, vo-tech teachers must help students find employment with employers that offer the best possible chance for a long-term, successful career.

Let's look back: organizer, placement counselor, purchasing agent, public relations coordinator, general counselor, curriculum development specialist, and job placement specialist. These are some of the major roles of an instructor in a vo-tech center health occupations program, besides being a teacher and a health care professional. This multirole requirement may present a very large challenge, but not one that a concerned and professional educator cannot meet. Most of the roles switches will be automatic and never even noticed; some may require diligent effort to perform. In conjunction with the task of full-time instructor, the VHO educator at a vocational technical center must be willing to accept any role that will benefit students and improve the quality of health occupations education.

COMMUNITY COLLEGE INSTRUCTOR

In recent decades, this country has seen much change in society, industry, and, ultimately, education. Although traditional educational structures may remain, the traditional student does not. Whether the reasons for this movement away from successive high-school-to-college progress be financial, geographic, or lack of motivation or desire for higher education, the change in student population is a reality for the educator in the nineties. The community college setting offers today's student alternatives through technical certificate, career training, and Associate of Science degree programs. More specifically, the health care industry continues to require education and training beyond the high school level for entry into health occupations. Because health professionals expect competent employees, it is our goal as VHO instructors to meet these demands through high quality education. The responsibilities and tasks of the community college instructor include, but are not limited to, these categories: knowledge and responsibilities to the institution; responsibilities to students during didactic, laboratory, and clinical sessions; and responsibilities within the community itself.

To begin with, in order to meet these responsibilities, the educator must understand the community college system. One example is a system operated by the rules established by a state, its division of community colleges of the department of education, and the board of trustees of the college. The chief administrative officer is president of the college and provides educational leadership and administrative direction for all the academic and business activities of the college and serves as the official agent of communications to the college for its board of trustees. Instructors need to know their supervisor and their responsibilities. In order to work effectively in this type of system, instructors must follow a chain of command. An example of this is: instructor, department chairperson, assistant dean of Vocational Health Occupations, vice president of Applied Sciences and Technology, and president. However, understanding the chain of command is not enough. It is important to learn more about the entire administrative structure. Open communication with direct administrators regarding a particular program is essential. A successful program is one that has the support of administration.

Second, faculty in community colleges are expected to serve on one or more college committees. Such committees are called, Academic Review, Admissions, Appeals, Associate Degree Program Review, Awards, College Safety, Curriculum, and the like. Because community colleges encourage all students to participate in campus organizations and in vocational student organizations such as HOSA, educators are also expected to participate in activities through chaperoning student functions or serving as a sponsor or an adviser.

Third, faculty members are expected to be active in one or more professional organizations or associations related to their field of specialization. Being a member of a local, state, and national organization affords the opportunity to remain current in the ever-changing health care field. Another area of involvement is through membership in a statewide educators' association, such as Health Occupations Educators Association of (your state). These associations allow educators to meet and share information with others in their field. The information may include political issues concerning a program, innovative teaching techniques, program leveling, tech-prep, accreditation standards, articulation, and textbook evaluations. If an educators' association is not currently in existence in your state, it will prove beneficial for program educators throughout the state to form one. Beyond participation in these types of organizations it is important for an educator to be involved on the state level in such areas as state articulation in vocational programs, core leveling committees, and any other committee that may affect a program.

Last in this category, educators are responsible for budget preparation. Because VHO programs are some of the most expensive programs operating in community colleges, it is imperative the instructor manage the budget effectively. This includes a method to inventory the yearly budgets in existence in order to prepare budgets for the next academic year. Institutional discounts, bulk ordering, and sharing program expenses with support facilities such as hospital are issues necessary to understand as a budget manager. Usually budgets are prepared by the department chairperson in conjunction with support faculty. Once prepared, a budget is sent to the appropriate dean for review at a college budget hearing. The educator may be called upon to attend this meeting if products or equipment requests are not clear. In addition to budget preparation and requisitioning for educational supplies/equipment, the program instructor may become involved in grant writing. The appropriate dean at a community college has information pertaining to health occupations grants. These are a few examples of the types of responsibilities a community college instructor has within the institution.

Most important to any educator, in any area of education, are the responsibilities toward students. This area of responsibility begins even before the student reaches the classroom — through the instructor's involvement in the recruitment process. The program instructor must gain community participation in this process by utilizing individuals or institutions who employ program graduates or completers through devoting time or money to recruitment. Area high schools must be willing to allow instructors into their classrooms to inform students of existing programs. The instructor should be a member of the college's speaker bureau in order to gain access to local civic groups. The Program Advisory Committee can play an active role in recruitment by offering innovative ideas on the subject, as well as personally participating in the process. The result of successful recruitment activities will be a pool of high-quality applicants. Students cannot apply to a program if they are not aware of its existence.

It is important to mention that selective admissions into VHO programs are essential to continued program success. The instructor is responsible for reviewing all potential student applications, interviewing candidates, and selecting a class. It is important to evaluate admissions requirements on a regular basis to ensure they coincide with the students' success in the program. In addition, it is essential for the potential student to be granted an interview. This is beneficial for both the instructor and applicant so that pertinent information can be discussed and any questions answered. Topics covered in the interview may include class schedules, program costs, financial aid and scholarships available, work experience, anticipated salary, job placement, evaluation of entrance examination, and the student's involvement in the college or the community during the program.

Of utmost importance to educators are the responsibilities in the area of instruction, which include, but are not limited to, course outlines, course objectives, course requirements, topic outlines, student schedules, the grading scale, attendance policies, and objective evaluation mechanisms. Also, both instructors and students benefit from knowing and utilizing library resources, such as reference books, journals, periodicals, and information that is accessed through computers, if available. Inform students of these. The instructor must prepare in advance lecture material, audiovisual aids, tests, the grading format, and the selection of clinical facilities and continually document student performance. The educator responsible for off-campus facilities must provide adjunct faculty goals and objectives as well as evaluation techniques. An adjunct faculty program handbook can expedite explanation of such policies and can include all the information contained in the student handbook.

The educator should provide students with a comprehensive student handbook upon entering the program. The handbook should include information on the following: protocol for infection control, needle stick, handling/

disposal of hazardous waste, proper technique for handling emergency situations, and any other program policies that students should receive in writing.

Counseling represents another responsibility that educators must perform. Meet with students when they are having a problem with a particular course/material, or address their behavior problems or nonconformity to a program policy, such as the dress code, as required. Also, plan counseling sessions with students at midterm and prior to semester's or quarter's end, even if no problems exist. This allows the instructor an opportunity to offer praise for excellent work/performance and to discuss the student's progress in the program. If a problem exists, early detection and problem alleviation are imperative for student retention. Aside from teaching responsibilities, plan activities for students and families to come together at the college with their instructors. Plan a Relative Night, when students can invite family members to meet their instructors and see the facilities in which they are learning. These supportive family members, whether they are parents, spouses, children, or friends, are essential to students' success in a program (support may be financial aid or encouragement along the way). A Relative Night allows the supporters to see what a student is doing.

To reiterate, much time and preparation are required for classroom as well as clinical and laboratory instruction. Lecture, testing, and evaluation of students' clinical experience represent only parts of the VHO instructor's responsibilities.

Program review is essential once students complete a program. A thorough, yet comprehensive review process in addition to information from past students, employers, and licensing or certification results is important.

One final area in which the community college instructor has responsibility is in the community itself. To begin with, the educator must periodically offer continuing education courses to past students and other professionals in the field of expertise. Surveys are an excellent method for evaluation of courses to be offered. Other instructors besides you may be enlisted to teach such supplemental vocational courses.

Finally, serve on community committees, or join civic organizations and give back to the community that supports your community college and your program. Without community support there will be no programs!

In closing, the role of the VHO instructor in a community college setting is multifaceted. Involvement in these types of programs requires time and dedication in the preparation and instruction of students. However, there is no greater reward than a student's successful completion of a program preparing for a career in a health care profession. Education is a challenge — for both the student and the instructor. As change continues in society and industry, so will change continue in our educational system. The community college plays a vital role in meeting the needs of students today. Through innovative programs such as the vocational programs already in existence and those to be developed in the future we will continue to meet the educational needs of the students of tomorrow.

☞ DEPARTMENT CHAIRPERSON

An administrator of VHO programs can assume numerous roles such as department chairperson, classroom faculty member, and clinical instructor. The size of the department along with its prevailing organizational structure determines whether the department chairperson is primarily an administrator or serves in the dual capacity of faculty member and administrator. By the very nature of a school, meaning, its purpose of serving the local community, the organizational structure will be related to the goals. Regardless of the assigned role(s), one of the key responsibilities of a department chair is communication, not only with you as a faculty member but also with the various levels of administrators. It is hoped, your chairperson will establish an open-door policy whereby you can drop in and discuss concerns. Moreover, a similar open-door policy should be offered by you as well. You need to feel comfortable if your chairperson drops by your office for informal discussions. This should not be viewed as an invasion of your privacy, but rather as an opportunity to develop a more collegial relationship with your "boss."

An additional responsibility you have is to periodically keep your chairperson up-to-date regarding how your classes or clinical labs are progressing. Remember that whatever occurs in your classroom, laboratory, or clinical agency, you are accountable to your chairperson, who must be informed about such issues as minimally performing students and problems with affiliate clinical agencies. Regardless of the problems, don't forget to share your shining star days as well. You are the chairperson's eyes and ears in the classroom and community. Your chairperson loves to hear about your successes!

Another important aspect of the department chairperson's job consists of the recruitment, hiring, and orientation of new faculty. As a new faculty member, you should expect an adequate orientation to your job. Your department chair should explain the mission of the school, the policies and procedures of the department, the curriculum, and your role in the assigned program within both the classroom and the clinical laboratory. Further discussion should include the evaluation and promotion or tenure system, as applicable. Each school has its own system to focus on your performance as a teacher and your involvement within the school and community. One of the measures of your success is the type of student and community feedback regarding their satisfaction as consumers of your course and program.

In addition, you should expect a thorough orientation to the affiliate clinical agencies. Ideally, you should be able to spend at least a week either working or observing in the areas where you will be supervising students. Nothing is more frustrating than being in an unfamiliar clinical setting with a group of students looking to you for instruction and supervision.

Another important issue is whether you are required to join the local bargaining unit that may exist within the school. It is common for such bargaining units to be affiliated with a national association. If you are employed in a unionized school, you will need to understand your faculty rights as well as those of your chairperson.

Your chair should review the expected level of participation on school and department committees. Because committees have a long-standing political and power structure, you may want to avoid the power games. Once you feel comfortable with your teaching role, seek membership on the committee(s) that interest you. Sometimes committee involvement is part of the promotion or tenure system. Moreover, as a word of caution, don't overvolunteer. Your first responsibility is to your students; when you spread yourself too thin, everything will suffer, including you.

A health occupations department that has a large faculty may be able to assign you a senior faculty member as your mentor. Don't hesitate to ask for assistance, especially when you are a novice to teaching. Team teaching can assist you in learning how to discuss a subject, develop lesson plans and test questions, advise students, and evaluate students in a clinical setting. Locate your institution's instructional resources such as the library and the media and tutoring centers, and determine the appropriate contact people. Also ask about curricular resources within the department.

Your mentor can assist you to set daily and weekly priorities as well as to develop realistic expectations. Discuss with your department chair or mentor your workload and the expected amount of preparation time for class. It usually takes 8 to 10 hours to prepare a 2-to 3-hour lecture for the first time. If you are taking twice this long, seek help immediately! Don't struggle in silence; help is always available, especially from your supervisor.

Once you have settled into your role, explore the organizational structure and determine how the department fits into the structure. Discuss the school's relationship with other local schools and colleges. This is particularly important when your health occupations program is articulated in order that your students be able to pursue further education. Your chair should also explain your department's relation to the state department of education. In some states this relationship is quite formal and is involved in regulating teacher credentialing and enforcing professional development requirements.

Your level of creativity is limited only by your energy and talents, provided that you promote and support the school mission and department goals. However, you have an obligation to inform your department chair of innovative projects that you are undertaking. When students complain about a new teaching method, your chairperson can be more supportive when aware of the experimental approach. Don't become misled about the concept of academic freedom. You must still remain responsive to your students' needs and the objectives of the program and school.

The chairperson is your strongest advocate; that advocacy may assume many forms. One example may be during a student grievance process in which you failed a student for poor performance in the clinical setting. The chairperson may need to mediate sessions between you and a student. Don't become defensive when at first the chairperson appears to be listening more intently to the student's side of the issue than to your concerns. This approach may be quite unsettling to you. Nevertheless, when the student has been treated fairly, the outcome, regardless of the consequences, is more palatable to the student. Remember, the student is a member of the community, and without community support your program will not survive.

Another example may be selling your request for a change to the divisional dean or dean of instruction. Now your responsibilities as a faculty member and those of your chairperson should merge. Although your chair may wholeheartedly support your idea, unless the idea can be financed, the request may be ignored. When you submit an idea, brainstorm all the strengths and weaknesses of the proposal. Think of alternative solutions. You will experience success when your administrator has more options to sell to superiors.

The chairperson is often viewed as a role model not only for the department but also within the community at large. Once you accept a position as a faculty member, you assume similar responsibilities. You were a role model within your health care profession; now, the role has simply expanded to include students, colleagues, and other members of the educational profession.

In summary, the chairperson and all faculty members are accountable to one another. When all who are involved understand their expectations, the job of teaching future health care professionals becomes fun!

☞ SCHOOL DISTRICT SUPERVISOR

The school district health occupations supervisor or consultant is a valuable resource for schools and teachers. The new teacher can feel overwhelmed by all the instructional, procedural, and administrative responsibilities. The school administration and experienced teachers can give direction, but the district consultant can provide specialized help for health occupations, guided by broad practical experience and by the school district's educational plan.

The school district health occupations consultant usually has a background in health care coupled with professional education. The position's duties and responsibilities may be directed at either a secondary or postsecondary VHO program or at both levels. These duties consist of teacher assistance, program development, technical assistance, professional improvement, assistance for school-based vocational health occupations departments, and liaison with the community of interest.

As with all leadership positions, the consultant's ability to work and communicate effectively with people is essential for success. For the new teacher it is important to know where help can be obtained quickly and with supportive reinforcement. The answer is the school district health occupations consultant.

Consultant Background and Preparation

The consultant suggests how to get started, what has priority, how to get materials, and who in the community can be helpful; these suggestions are especially important for the new teacher.

The VHO consultant has experience as a health care professional, just like the new teacher. This past work should help form a professional bond between consultant and teacher. In addition, all VHO professionals need to stay current in both their specific disciplines, maintaining appropriate state licensure and educational certification requirements as required.

The consultant has had successful teaching experience in the classroom and skill performance in the laboratory and at the clinical site. Many have also held responsible positions at the college, in the school district, or at the state level and bring these experiences with them.

As a health care professional, the consultant must stay active in professional organizations, such as the American Vocational Association, the state AVA affiliate, a professional organization (in the health care field), Health Occupations Educators, and other educational societies. All of these professional activities provide the consultant with a tremendous network of colleagues and resources that can be tapped as needed.

Educationally, the consultant has training in a specialty, generally has both a baccalaureate and a master's degree, and may have a doctoral degree. A major educational consideration for the consultant is state certification, which is the state regulatory method to ensure that an individual meets standards of practice. The consultant must in most cases be certified as a VHO teacher as well as in administration and supervision, as required by a state.

A school district consultant has worked in health care, taught, and navigated through the education maze. The new teacher in particular can and should take advantage of this expertise.

Consultant Duties and Responsibilities

It should be recognized that an overlap of duties and responsibilities may exist between the district consultant and the school. Diplomacy and positive communications are hallmarks of an effective system so as to avoiding conflicts. Also, depending on the school district's organizational structure, these duties may be spread among several individuals, or the responsible person may have a different title. In some districts, one consultant may have responsibility for more than one vocational area or for all the vocational areas, including health occupations. For the sake of completeness, a global view of duties and responsibilities will be addressed without regard for actual authority.

In terms of teacher assistance, the school district will have policies and procedures for orienting new teachers. This is often called a new-teacher program, which incorporates district and school policies with state legal and regulatory considerations, including health care worker professional licensure, teacher preservice, teacher certification, and college course work for teacher certification. The consultant can be involved in orienting new teachers, both officially and unofficially, through the contacts encouraged by the system. For example, the consultant can advise the teacher in classroom management activities, including problem solving and with pupil placement issues. In addition, the consultant may observe the teacher in the classroom for teaching and program improvement purposes.

State teacher certification laws regulate educational practice by establishing standards for teachers and administrators. Teacher certification mandates educational and work experience requirements for VHO teachers. For the new VHO teacher, the number of years employed as a laboratory technologist, respiratory therapist, radiological technologist, registered nurse, or the like is a stipulation for teaching qualification. Specific college or university course work is also necessary for initial teacher certification, which lasts a specific length of time and requires course work, continuing education units, and/or inservice points for renewal. The consultant can be extremely helpful to the teacher in obtaining certification and for renewal thereafter.

School principals or directors can call upon the district consultant for assistance in finding and selecting new teachers. The consultant often will have the names of individuals who are interested in teaching and can match these with schools that need additional instructors. The consultant's professional contacts can be very useful in this instance.

Regarding program development, consultants will use all of their background experience and networking with others in program planning, development, and monitoring progress. Working with school principals, district staff, teachers, and local professional groups requires a high degree of administrative skill. New programs need to meet all state department of education requirements for facilities, equipment, and curricular materials. Resources can be obtained from schools that already have the program and have taught it, as well as from state and national sources.

Program expansion and/or improvement can be supported by the active consultant. Careful planning and marshaling of support for these activities are part of the art and science that the successful consultant must apply.

Technical assistance in health occupations education is the most varied of the consultant's duties and really means providing help for the programs and teachers involved. In this section, the following duties and responsibilities will be presented: curriculum issues; equipment and materials acquisition; educational specifications; vocational student organizations; program review, audit, and accreditation preparations; and review and recommendation of textbooks and other instructional resources for schools.

Curriculum has many definitions, but it can be thought of as the educational plan that is written before the instruction is carried out. Health occupations education is a subject-oriented set of disciplines that often have identified student learning outcomes or endpoint behaviors. There are many sources for curricular guides, including state and national models. In addition, the school district or school may have curriculum available. Taking this curriculum and specifically developing lesson plans or lab demonstrations using equipment and media are necessary for curriculum implementation. The consultant can lend experience to the new teacher and help bring the curriculum to life.

Frequent curriculum revision is essential for all of the health occupations. Continual technological developments in equipment and medical procedures plus changes in personnel legal requirements demand that the curriculum be updated regularly. The consultant may be able to coordinate funding for curriculum revision activities. Equipment and material acquisition represents an area in which the consultant can be very helpful. The sources for acquisition are local, state, and federal and require the completion of specific forms. These are usually called requests for proposals. They consist of a time-consuming, procedural process with deadlines to be met for approval by the school and the district. Often the state will be involved in approving the funding. The requests must have current prices for ordering purposes and may have to go through a competitive bidding process. Grants from other sources are also available requiring many of the same procedures as outlined above. When these proposals are funded, the consultant may be responsible for preparing requisitions, maintaining records, monitoring progress, and communicating with the funding source. The teacher and school are valuable allies for the consultant in this process.

Gifts and donations are also available from the community and can be valuable to health occupations programs. Local school district policy must be followed in accepting them, and the consultant can help.

The consultant also assists schools with both their educational specifications and their facility design input. The specifications are needed to ensure that new or renovated classrooms meet local or state requirements and provide students with the opportunity to meet their program objectives.

Federal vocational money (Carl Perkins Act) is provided to the states to fund vocational student organizations, among other things. Health Occupations Students of America (HOSA) promotes leadership development, and health occupations teachers are encouraged to become their student's sponsor. One of the highlights of HOSA activities is the skill competitions held locally and at the state and national levels. The student growth and accomplishment that are realized through HOSA membership are extremely rewarding for students and their advisers. The consultant can be a valuable resource in HOSA coordination and participation.

Program Review, Audit, and Accreditation Preparation

The consultant is usually responsible for ensuring that health occupations programs are effective and meet regulatory standards. These requirements are assessed by various agencies and necessitate proactive preparations. The consultant should be involved in report preparation and record maintenance, which are essential components for successful program review and audit outcomes.

The state may regularly conduct compliance audits for attendance records or vocational program review. Vocational program review is carried out to check that the program is meeting specific standards. Legal requirements must be met, or the district and school can be penalized by having funding withheld or having to pay back the funding. The new teacher will want to use the consultant's expertise to be prepared for these reviews.

Audits of registration forms, attendance records, and the funding elements of grants will also be conducted. These require attention for compliance.

Many of the VHO programs have mandatory or voluntary accreditation requirements that are tied into student eligibility for credentialing examinations. A primary example is a nursing program that must be approved by the state board of nursing, allowing graduates to apply and take the nursing licensure examinations that permit practice as a nurse. Other health professions have accreditation through the American Medical Association Committee for Allied Health Education Accreditation (CAHEA). Under CAHEA each profession has a Joint Review Committee that conducts the actual accreditation process and reports its findings to CAHEA. CAHEA then decides to grant or withhold accreditation to the program.

A sometimes controversial duty for the consultant is the evaluation of state or locally recommended textbooks and instructional resources for school use. This activity should be conducted according to district policy.

Publishers and media experts can be useful to the consultant in providing information on the texts available. This information can be shared with health occupations teachers for their input. Often publishers' representatives will allow new texts to be reviewed and kept by the reviewer in exchange for a reviewer's comments. This can be an inexpensive way to build a library, especially for the new teacher.

Professional Improvement

Inservice and staff development activities are usually coordinated by the district consultant. These are useful to update teachers on policy and procedure, teacher certification issues, and specific health occupation information. The consultant may also be required to attend regulatory meetings or conferences to remain current. Teacher travel and registration for professional meetings may need to be coordinated through the consultant's office.

Topics for inservice can also be identified from local needs and from state and national trends and can center on specific issues requiring attention. These activities can provide points toward teacher certification renewal and may be coordinated by the consultant.

With regard to planning, the school district may have the consultant work with the schools on planning issues, including budgeting for activities and capital expenditures. Planning activities may include both short-term and long-range planning. Short-term plans are usually for the current school year and are made for less than one year into the future. Typically these are related to what is needed this term, how to meet goals, and how many students must be provided for. Typically, supplemental or part-time courses are also coordinated with the consultant.

Strategic planning looks at longer-range needs and tries to match resources with them. The consultant can provide input on what the future may hold and how these needs may be met next year and the year after that. All of these plans must fit a school's mission and that of the school district.

Course Offerings

The consultant can help the school with selection of course offerings, including those to be added or deleted for the school year. These course offerings may be in response to state or local requests.

Interpretation of State Standards

Interpretation of state standards or requirements is a service that the district consultant can provide for a school. Standards may cover facility and educational specifications, teacher certification, minimum student grade levels, and curriculum materials. These standards are often legally mandated. The consultant who networks with professionals throughout the state and nation represents an excellent resource for interpretation and preparation activities.

Schools and their programs must respond to the needs of the community. The district health occupations consultant can help organize a health occupations advisory committee comprising key people in the area. These key individuals can assist with locating support for new programs, secure equipment and services that may be beyond the school's means, and help identify special needs to be met. Surveys of needs can be conducted using key community leaders as facilitators. Membership should include representation by health care facilities personnel, members of professional organizations, educators, and lay people. In addition, alumni and current students can give the program's target population — students — a voice in their future.

The consultant will probably belong to various community advisory committees and professional organizations. These are good resources for a school and encourages active communication with the area's leaders. Student scholarships can be promoted with these groups as a means to ensure that area leaders continue their involvement with the health occupations programs.

Because health occupations programs usually require clinical rotations in local health care facilities, there is a need for legally binding contracts between the district and those facilities. These agreements must be negotiated for newly conducted facilities, and all should be updated regularly. The consultant will have to work closely with the district's legal department and the health care facilities on specific requirements.

The consultant also can represent the district on local planning agencies that have articulation committees with a view toward teacher-school problem resolution and local university matters (student intern placement, preceptor assignment, research, teacher certification). The consultant may also provide input on policy development or revision for the district.

The school district health occupations consultant is a valuable resource for the teacher, the school, and the school district. Educators are encouraged to develop a positive working relationship with the consultant.

☞ STATE DEPARTMENT PERSONNEL

Education—Big Business

On your path of changing from clinician to teacher, you have been or will be exposed to a large number of people with different titles and responsibilities, not to mention an entirely new vocabulary of acronyms. Education is big business, and it requires a large cadre of individuals to manage it. It is not so different, however, from large medical centers with their chains of commands or mazes of communication lines. Keeping that comparison in mind should assist you in understanding your state department's relation to you.

Mission, Purpose, Structure

While each state's structure may vary, each does operate a state department of and for public education. Vocational education's structure is a part of the state's organization (Figure 16-3). One of the common missions of state education departments is to offer all citizens a fair and equal opportunity for an education. It carries out this mission primarily by influencing legislation and labor-setting policy and by assisting in managing all levels of public education. "Public" refers to those institutions and programs supported by both state and federal tax money, including public schools (kindergarten through twelfth grade), area vocational/technical centers, community colleges, technical institutes, and state colleges and universities.

Each state department is governed by laws and at least one board of education. The board is generally composed of private citizens, politicians, and educators who are frequently appointed by the state's governor or elected by its citizens. A state superintendent or commissioner, either elected or appointed, serves as the "CEO" of the state department of education.

The manner in which public education is implemented and managed in each state is determined by the organizational structure, which is established

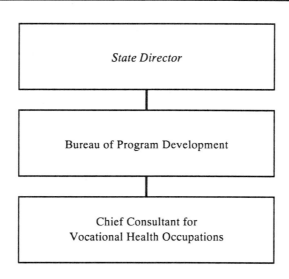

FIGURE 16-3: *One Model of a State Division of Vocational and Technical Education*

by its leadership. Your school, your department, your HOE program, and your job exist because they are parts of an overall organizational plan most likely established at the state level. It is considered to be an effective and efficient manner for delivering a fair and equal educational opportunity to all students, including the ones you teach. In essence, this constitutes the initial relationship your state department has with you.

Expectations

Because a state department is composed of numerous divisions and subdivisions, it is important for you to know exactly what you can expect from its many employees. That's right — what you can expect. And though you may feel your state department is far removed from where you are, it exists to serve you, local and regional administrators, and students. Whether you teach in a local high school, area vocational-technical center, community college, technical institute, or college or university, the state department employs administrators, specialists, consultants, and supervisors whose expertise may be relied upon. They are accountable to the success of your program just as you are. Thus, your relationship with them should be a positive one.

Keeping in mind the diversity of state department personnel, for our purposes, let's discuss expectations you might have of most any HOE program administrator (specialist/consultant/supervisor). These individuals are generally housed under the division of vocational-technical education within a section referred to as health occupations education. Office locations may include the state capital and regional locations. This dependents on the number of available administrators, specific job descriptions, and a state department's organizational structure.

HOE Program Administrator: Role and Function

The primary role of most HOE program administrators is to establish accountable policies that influence the manner in which programs are delivered statewide. Essentially this includes a number of functions through which this role may be performed. For example, the following may be performed.

1. Establish program standards.
2. Establish curriculum standards.
3. Provide professional development.
4. Determine teacher and student certification/credentialing standards.
5. Provide regional and local technical assistance for both administrators and teachers.
6. Serve as state adviser to the Health Occupations Students of America (HOSA).

7. Establish/implement program accreditation/evaluation/performance standards, sometimes inclusive of state university HOE teacher education programs.

This role and its function may seem broad, but what it means to you as a teacher is the basis on which your program operates and on which you are held accountable. And it is determined primarily at the state level by HOE program administrators. Understand, however, that such standards more likely are jointly agreed upon or even developed by a state HOE advisory board composed of health industry representatives, educational administrators, and possibly parents and students. In addition, such standards must (may) be approved by the state director of vocational education or a state board of education. Program administrators may also involve local teachers on management teams/committees that assist in developing such standards. This is an effective participatory management technique and affords teachers ownership of the statewide program. You are encouraged to volunteer or agree to serve on such teams/committees. The experience offers you a broader perspective of HOE as well as valuable information and resources for your use.

You may be surprised to know that before you were employed to teach or manage your HOE program, your state program administrator probably was involved in its planning, development, and implementation. The state supervisor is generally aware of you even if you have not already met.

Perhaps you are asking at this point how does knowing the state's HOE program administrator's role and functions specifically relate to you? After all, this person may be miles away, and you need answers now! Do not panic! Education has a creditable reputation for having individuals within your department or school who can advise you. Even they, however, may suggest that a state HOE program administrator should be contacted for detailed information. This may be arranged through teleconferencing or an on-site visit. Most local administrators are agreeable when a teacher contacts the state HOE program administrator. Most state HOE program administrators welcome such contact. However, do not become discouraged if such individuals are not immediately accessible. Their responsibilities have them frequently involved in meetings and on field visits. If telephoning, leave your name, number, and message with the professional office person, who may even be able to assist you. If your need calls for an immediate response, the program administrator will be contacted and will return your call. If you need on-site assistance, expect to wait at least two weeks. Most important, if you are in doubt about any facet of your program, feel free to contact the HOE program administrator, who seeks as much as you do your success as a VHO teacher. This constitutes the foundation of your relationship with the state department. Right now, confirm the HOE program administrator(s) in your state.

Situations that Relate a Program Administrator to a Teacher

Earlier it was recognized that when you need answers, you need them immediately in order to feel more comfortable delivering your HOE program. One of the greatest frustrations new teachers have in their transition from clinician to teacher is whom to ask about what. The following are examples of situations a state HOE program administrator should be able to help you resolve. Keep in mind that most states provide an orientation for new teaching personnel that includes these general areas, or the issues are covered during completion of a college- or university-based HOE teacher education program. You are encouraged to ask questions about:

1. Meeting teacher certification requirements if applicable to your employment.
2. Managing/teaching competency-based education.
3. Managing/teaching the approved curriculum, implementing a total program scope and sequence, organizing/presenting information, assessing/diagnosing student needs.
4. Ordering equipment, supplies, instructional materials, textbooks, computer software/hardware, audiovisual aids.
5. Developing/managing a program budget/inventory.
6. Managing an HOE advisory committee.
7. Administering student competency testing (written and performance).
8. Managing a local HOSA chapter, preparing students for competitive events, providing leadership development opportunities, integrating HOSA into the HOE curriculum.
9. Preparing students to meet credentialing requirements.
10. Preparing for program accreditation/evaluation.
11. Integrating academic and vocational education (e.g., science and HOE).
12. Integrating HOE within a technology education model.
13. Using a variety of teaching methods.
14. Applying education research to classroom instruction.
15. Disciplining students.
16. Negotiating industry-education-labor partnerships.
17. Managing clinical internships/practicums/mentorships.
18. Arranging/managing classroom/laboratory facilities.
19. Preparing for teacher evaluations.
20. Marketing HOE.

Please note that local administrators of vocational education have access to budgets/financial resources to support their local programs. Requests for such resources should be submitted to these individuals.

Public education is big business. It is managed by a multiplicity of individuals. For the clinician making a transition to becoming a teacher, it is important to take advantage of as many of these human resources as possible. State departments' HOE program administrators can be a most valuable resource. It is their specific role and function to offer leadership to the most effective and efficient delivery system possible based on accountable standards. Their expertise can afford both local administrators and teachers a successful collaborative effort that supports a successful program and teacher.

TEACHER EDUCATOR

This section focuses on the university educator and the roles defined by that position. In most universities, there are three broad categories of assignments: teaching, service, and research/creative activities. This section will describe these responsibilities as related to Vocational Health Occupations.

Areas of Responsibility

This role of teacher is the most obvious one attributed to being a teacher at any level; however, at a university the weight of this role is different from the one assigned in middle school, high school, a vocational center, or a community college.

It is assumed in some cases that you are already a good teacher, and unless proved otherwise, that is the situation. Now this does not mean that teaching is not of prime interest to the VHO teacher educator, because most of those in this area love teaching. What it does mean is that the emphasis is not generally on teaching for advancement in the system. The levels of promotion — from assistant to associate to full professor — are usually dependent on one's success in the research or creative scholarly area, not teaching or service. The first step to becoming tenured is based on all three areas, especially the research/creative area but to advance from associate to full professor, however, the emphasis is more heavily on research/creative scholarly activities than on teaching or service.

Our teaching focuses on the educational component — those skills that develop practitioners into teachers — called education content or pedagogy. Broad areas include teaching techniques, curriculum development, media, and vocational education topics. In other words, the contents of this handbook are the subjects we teach in our courses.

Programs available in universities for VHO teachers are preservice or inservice by nature; that is, courses are completed prior to being hired as a teacher or after being hired. Most VHO teachers are hired because of health care field expertise and then are taught how to teach. This is where you will meet one of us.

It is our responsibility to assist you in making the transition from practitioner to vocational educator.

The service category is the area in which participation in state and national associations is included, such as in HOE/AVA and HOSA. In the reward system at universities, this area usually receives the least weight, even though we often do a great deal of service. Participation on program and school advisory committees is also a responsibility, and we try to be as involved as possible.

The area of research/creative scholarly activities receives the most emphasis in the university system in terms of achieving tenure and especially promotion to a full professorship. Research — adding to the knowledge about a targeted subjected — is the prime area of focus. In that area you as a teacher may be contacted by survey or in person to participate in a research project. Your support in such endeavors is appreciated because of the newness of VHO and as a field in which little research has been completed and much needs to be done.

While research is of utmost concern, other creative activities also fall into this category. This book is an example of a creative activity, as would be the application of new technologies to deliver instruction.

Characteristics of VHO Teacher Educators

Generally the background of VHO teacher educators is similar to that of a VHO teacher. We, for the most part, have been health care practitioners, and many of us were also VHO teachers who continued our education. Now we teach teachers and are still teachers, but with a different audience. Historically, most VHO teacher educators were women with nursing backgrounds, but, other health fields are represented now, and men are entering the arena. The responsibilities are generally not health field related but are in education, vocational education more specifically, and health occupations in particular.

U.S. DEPARTMENT OF EDUCATION PERSONNEL

[Editor's Note: This section is dedicated to the memory of the life and work of Catherine Junge.]

The U.S. Department of Education (USDOE) is another dimension of local and state education structure. As a teacher, however, you can be proud that our nation views education as a major means for effecting change in its population. As a voter, you have the responsibility to ensure that knowledgeable and competent leaders make such decisions, because education and health care are also political arenas. This is especially true at the federal level. It is in Washington that significant legislation related to education and health care is initiated. There is no doubt that what is accomplished in Congress affects individual states and how each will be able to implement or continue effective educational and health care delivery systems. Moreover, the various federal branches of government influence public policy in a manner that can even determine how your health occupations program is implemented. But given our focus on education, this section will address the USDOE.

Governmental Branch

Printing an organizational chart of the USDOE would take several pages. The division most closely allied to you is the Office of Adult and Vocational Education, led by an appointed assistant secretary (Figure 16-4). It should be understood that such appointments determine, from one USDOE secretary/assistant secretary or presidential administration to the next, that roles and functions can and do change. Consequently, this can affect the USDOE's relation to you as a teacher.

Role and Function

The overall role and function of the Office of Adult and Vocational Education is to serve at the pleasure of the president of the United States and an appointed secretary. This depends on the president's and secretary's political agenda or goals, which, in general, may be interpreted to mean that the assistant secretary and staff serve as advocates for the adult and vocational education system. They demonstrate this advocacy through support of legislation that affects adult and vocational education. Establishing rules and regulations that guarantee appropriate implementation of the legislation is a major function of the office. Moreover, various educational standards may be developed if in keeping with the secretary's goals for the USDOE.

In past years, the Office of Adult and Vocational Education has employed program specialists to give leadership to specific vocational program areas, for example, HOE. Such individuals may or may not have relevant educational backgrounds or experience.

Program Specialists

Program specialists are expected to keep abreast of education and industry trends and communicate such information throughout a nationwide network. For example, an HOE program specialist might represent all health occupations educators on national committees, attend education and health-industry-

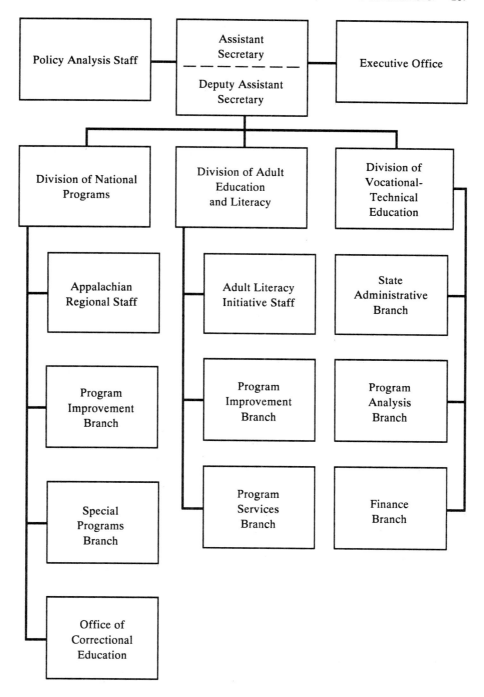

FIGURE 16-4: *U.S. Department of Education Office of Vocational & Adult Education*

related conferences, keep up-to-date on critical issues, utilize networks to effect change, actively participate in the American Vocational Association and its Health Occupations Education Division and the Health Occupations Students of America. Because this perspective is a national one, the program specialist can be extremely helpful in sharing information about exemplary programs, curriculum materials, and innovative delivery systems.

More specifically, your relationship to program specialists is crucial to their effectiveness. "Why is this true?" you may ask. Specialists can be no more effective in communicating than the information shared. Likewise, they cannot represent you successfully if they are uninformed about critical issues influencing your specific career area. Because federal government is so very complex, each level needs its networks. You can make a difference by helping to keep USDOE program specialists informed as they seek to keep you informed.

Like state program specialists, federal program specialists have limitations. Consequently, the following represents some areas in which you could rely on their assistance. It is advisable to keep state program specialists informed of your needs or interests as well, because they can also be helpful, given specific information forwarded to them by the federal program specialist. Such information may consist of:

- Developmental legislation that may affect the credentialing requirements of your students
- Projected health care worker needs
- Programmatic statistical information — national statistics
- States that have programs like yours, for which a contact can be identified
- Current general education legislation that might influence funding of your program

The USDOE-HOE program specialist is a valuable information source, and you are encouraged to write or call.

Health Occupations Education Program Specialist
OAVE/DVTE/PAB
4325 Switzer Building
Washington, DC 20202-7322
202-732-2427

The relationship that a teacher has with the USDOE is generally based on the current presidential administration's goals and national agenda. This does not imply that the USDOE staff is inaccessible to you as an HOE teacher, however. The entire USDOE staff serves as advocates for all of education. The Office of Adult and Vocational Education and the HOE program specialist within the USDOE are more closely allied to your needs and interests. Because it is the role of the office and the specialist to keep abreast of the movements, trends, legislation, and standards related to HOE, teachers are encouraged to communicate directly with them if needed. It is also the function of the specialist to communicate through a national network of states and territories any information and materials that can be useful and usable. Before contacting the USDOE program specialist, you might discuss your concern with your own supervisor or state program specialist. Needed information may have already been communicated. Information you would like to share at any level is always encouraged.

References

AVA. American Vocational Association: Constitution, Bylaws, Program of Work, Organization Chart. Alexandria, VA: author.

AVA (1991). AVA-HOE Division Management Action Plan. Alexandria, VA: author.

Bywaters, D. R. (October-November 1985). "Total Marketing: An Approach for the Future." *A&SM*.

Dade County Public School System. (1991). Position description: Instructional supervisor, health and public service education. Miami, FL: author.

Hillsborough County Public Schools. (1991). Position description: Supervisor of health, public service, and cosmetology occupations education. Tampa, FL: author.

Katz, D., R. Kahn, et al. (1980). *The Study of Organizations*. San Francisco: Jossey-Bass.

Myers, E. M. (March 1990). "A Future Vision." *Association Management*.

Orange County Public Schools. (1990). Position description: Program consultant for secondary home economics and health occupations. Orlando, FL: author.

Public Law 101-392. (1990). Carl D. Perkins Vocational and Applied Technology Educational Act Amendments. Washington, DC.

Rosenberg, K. (1985). *Organization Management* (4th ed.). New York: McGraw-Hill.

U.S. Department of Education (1991). *USDOE – Office of Adult and Vocational Education: Organization Chart*. Washington: author.

Webster's New World Dictionary (2nd ed.) (1908). Cleveland, OH: William Collins and World.

17

Uses of Current Technology: What's Available Now?

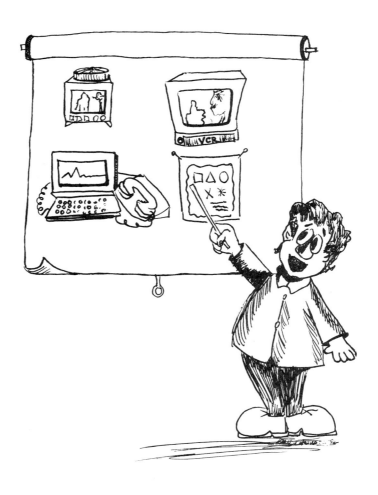

Vocational education cannot afford to be behind in technological advancements, because the health care industry has always been in the forefront of technological advances and the educators of health workers must keep up with technology in order to produce a hirable product.

Prosser stated in his *Sixteen Theorems on Vocational Education* that "vocational education will be efficient in proportion as the environment in which the learner is trained is a replica of the environment in which he must subsequently work" (1949). Changes in procedures and technologies within the industry require that health care students receive intensive clinical exposure to patients, specimens, and hands-on activities. Education must follow suit, with exposure of the same trainees to technological advancements that they will be required to use.

AUDIOVISUAL EQUIPMENT

Traditional "AV stuff" . . . Can It Make a Difference?

In these times of high-tech here, high-tech there, high-tech everywhere, what's one to do? This chapter examines your options in the midst of technologies flying hither and yon and lets you be the judge.

The premise, faulty but increasingly popular, holds that when we speak about technology in today's classroom, we mean computers! Even in the best of technology-based worlds, however, there remains much, much more than just computers.

Assume that we proceed into a future in which all teachers and learners have access to desktop versions of the NeXT computer, Steve Jobs' mystical "black box" technology cube PC in which all things for all people seem evident. There will still remain a need for us just-plain-folks to know something about what we call "traditional AV stuff."

This section examines a number of ideas about traditional audiovisual (AV) materials and equipment and will help each of you to make a real and lasting difference to your students.

Sections on the following areas are included:

- The umbrella concept of instructional systems design (ISD)
- Teacher as medium
- Medium as teacher
- Stuff that doesn't get projected
- Projected materials that don't talk back
- Projected materials that do talk back
- Adding movement to the mix

- Putting it all together
- Stuff they never told you in college
- Case studies of real people using AV stuff

Generally, the overall tone of this section will mirror informality, as if you were sitting down with a friend at lunch and what's in this chapter arose in the conversation. Now then, relax, and let's begin.

The umbrella concept of ISD: preplanning pays off. If you know where it is you are heading and have a clear picture of the target, that increases the likelihood you'll reach your goal.

ISD provides us with a paradigm for ensuring that we get where we want to, and know when, how, and why.

Most ISD models have five parts: analyze, design, develop, implement, and evaluate. That's ADDIE for short. Basically this means that first you conduct an analysis of every possible aspect of why and how you are planning to conduct instruction. The old saw holds that you are justified in developing instruction if there is a gap between what is and what should be. For example, among your learners there exist wide differences in knowledge of safe clinical skills. This is ample justification for you to begin to develop instruction that will reduce that gap. The analysis stage involves looking at everything, from what your learners already know to the physical site where the learning will occur. It looks at levels of learner readiness, of learner abilities and learning styles, and even motivation. It also seeks to locate materials on the topic you are to instruct. No need to reinvent that particular informational wheel if it's already been done!

Assuming no materials cover the topic, the next step is to design them. At this stage you'll have to make choices: type of media format, available resources, available talent to produce the materials, available expertise. Why, just about "available" everything.

Once your materials have been through the design stage, they must be developed, in addition to the methods for using them. It is not enough that one merely produce a set of overhead transparencies on a topic; one must know the order in which they will be used, the appropriate manipulation of overlays, and how the materials presented via transparencies relate to the curriculum in its entirety. The more complex the design, the more attention must be paid to production.

Implementation follows development in a logical progression from design and development to actual use of the materials in instruction. Here is where the proverbial rubber meets the road in that the act of teaching now occurs.

Evaluation, in its final or summative form, now takes place. Did you and your materials actually close or eliminate that gap between what was and what should have been? If not, back to the ISD drawing boards, for something went awry.

We just used "summative" and now, to add to the mix, we'll throw in "formative," for those two are the saviors of our hide, if we remembered to invite them along for the ride.

Simply put, what we're saying is that, within the ISD model process, you've got to evaluate every step of the way (termed formative evaluation or forming it as you go). Revise on the basis of what your continuing evaluations tell you rather than wait until the end (summative), when it may be too late!

With this instructional systems design model down pat, some may say it's too complicated to use. Don't you believe it, not for a single moment! What has just been handed to you is a systematic means through which you can conduct instruction, be it face-to-face sans technology or laden at every turn with this or that new gadget.

Your main goals are to get a handle on how to write a decent behavioral objective (Mager, 1984), to decode ISD (Gagne, Briggs & Wager, 1992; Kemp, 1985), to learn how materials are produced (Kemp & Smellie, 1989; Marsh, 1983), to then learn how and when to use a bunch of media when the time is right (Heinich, Molenda, & Russell, 1989), and, finally, review just a few basic presentation tips to give you that polished professional look.

Teacher as medium: The late Dr. Eugene Oxhandler used to say with delight, "If technology can replace a teacher, it should!" He would then go on to say that technology, properly used, will "re-place" teachers, putting them to the side of the podium rather than having them continually occupy center stage. Oxhandler was making a case for the increasing role change on the part of the teacher, from that of omnipotent dispenser of knowledge, to facilitator, one who allows and encourages rather than makes things happen. He spoke those words some thirty years ago, and his prophecy rings truer as each day passes.

Oxhandler and a number of the author's (R.C.) other mentors (Drs. Don Ely, Jim Finn, Howard Hitchens, Jerry Mars, Sherm Swartout, and Des Wedberg) would each, in his own definitive manner, have said "You, the individual, the living, breathing, talented, dynamic, self-motivated, creative teacher, are still the best medium around!" And you know what? They were right!

Medium as teacher: Increasingly, especially as more sophisticated technology-based delivery systems emerge for use in the schools, the decision has to be made as to who is actually doing the "teaching" — the teacher or the material on the video, videodisc, or computer?

If "control" is where you're coming from, then whatever materials you employ, no matter how good they might be, will always take a back seat to you and your role within the instruction being proffered. Conversely, if the materials being presented via the media are of high caliber, the wise teacher knows that this is the time to stand aside and let the "content do its thing."

Clearly, as the quality of technology-based materials continues to improve beyond what any of us were able to foresee only a few years ago, it quickly becomes apparent that the content being delivered may be well beyond the scope of the classroom teacher. Wow! Now what? The simple response "I don't know" should suffice for most. Where is it written that teachers cannot, nor should not, utter these words?

As the spiral of information descending upon each of us continues to quicken and expand, there is practically no way in which any of us can possibly keep up with what is happening in our own field, let alone that of anyone else! The problem then becomes one of, "How do I let this 'dumb' machine outteach me, outlearn me, and, worst of all, have my students asking for more?" Don't even try. Realize that there are just some things over which we have no control. The information explosion is one of them.

So much for philosophy, future trends, and the like. Let's get down to cases and look at some of that traditional AV stuff.

Stuff that doesn't get projected: In the classroom, be it an elementary school or adjacent to a corporate suite, the one thing we can count on most is that there will be a writing surface somewhere in the room. Many call it a chalkboard; some call it a dry-erase board; a few call it an easel with a pad of paper attached; and on occasion some call it an "electronic chalkboard." All are viable options for teachers to demonstrate their prowess in unimagined ways.

Preparation, as in all examples we can envision, is the key to success in using media of any kind in any format. This applies equally to the old tried-and-true traditional chalkboard as much as it does to the computer. If you tear into your classroom at the last minute and expect that you'll be a chalkboard wizard . . . you're wrong.

Assuming you are no van Gogh of the chalkboard, admit that you're not even close. Fake it! Go in ahead of time and project your intended diagram or work of art onto the display surface, using an opaque or overhead projector. Very lightly, trace the outlines of your schematic, artwork, or whatever. Then pull down the screen in front of it until you're ready to discuss your chosen concept. No screen in the room? Use a sheet of newsprint to cover your drawing until needed.

If you have a screen, stand to the side of it and begin to describe your idea. After pausing for dramatic flair, pull up the screen and begin to rapidly chalk in your drawing, simply following the very light outline you've put in place ahead of time. The same goes for dry marking boards and paper pads on easels. Planning makes artists of us all!

A relatively new device is the electronic chalkboard. It is rarely seen in schools for a variety of reasons. Money is part of it, but resistance to change is the bigger part. The electronic chalkboard is an electrified dry-erase board that allows you to use any of four movable writing surfaces to print in hard-copy (paper) form what was on any of them and to collapse the four screens of data to one hard-copy printout.

Imagine such a device being used in a brainstorming session at a given location and then, via fax, transmitting the hard-copy results thousands of miles in a few seconds. Makes distance education an affordable reality.

In considering nonprojected materials, don't forget the wonders of bulletin boards, exhibits, posters, and the wide variety of other traditional formats that learners continue to enjoy and teachers continue to employ.

Projected materials that don't talk back: Used in their simplest form, the following are categorized as mute projected visuals; that is, they don't require electronic amplification.

- Overhead transparencies
- 2" × 2" slides
- Filmstrips

Because there is less and less dependence on filmstrips in schools these days, let's discuss them first. In times past, filmstrips were the media workhorses of many VHO teachers, no matter the particular subject taught. Sometimes they had sound accompaniment; at other times they didn't. In a progressive format, they allowed the teacher to unfold a concept in a logical fashion. They did not, however, allow for much flexibility, given that the visuals were all physically connected and followed a very specific order. Therein lay an interesting contradiction.

Filmstrips remain in use in many schools. This is in large measure because there are simply not enough funds to replace the old filmstrip collection with more contemporary formats and, more important, contemporary ideas and information.

It would be sage advice to "salvage" the remaining filmstrips you may still have by cutting them up and mounting them in slide frames especially designed to hold the half-frame filmstrip format. In this way, at least you'll have some additional visual materials you can arrange and rearrange to suit your needs — until your school can afford to replace the materials, that is. Word of caution: Check with your media specialist before attempting this exercise.

Overhead transparencies are alive and well, thank you very much! They are a more contemporary form of "instructor's notes," which just take a bit longer to yellow with age. (Already we see the emergence of the "traditionalist" AV user, yes?)

Certainly the operative word when using overhead transparencies, assuming they are used correctly by the instructor, is control. You, the teacher, are definitely in control.

Suffice it to say that, with today's substitute for the chalkboard—the overhead projector—few miscreants can escape the penetrating vision of you who teach them. After all, if you are using the projector correctly you are facing the class and not the wall!

To any who might be even a tad technophobic, the overhead projector is by far the easiest device to use. It lets you look somewhat "with it" in technological terms, and it may even appear as if you enjoy using such devices in your teaching. There are innumerable sources for overhead transparencies, but, barring access, you can make them quite easily.

Overhead transparencies store nicely in file drawers, assuming you've mounted each onto a cardboard frame, and there are increasing means through which they can be produced. The advent of computer-based production of overhead transparencies exists now.

We'll save discussion of various and sundry presentation boo-boos until the last part of this section.

An earlier cousin of the overhead transparency is the 2" x 2" photographic slide. Ask around, and you'll find numerous camera owners, should you not have one of your own. Slides are flexible in terms of arrangement, and they're fun to make. Slide making can be involving, sometimes to the point of becoming an obsession, because making them forces you to explore the notion of visual literacy so that what you photograph can be used as an exemplar.

Properly produced (crafted) slides can be woven into instruction at innumerable places and can be obtained within a single day, assuming you use the right type of film (Ektachrome) and either know how to use E-6 processing or know someone who can do it for you.

The major requirement to keep in mind when producing slides is to understand visual composition. Mastering the mechanics of focus and exposure will follow with experience, but having a good eye for what makes a memorable shot sets one apart from another.

This author suggests to students that, whenever possible, they shoot using a horizontal format rather than vertical. The simple reason for this is that, should you go on to fame and future glory, and the local television studio asks to use some of your slide work, only those shot in horizontal format will be usable. Let's think fame, now!

Projected materials that don't talk back: It is very possible that sound could easily be added to any of the materials discussed thus far. Not only does sound add interest for both teacher and learner, but also it is just more natural. The sound you add may originate only from within you or another, or it may be electronically reproduced and enhanced via tape or compact disc musical inclusion.

As with all production and use of instructional materials, the caveat of adherence to copyright procedures must necessarily be stated. Simply put, that means don't rip off your artistic neighbor by stealing his or her stuff. Either get permission, compose your own audio additions, or don't use one unless the source has been dead for no less than fifty years. Even then, be cautious, because your source, although taken from one who has perhaps long since passed on, may have been adapted by one or more individuals who are very much alive and with us. If in doubt, ask.

Of course, when we think of sound and visuals, we also begin to think of motion, our next area of discussion.

Adding movement to the mix: The time will come at last when you begin to go beyond the pale of just using simple media and become adventurous. Go for it with video! Or film! (Much of what follows in this section applies to both film and video.)

In today's classroom, the use of film, like filmstrips, is on the wane. Videocassettes are just too easy to use, so why bother with that bulky projector! The purist filmmaker will be fuming, but, face it, folks, unless you're really into the culture of film, the expedient choice is video. To be sure, in film production there does still lie a totally involving experience, one that should not automatically be shunted aside, especially if you happen to be the one so skilled. However, video, with its ease of use and immediacy of production, is probably the medium you will find most readily available and thus will use.

Check your sources before renting the nearest sound stage. It is likely that the great epic you wish to create is already "in the can." See what's already been done before you shoot even a foot of video. If nothing exists, or that which does is so shabby that even your in-laws would blanch at using it, then consider video production as an alternative. Like so many other aspects of producing and using some of these traditional media formats, videomaking is also fun! It is, as has been stated earlier, a whole lot more involving than is viewing what someone else has done.

The simplest advice to you, the budding video producer, is to check with your school to learn what talent and facilities might already exist. In some schools, there are quite sophisticated video facilities in place in addition to talented professionals who know what to do with them. Tap that resource, and you're miles ahead of the game.

Putting it all together: From our point of view, this means remembering to attend to all the little details that constitute successful instruction. It also means remembering to evaluate whether the final product did, in fact, achieve the change in behavior you were seeking in your learners. If it did that, then it was all together for you . . . and them!

Stuff they never told you in college: There resides in all of us that secret desire to share those things the administration held so cherished, so inviolate, that you'd have given anything to tell your class. Such is the situation with me as well, especially regarding those little secrets of presentation that can make the difference between having egg on your face and bowing to a standing ovation for a presentation extremely well executed.

Case studies of real people using AV stuff: Let's pry open that previously unattainable Pandora's box of presentation giving and see what might emerge.

In terms of Boo-boos, perhaps the one presentation gaff that always sends me ballistic is the white-screen phenomenon. This is the one in which the presenter, about to begin the address, turns on the overhead projector (slide projector, etc.), and, lo and behold, naught but a blinding white light pierces your vision. If you've been partying the night before at your convention, this is the last thing you need at 8 a.m. If you haven't, it makes you wish you had.

As long as we're on the case of the wayward overhead projection user, let's add to the list the practice of block-the-screen-from-view syndrome. Here you have a hulking person standing between the screen and the projector, successfully managing to exclude from view all but the smallest corner of what is supposed to be seen. Oh yes, one need not be hulking to accomplish this feat.

Then there's the one who, to be certin each student sees what's on the screen, stands beside it and, line by line, reads down the list—verbatim. This instructor uses a pointer and, depending upon his or her mood at the moment, a soft and delicate tap or a resounding boomer, the latter mostly for effect.

Administrators know that the power of a good, loud school buzzer will stun the class long enough for the teacher to once more regain control of the class; so too does the media buff know the value of crescendo appropriately timed.

Then there is Mr. Fuzzhead, totally and blissfully ignorant of the fact that the transparency is being shown upside down and possibly even backwards to boot. And that selfsame visual, being of such stellar quality that it merits special acclaim, remains on the screen for the next ten minutes . . . or more!

His associate, Ms. Technoglee, has taken every possible media-use class ever given and knows that one sits beside the overhead, turns the projector on only after the visual has been placed on the stage, and turns it off when not needed. She also arrived at the class well in advance to ensure that focus, screen size, and alignment of image would be correct. Unfortunately, however, she was asleep at the wheel when her instructor cautioned about violation of accepted graphics conventions, as well as keeping in mind the KISS principle (keep it simple, stupid!). The result is that Ms. Technoglee's transparencies resemble road maps you'd get from your auto club, laden with all kinds of information and done in letters even your cat couldn't read with his face upon the transparency.

Your own transparencies will be greeted with accolades if you follow a few basic rules.

- Restrict yourself to one basic idea per visual.
- Make sure any letters used can be easily read even a hundred feet away from the screen.

Remember the KISS (Keep It Short & Simple) axiom by dealing with a single visual concept. Overlays are fine, as long as you don't use so many that they cause the screen to go dark.

Use both color and icons to good advantage but sparingly.

Mount your transparencies in frames so they don't curl on the projector stage. This allows you some space for "cheat sheet" notes on the frame's margin and makes the class think you're quite erudite.

In summation, regarding the noble use of overhead projection and aside from areas already mentioned, attune yourself to the next paragraph.

Sit beside the projector, cast occasional glances back at the screen to be sure that focus and alignment are correct, use a pen or similar item to point to items on the transparency (not on the screen), and keep most of your attention on student eyeballs, because that's where you'll get real feedback as to how you're doing.

Given that we made such a big deal over photographic slide use, there are some items that, if one is aware of it, will make life in the slide lane far easier.

We repeat, get to the classroom earlier than students, and see that your equipment is set up and that it works.

The philosophy of yesteryear always went that, to load slides into a tray, you should put them in upside down and backwards. Wrong! The Cornellian foolproof, goofproof way to succeed in using slides, assuming that your camera eye was not too far askance, is very simple. (We also assume, by the way, that you've created the slide set to help you achieve a specific behavioral objective and that using slides is not just a chance for you to share last year's summer holiday with yet another captive audience.) To begin, place all of the slides on a light table or other surface where you can see them clearly. Cull out the poor ones. Better not use any visual rather than include even one shoddy shot.

Put the slides in the order in which they will be used. At this stage, each slide should be on the light table so that it is right side up and as the scene looked when you took it.

Not sure if the scene is backwards or forwards, for example, a shot of flowers or a landscape without any identifiable cues as to correct or incorrect side of the slide? Gently pick up the slide and tilt it a bit so that light reflects off the film surface. If the surface being reflected is totally shiny, you have the side right. If, however, you can see slight ridges on the film's surface, the slide is backwards. What you're seeing are the layers of chemical emulsion that coat the slide. That side always faces toward the screen, or away from you.

Once you have all slides arranged on the light board the way you want them projected, the big moment has arrived—loading the carousel. Pick up slide number 1, turn it upside down, and insert it into the number 1 slot in your slide tray. Keep on going until you reach number 80.

If you are using a carousel-type of slide tray, load your slides and then number them or put a "thumb spot" on the upper right corner of each slide. Just gently ease each slide up about halfway out of the slot and make your mark. This assumes that all slides are in sequence and properly placed into the slots. Why do we do this? If you accidentally drop the slide tray and they spill onto the floor, having them all numbered saves you beaucoup time; all you have to do is order them numerically, grab each slide by its number, and slip it back into the slide slot. No need to hold up the slide to see if it is right side to or vice versa; the numbering system has taken care of that for you.

Don't mess around with those 160 slide trays, because the slides always seem to get hung up and then where are you? This, by the way, is especially true in humid climates such as in Florida, Hawaii, Brisbane, or Cannes. (Just threw these in, should the wanderlust attack and should you find yourself having to present in an exotic locale.)

If you have followed your media doctor's orders as described above, you should now be collecting rave reviews from your critics, read, students. At least the slides will have been projected correctly. As far as their content, that one rests with you.

Remember, once more, no white screens! A simple way to avoid that problem is to put a logo slide at both the front and back of your presentation. When you turn on the projector, there's your school logo, and when you see it again, that's your cue to off the projector. Not complicated at all, just requires some semblance of memory.

Video, just like film, longs to be cued to the exact spot where it is supposed to begin. Now that may well be the title and opening credits, or it may be a spot in the middle—that precise place where you want to make a major-league point. If either is the case, get it cued in advance. Don't fumble here and there searching in vain for the lost frame. (Lost chords we can handle, but lost frames take more patience.)

Like any good showperson, you've seen, also in advance, that the volume is where you want it, and that there are sufficient television sets to allow all to view the masterwork . . . comfortably. If a film, you've also seen that the focus is accurate and that there are no frames out of sync.

Once more a "rule" emerges: Cornell sez, as do infinite numbers of others, that there's no direct correlation between the running time of a given film or video and the number of minutes in a class period! Or at least, there should not be. There is no rule that says that, if the urge strikes, you should show only those magical few minutes (or seconds) of the work and let the rest remain dormant within the VCR or projector.

There are innumerable other axioms that could be thrown your way, but there's only one to which I cling, and it may well answer your nagging, yet unspoken question about why I make such a big deal about all this presentation stuff. (Cue drum roll, klieg lights, wet cement.) If you are going to use a medium, no matter the form, use it properly and use it well! You are a professional in every respect, and that professionalism must extend to when, why, where, and how you use media to deliver ideas. Media can make it happen, if properly used. If misused, media can make you look like a jerk. Take your choice.

A VHO Teacher's Perspective

Those who are new vocational teachers use media as a method to gain students' interest, present educational material, and manage the classroom environment. Teaching without formal educational preparation is a challenge; however, a background in health care presenting self-care instruction and presenting educational programs for continuing education helps. Continuing university course work toward teacher certification complements the need to use media effectively. Using prepared media allows lesson planning to take place prior to class presentation. The first year of teaching is a crush of activities, in new settings and with the need for a tremendous amount of outside planning. Matching media type to the lesson represents a learning experience of its own.

The types of media used are films, filmstrips, overhead projection, coloring book projects, and video (professionally prepared or self-prepared). Each of these has advantages and disadvantages for classroom use. Equipment and time costs must be considered with the use of each type, but cost is not a major element of this section.

Common media. Films (16 mm) require a projector and a screen. An advantage is that they are already prepared; disadvantages are that they are commercially prepared, expensive, and possibly outdated, and the content may not exactly meet your needs. Also, equipment problems can arise at any time, causing interruptions. Distractions can be the datedness of the film, with old-fashioned clothing and hairstyles interfering with the content.

Filmstrips can be used to introduce a subject or reinforce a concept. Major disadvantages are that they can be very boring and that students can lose attention. Also, whenever the room lights are lowered, students can wander mentally, fall asleep, or become disruptive.

Overhead projectors have numerous advantages for classroom use. The lights can be kept on and the pacing is set by the teacher, depending on student progress. Teachers can prepare their own overheads using a marking pen and clear transparency sheets. A cover page can be used to allow "discovery learning" to occur. Overheads offer flexibility in preparation and can be used both to present information, graphics, and charts and for quizzing students. A disadvantage is that the teacher must manually change the overhead, and therefore the presentation is teacher dependent.

Focused topic video production. Teaching health care skills to secondary students requires getting the students' attention and retaining it. Because of limited use of video taping from television, additional video production is necessary. As this is the "visual generation," with students relating to videos, the author's home has become a limited production studio. The commitment for equipment (camcorder, VCR), supplies (blank tapes), and time (6–8 hours per 30 minutes of video) can be costly, but it has been a positive investment.

Three videos have been prepared to date ranging from 20 to 30 minutes in length. They cover home safety, bandaging wounds, and fitness using a home exercise machine. The students ask, "Is this another homemade video, teacher?" When they hear, "Yes!" they know what to expect. Students have said that the videos are getting more interesting.

Preparation to produce a video demands attention to detail. The video must either fit into an existing lesson plan or become a video lesson plan. Video can be used to present skill demonstrations for student introduction, preparation for skill practice, self-check of skill performance, and remediation of weaknesses.

Production components include a camcorder with charged batteries, blank tapes, storyboard layout for content and sequence, lighting, information placards (titles, definitions, terms, etc.), background music, and props. For our example, the bandaging of wounds will be described.

The storyboard is developed, constituting an outline of the scenes to be shot during production. The terms with definitions are placed on placards for use with the corresponding shots. Lighting is set up and tested for each shot. Props (in this case, stuffed rabbits with long ears and limbs) are obtained and positioned for shooting. Bandages are prepared to size for application, and public domain music is selected for each shot to gain student interest.

During the shooting of a scene, direction of the elements is necessary. In our example, the following steps are utilized:

Lighting is set up and checked.

Rabbit's leg is extended for bandaging.

Placards with the names of bandage types are placed in background.

Music is started before each shot begins.

Rabbit's leg is bandaged in steps, showing each fold and movement with a separate shot.

Review of the shot is done to determine if it is acceptable or needs to be reshot.

Reshoot as necessary.

Editing of the piece, using the camcorder and a VCR, is carried out following the completion of shooting. Having an outside person review the product for mistakes or perception problems is an important final screening step before presentation. Reshooting and reediting are accepted parts of production to ensure high-quality instruction. Once the production is acceptable, it can be copied and used.

The production of videos has been a creative outlet for the author and a way to gain students' attention during class. The students have enjoyed the productions and have provided feedback for making them more interesting. It has been fun and rewarding to produce videos for classroom use. Many schools have video cameras and in some cases video-editing equipment for that professional quality. Give it a try — use the media and make your own videos.

USING COMPUTERS

The computer and its associated technologies have begun to be infused into the hands of the teacher. Using these tools, the teacher has an opportunity to be creative and dynamic. Some of these technologies look complicated and could be intimidating, but they are designed to be easy to use even by the most inexperienced individual.

As a new teacher, you might feel overwhelmed by the many new electronic technologies available, but as you mellow, you will become more aware of the tools available to help you develop from a good teacher into a dynamic one. For the most part, these new technologies are not as difficult to use as they first appear, and they can be extremely useful tools in your teaching career.

Computers are functioning in our world in many ways, some of which you may not be aware of because they are transparent to the user. In the 1990s, very few individuals can escape interacting with computers, because they have become a part of just about every industry. The airline industry, the grocery store industry, the banking industry, the telephone system industry, the transportation industry, the automobile industry, and the health care industry are all heavy users of computers and other electronic technologies.

Computers have become popular tools to assist professionals with their job tasks. The same is true for teachers. The computer can be used to help you present subject matter, as well as to manage what you teach with a few other activities in-between.

There are two basic types of computers used in schools today. They are the Apple II and Apple MacIntosh–based machines and the IBM or PC-based machines. Although a computer is a computer, differences in their individual operating systems make taking a course in learning how to use computers a must for new teachers.

If in your career as a health care professional, you had an opportunity to use computers, or you are simply interested in technology, you will find computers in education just another extension of the applications with which you are already familiar.

Computer Applications

Computers are used by professionals, including teachers, to complete applications (a particular use of software program) of word processing, spreadsheets, and databases. Perhaps the most common use for teachers consists of word processing. The computer is a word processor when you are using it as a typewriter, but it has the advantage over a typewriter in that you can make corrections (editing) easily and move text around (cut and paste) as needed without having to retype the entire manuscript or use correction materials. Typed lessons are neater and more easily read as opposed to handwritten ones. Word processed materials presented to students reinforce the professionalism of the instructor and the extreme importance of the lesson. There are many word processor programs available to select from; some are very simple, and other, more complicated ones include spelling checkers and thesaurus modules. Once you begin to use the computer as a word processor, you will wonder how you ever got along without one, because the uses are endless. For example, this entire book was word processed using a program called WordPerfect 5.1. It was checked grammatically using RightWriter.

Spreadsheet applications are probably less frequently used by teachers because they apply best to the accounting activities necessary for budgeting. Most teachers have such a tiny budget that they feel spreadsheets are too much trouble. Spreadsheets can, however, be used to keep student grades.

Database applications are used by teachers to manage all sorts of information. Keeping track of student emergency information, inventories, and purchases are simplified by the use of database programs. Information is kept in identified "fields" and "stored" until it is needed to generate a "report." A report can be printed using some or all of the fields anytime you desire. A report may be as simple as generating mailing labels or as complicated as producing a complete medical profile. Although it takes some time to get a database established, maintaining it becomes routine after a while and represents a timesaving tool for busy teachers and practitioners.

Students can also be taught word processing for creating a résumé and job application letters, as well as for printing term papers that you can actually read. They could use spreadsheets for projecting lab results and databases for keeping track of information that is important to them such as drugs and drug reactions, job options, and hospital staff data. If you have sufficient computers in your school, once you are comfortable using them, you will think of many creative ways to involve your students in using them for various applications.

Recordkeeping

Computers are used by teachers to "input" students' grades. Many of the programs on the market perform a variety of mathematical formulas to calculate averages, standard deviations, and means. Some let you drop the lowest grade. Most enable you to establish grade standards and to weight individual assignments. For example, some school districts consider a 93% as the lowest A; others use 90%. Some programs are equipped with graphics capabilities that can print a graph of your grade distribution. Using a grade book program allows you to help students calculate the minimum grade they need on any particular assignment or test in order to obtain the grade they desire for the term. Such a program also enables you to give written progress reports to your students as often as you like.

For Teaching

The computer offers many useful ways in which teachers can become better teachers. This chapter will present several ways that computers are used in teaching and classroom management.

The most common way to use a computer in education is in the computer-assisted instruction (CAI) mode. In this way the computer is used along with appropriate software (instructions that tell the computer what the operator wants to do) to assist students who are learning via a drill-and-practice process or to tutor students who need additional learning activities. Simulation is a common use of computers in VHO instruction. Games also are occasionally used as teaching tools.

Perceiving a computer as the tool it is makes learning to use one simpler. In most cases, you select the software, insert it into the computer, sit students in front of the computer, and turn it on. In many schools, a media specialist or computer instructor is available to assist both you and your students in becoming computer literate.

The hardest part of CAI is selection of the appropriate software to use to teach your students what you want them to learn. There are many software packages on the market to assist the health occupations education student in learning vocabulary and math facts. Popular topics for software would be anatomy and physiology, drugs and solutions, science, and nutrition. A list is provided for you in figure 17-1 to help you see what is available; national companies who distribute vocational education software distribute catalogs to all schools. Of primary concern is that you as the teacher must first review the software to determine if it is appropriate for your use. A simple procedure for this is to first locate or develop some way to keep track of your software reviews. Index cards or a database program will help you keep your reviews organized. List the title, author, vendor, cost, and type of equipment needed to utilize the application. A thorough review will take some time but will be time well spent when you prepare your lessons incorporating computer instruction. The following steps are suggested as a method for reviewing instructional software.

1. Preview the program for enjoyment. The first review will help you determine if you want to continue the review process. If you can't use the software, admit it and try to find something else that can be used.
2. Rerun the program as if you were an average student. If you like it and learn from it, so will your students.
3. Rerun the program for evaluation. Consider your best student and your worst student. Can they both benefit from the software?
4. Develop lesson plans using the software. Develop worksheets that will support the software and assist in the learning process of students. If you have a limited number of computers, you will want to develop worksheets for students to complete before they work on the computer, another to use while they are at the computer, and a third to use for reinforcement following their time on the computer.

As you can see, the process is time-consuming, but you will probably agree that it is worth the effort when your students learn their subject faster and more thoroughly. Computers are not designed to stand alone as the sole teacher; they need the teacher to facilitate the process.

Test Construction

Computer programs are also available that will allow you to develop a test item bank of test questions, keyed to objectives if desired, that can be used to generate tests at random for any occasion: quizzes, midterms, finals, and comprehensive examinations. It takes some time to enter the test items, but once they are in your database, all you have to do is select the questions.

Some computer test item programs also allow you to administer tests to your students using the computer. The student takes the test and receives immediate feedback as to the grade. This grade can then be saved to a teacher file, from which it can be retrieved at a later date and posted in an official gradebook. Some programs are even able to tell the teacher which questions the student missed. If your program uses individualized, paced modules, having and using a test item bank program will be an asset to your teaching.

The computer can also be used to prepare your lesson plans and all of the handout materials to be used in your instruction. You will find this application of the computer extremely valuable. As you become more proficient using the computer, there are many presentation tools that will help you to create overhead transparencies and illustrations. Lessons become very easy to revise and update as information changes or if you just want to try a different technique.

There are many ways that the computer can be used to manage your instruction and to help you become more efficient in your teaching.

INCORPORATING THE TELEPHONE

Teleconferencing is a variety of media that can be used over telephone lines (using the common RJ11 or RJ14 modular phone plug) to confer with other parties. Teleconferencing may use speaker phones and bridges, computers, freeze-frame video, audio/graphic methods, and facsimile machines joined together over phone lines — the RJ11 connection. Many of these technologies are probably already in place in most of the facilities in which medical care and health care training occurs. Certainly the facilities have a phone and phone lines.

A student entering a new profession at a new work site with unknown coworkers does not need to contend with the sudden culture shock of being forced to operate unfamiliar equipment. The student needs to be as well prepared as possible for the use of the technology prior to being hired.

Audio Teleconferencing

The simplest of teleconferencing is easily accessible for all telephone users. All that is needed is a telephone capable of connecting two or more parties together. Most office phone systems have a built-in conferencing capability. An operator-controlled switchboard is usually able to conference several calls together at one time. Speaker phones add to the convenience of audio conferencing by permitting many people in one room to hear and speak over a single phone line or permitting the user to freely take notes or access materials in the room by moving about.

The conference room environment is of great importance for the moderator/instructor to consider when setting up the conference. A room close to the welding lab, near the secretarial pool, or with a noisy air-conditioning system can destroy a multiparty audio conference. The physical decor of the facilities must not be so busy or elaborate as to distract the visual attention of participants. Audio conferencing is predominantly nonvisual in nature and requires the undivided attention of participants. Accompanying notes, memo pads, copies of outlines, and pictures or résumés of participants can help members to focus on the topic at hand.

Facsimile

Visualize an ideal multimedia teleconference that would require virtually no capital outlay based on current technological capabilities. Even the smallest of health care offices and clinics today have multiline phones, facsimile (fax) machines, and copy machines. These simple machines could produce an excellent foundation for inservicing and for educating the staff or for merely holding multioffice brainstorming/staff meetings.

Storing the fax machine and the copier in a room adjoining the conference area permits easy access to the equipment and yet maintains a quiet atmosphere in the learning area. The copier permits the copying of text material, notes, outlines, and visuals to be transmitted over the fax machine to the other locations as needed. Roll call can be taken swiftly (without taking up class time) by faxing a sign-up sheet to the facilitator's location.

Participants' photos and résumés can be faxed to the other sites at the beginning of the session to give the group a sense of familiarity and camaraderie. Preprogramming all of the fax machines for the numbers of each of the other sites will facilitate automatic forwarding of the materials when needed. One person at each site should be familiar with the phone system, fax machine, and copier in order to ensure that inevitable technology problems can be swiftly surmounted.

The computer fax/modems now available can save a great deal of time, money, and supplies. The conventional fax machine receives a paper image on one end and outputs a paper image on the other end of the RJ11 line (Figure 17-1). With the use of a fax/modem, paper is merely an added bonus that is used to make documentation copies or for mass reproduction. In a fax/modem setup, the sender may upload a file from disk through the modem to a conventional fax machine or to another fax/modem. The conventional fax machine will reproduce on paper but the fax/modem will download to a file that can be saved or printed at a later time. A paperless communication process can occur when both sender and receiver use the fax/modem system in the computer system.

This system can be expanded by purchasing a phone bridge that permits multiple sites to call in to a single number and be connected to each other automatically (Hudson, 1987). No operators or line swapping/holding is necessary. Audio conferences can be planned within minutes and require little preparation or training. Emergency sessions are possible, allowing for learning in "real time." Just dial the number and turn on the speaker.

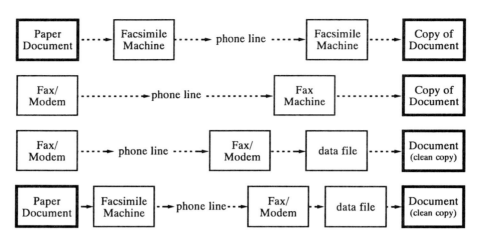

FIGURE 17-1: *Facsimile Methods*

Freeze-Frame

There are various other methods of using existing telephone lines. Freeze-frame video is the transmission of visual images over telephone lines intermittently with audio signals. Pictures of participants, visuals, or facilities can be projected to the other locations, allowing for greater visualization of the circumstances. The equipment needed for freeze-frame video may limit the facilities and require greater planning for the presentation (Hudson & Casey, 1985).

Recently the video phone has been made available to the general public, again, using regular telephone lines. It permits semilive motion to be sent over the telephone. Think of the applications for this technology—between two sites or between multiple sites using a telephone bridge.

☞ COMBINING THE TELEPHONE AND THE COMPUTER

Integrating the standard telephone connection at home or work with a computer, communications software, and modem offers you and your students access to the world. Usually, this access is free or at very reasonable cost.

Electronic Mail

Electronic mail systems permit communication with individuals or groups. To get started you must have a computer and a modem. The computer may be almost any flavor that you have available. Both Apple and IBM compatibles are popular computers that accommodate electronic mail. If you already have a computer, a modem can be added for $75–$150. You will want to purchase one that communicates at 2,400 baud or faster. The modem can be internal (inside the computer) or external. For a nominal fee, a local computer store (perhaps where you bought your modem), will install and set it up in your computer. Once it has been installed and properly configured, it is relatively easy to use. You will also need a communications program such as Qmodem, Telix, Procomm or one of the other fine communications programs available. Many times a basic communication program is even included with the purchase of the modem.

To get the modem running properly it will be necessary to configure it to run with your computer. Read the documentation that came with the modem and the communication program. Again, you may want to rely on a local computer dealer to set this up for you. You may leave behind questions and answers to problems when other students or the instructor are unavailable. This means of electronic communication is termed asynchronous because users can send and receive "mail" at any time. One example of a public education network is the Florida Information Resource Network (FIRN). FIRN permits any teacher in the Florida public school system to use the network at no cost. An excellent network, FIRN is used for both professional communications and course offerings (Hudson, Paugh, & Olmstead, 1990).

Computerized programs require personal exploration of the system as well as self-motivation. It is easy for an instructor to tell which students in the program are putting sufficient effort and planning into their educational endeavors. Electronic mail for individual and group messages or discussion of topics empowers students and teachers to manage their time more efficiently.

Bulletin Boards

The 1990s have developed into an age of electronic communication, and one of the fastest-growing areas of communication is the electronic bulletin board system (BBS). By harnessing the astonishing power of the personal computer and linking it with a phone line, BBSers are able to exchange information with each other, reaching out to all corners of the globe.

There are over 10,000 bulletin boards operating nationwide, with about three new boards going on-line daily. FidoNet, one of the earliest bulletin board networks, was started in 1984. Within a year, the network had grown to 300 boards; by the end of 1990, there were over 6,000 FidoNet boards located in thirty-five countries. These boards are generally operated from a home or small business by one or two individuals who began these as a hobby. There are several commercial data banks, or information resources, which also provide bulletin board functions. These include data banks such as CompuServe, DIALOG, America Online, and Prodigy, to name a few.

There are many government-operated bulletin boards that BBSers may tap into. The U.S. Information Agency, the Government Computer Network, the National Weather Service, NASA, the National Science Foundation, and the Department of Commerce are among the agencies that make bulletin boards available to the public. Some cities are establishing community-focused boards. Cleveland's Free-Net is an outstanding example. There citizens can obtain local news, chat with one another, or consult health care or educational professionals without leaving their home or office.

For educators there are education bulletin boards, such as the National Education Association bulletin board, and state educators BBS, such as FIRN. These boards not only provide electronic mail services but also allow educators to keep abreast with educational developments, legislation, and lively discussions of interest to educators.

Local bulletin boards are often free to tap into or charge a moderate yearly fee. Many larger cities have 100 or more active boards that are just a local phone call away. Many have literally thousands of "freeware" or low-cost "shareware" programs that are offered for downloading (taking it down from their bulletin board and sticking it in your computer). Many of these are offered free by their author; others ask for a donation if the program is used. For teachers there is a large selection of educational software, which may be of value in the classroom. Some software programs have been written just for teachers, such as electronic gradebooks and lesson planners, in addition to interactive programs for students. These programs cover almost every discipline.

Both Rime and Interlink offer an educational conference with many active, lively discussions concerning education. Often students log on to these conferences and give input from their perspective. For teachers in the health-related fields, there are medical conferences in which health-related topics are discussed. These conferences not only discuss many of the newest techniques but also follow the latest legislation that may be of concern to participants. And there are local bulletin boards run by health care workers specializing in certain medical areas.

With the relatively low cost of bulletin boarding, many educators now are tapping this new technology for both fun and education. There are many different types of BBS. You'll find several that are just right for you, but to do that you have to make that first call.

To call a BBS you will have to know its phone number. Many times the numbers are available from local computer dealers, friends, or network administrators. Some of the more popular bulletin board numbers may even be included with your communications software. Once you log on to a BBS, you will find numbers posted of many other BBS's in your area. By calling a few different local BBS's, you can find out which ones are right for you.

You enter the BBS phone number into the dialing directory of your program. You then instruct it to dial that number for you. When the two computers connect, the other computer, called the host computer, will ask for your name and password. The first time you log on, your name will not be in its database because you have never called before. The host computer will then ask if you would like to log on as a new user. You will need to type "yes" at the prompt. The host will then ask a series of personal questions, which you must answer honestly. The questions will include your name, address, and phone number. The systems operator (SYSOP) of the host computer may also want to know your age, work phone number, and type of computer you use; some even ask if you have any hobbies.

The reason that the SYSOPs ask these questions and store the answers in their database is to ensure that you are not a hacker trying to ruin their computer. Remember, you are roaming around in very expensive computer systems, and until they know who *you* are, they are going to limit your access.

Often a personal BBS will go through a callback routine. The host computer will ask you to verify the phone number you are calling from and then will hang up on you and call you back at that number. You will then have *your* computer answer the phone when the host computer calls, and you will send your password back to the host computer. This is quite easy to do, and what is about to happen and what to do when you are called back are explained clearly to you. With this completed, your security level is usually raised much higher so that you may join conferences or upload and download files.

A BBS is laid out like a house. When you call and log on, you will be in the Main Room. There you can check your mail and get the latest news. There are also doors from the Main Room that you may open, which will put you into a completely different area of the computer. There you are free to explore that room or roam to another area of the computer by opening another door. Throughout the whole process you are given directions so you don't get lost.

There are two areas of primary interest to you as a teacher. One is the files area and the other the message area. The directory of the files area usually shows you a large number of shareware programs that are available for you to download. There are many educational shareware programs available for downloading. Many of these programs may not fit your need at the moment; perhaps some of them will. There are ones such as gradebook programs for teachers as well as learning programs for students. When you decide on one or more of these programs that you would like to look at, you may immediately download them, and when you have finished your communications session, you may use them. The program has been transferred into your computer just as if you had gone to a store and purchased it.

The nice thing about shareware is you may use the programs to see if they are of value to you. If you decide to keep and use a program, you are expected to pay the author for the work he or she has put into it. Documentation comes with the program telling you what the author expects from you. This is all on the honor system, but by registering your software you allow the shareware system to work. Most of the time the program fee is nominal ($10–$30). This is considered an excellent value compared with the cost factor of commercial software. Some of the programs are even distributed free for all to use.

Another area that you will need to explore is the Conference area. Like in a large file cabinet, messages are stored in an orderly fashion. You can access only the areas that you are interested in and read those messages. There are over 200 conferences defined on the Rime network alone. Some have as many as 150 or more new messages per day. The Education conference has an average of 15 messages each day. On the Education conference on the Rime network, you are free to discuss teaching problems that you may be having, or you may help others with problems they may have posted. You may want to ask another teacher about a computer program that you are looking for and get recommendations from the trenches on what works for them. It's people helping people. Be forewarned: bulletin boarding can become addictive, but you will meet many new friends.

Another area that primary and secondary teachers may want to explore is setting up a BBS in their own school or classroom. Of course a computer would have to be available along with a modem and phone line. This is becoming more popular every day. Once you become proficient at bulletin boarding, you will find that a BBS is relatively easy to start and maintain. If your school isn't in a position to accommodate a BBS, it doesn't mean that you cannot still have your students involved in BBSing.

Most BBS's have an easy way for you to quickly download a new days' mail (messages) and read it off-line at your leisure. If you have even one computer in your classroom or have a laptop you can bring from home, you and your students can read and respond to those messages. It is easy, under your direction, for students to type messages to each other and discuss things among themselves. The messages can then be uploaded through the BBS when you return home from work, and a new package of mail downloaded for the next day's class. Getting students involved in reading and responding to messages can be a powerful learning tool. It will certainly familiarize them with computers and improve their keyboarding skills. Perhaps of even greater value will be the improvement in their communications skills. Young minds benefit from putting their creative thoughts into words. With your help, students can be taught to write well-thought-out messages with the tact and finesse that are often missing today.

Health Care Resources

Many communities have computer-based help lines for local citizens to call to receive emergency and nonemergency advice 24 hours a day. One such program provided by a hospital is ask-a-nurse, which is available for contacting a local nurse, who can input symptoms, medical conditions, or prescriptions into a database and recommend a course of action. The caller may be referred to an emergency room or advised to call a physician immediately or give the situation some more time. A log (database) of the interaction and the "patient" receives a checkup call the next day to see if the help was useful or if the caller needs additional help in seeking a solution.

Cleveland Free-Net is a public-access computerized health care assistance program. It provides the community with information in the areas of diagnosis, symptoms, treatment, medications, testing, and prevention (Hekelman, Kelly, Grudner, 1990). People who are unable or unwilling to consult their regular medical provider can access confidential assistance about their concerns. This program may provide medical facilities with a screening method that prevents minor problems from monopolizing the valuable time and talent of the caregivers and permits more time to be devoted to the seriously ill. In addition, escalating health care and insurance costs may be contained when unnecessary trips are eliminated.

Portable equipment, such as electrocardiograph (EKG) units, is used in conjunction with phone lines to automatically send readings to health care facilities from patients' homes. A life-threatening situation can be handled quickly and with little effort even before emergency medical care arrives.

One such incident was portrayed on a national emergency television show. The patient had had a heart attack and his wife hooked up the phone to his briefcase-enclosed EKG machine. The hospital read the incoming tape and advised the wife to administer a shock from the instruments enclosed with the EKG unit. The patient was revived prior to the emergency squad's arrival.

Many databases are available for both instructional and noninstructional purposes. There are Chemical Industry Notes, a Pharmaceutical News Index, Chemical Exposure, Chemsearch, Chemzero, TSCA Initial Inventory, Foundation Grants Index, Grants, Chemlaw, Drug Information Fulltext, EMBase, Health Planning Administration, International Pharmaceutical Abstracts, Life Science Collection, Medline, Mental Health Abstracts, Telegen, Scisearch, Child Abuse and Neglect, Family Resources, and PsycINFO, to name several (Lewis, 1984).

Educational Resources

Another resource used frequently in Florida for educational purposes is the State University System of Florida's Library Users Information Service (LUIS), an electronic card catalog. Many state university systems have this type of program in place. And some local public libraries have added the technology for use by their clientele.

The LUIS on-line library media database is a program provided by FIRN. Users may access media by title, author, or subject. They receive by way of response an index of books with that title, by that author, or on that subject. A subindex may be presented for more detailed titles on subjects or by authors. The choice of a particular title results in viewing a bibliography, subject headings, the location in the library, the call number, and the availability of the material.

This information will provide long-distance learners or medical personnel with a means of preparing a shopping list of materials to investigate or check out. They can arrange their selections by stacks or floors, according to the information they received on LUIS, leaving off their list those materials that are checked out or missing based on the availability note. The ability to organize and plan library "junkets" increases the availability of research and clinical time. Time compression is extremely important to the full-time employee/parent/student.

A current Educational Resources Information Center (ERIC) microfiche database is available over the same FIRN LUIS system. A similar process to using LUIS provides the user with a listing of ERIC files available on microfiche at a local ERIC depository and presents an abstract of the research material requested.

ADVOCNET, an electronic communications system on a national level for networking in vocational education, is managed by the National Center for Research in Vocational Education. This system provides access to the national database Bibliographic Retrieval Service (BRS), which provides Vocational Education Curriculum Materials (VECM), ERIC, RIVE, Dissertation Abstracts, and other databases for research and curriculum development. All database information is available for downloading to a disk file or printer for future reference.

Computer Conferencing

Using computer conferencing as a medium for education is a step beyond electronic mail and VHO bulletin boards. This medium permits discussions by topics, again an asynchronous activity. Persons at distant sites are able to access each other and discuss topics at their convenience. Imagine a group of VHO teachers who could revise curricula and not be required to travel to meetings.

Another example is that students in remote areas would be able to obtain course work that is not convenient or accessible in the conventional sense (Harrasim, 1991). Health care providers who work full-time are sometimes unable to attend recertification or degree advancement courses unless they are within an acceptable driving distance of a major university or off-campus facility or unless they are scheduled on a compatible shift. A student registered for a computer conferencing class must learn computing in a very short time frame, as there is no time to waste and superficial attention to the subject would be detrimental.

The novice computer user will need to network with other students and computer users in order to make it through difficulties. The technology bug will then perhaps bite most of them, and they will look for every computer conferencing course they can find.

Experience in computer use, computer conferencing, and computer-based research can be beneficial for early success in a computer conferencing course but is not a prerequisite. Students may vary in experience from no exposure to computers, to daily use of computers on and off the job.

TELEVISION

Local, state, and national broadcast television constitute yet another technology for delivery of instruction. It can be via cable, microwave, or satellite as the delivery medium. Video, in most cases, is one way, whereas audio may be two way or multisite using a telephone conferencing service or a telephone bridge.

Guest speakers, field "trips," special programs, and entire courses can be offered using this technology. Preplanning is essential, just as one sees to for traditional classes, for effective programs.

Cable television requires hardwiring among sites and in the public sector is typically a subscription or pay-for-view service. Microwave or Instructional Television Fixed Service (ITFS) uses a beamed signal without the cable to transmit programming between sites. Satellite, of course, uses orbiting satellites that beam signals over a wide area that can be received by ground satellite receiving stations, or dishes.

In VHO education, you may be a television instruction participant in your teaching role, either as a guest speaker or even as a student (Arnold, Adkins & Hudson, 1992). As a presenter, it is incumbent on you to be prepared, provide appropriate visuals, and promote participation by students; you do not have to be a technology wizard, but you must teach and involve students. As a student, be an active participant, and study the process as well as the content.

Through long-distance education, students can actively share their experiences with fellow students and teacher educators. A combination of audio and computer conferencing media provides access to the educational community and empowers the adult learner.

References

Arnold, B., A. Adkins, and L. Hudson (1992). Using distance learning technologies. In *Proceedings of the 1992 SALT Conference*.

Arms, C. (ed.) (1988). *Campus Networking Strategies*. Digital Press.

Cohen, A. (1991). *A Guide to Networking.* Boston, MA: Boyd & Fraser.

Cornell, R. A. (Spring 1992). Style over substance or vice versa II: How'd we do in D.C.? *The DEMM Perspective,* 19 (4)

Cornell, R. A. (Winter 1992). Style over substance or vice versa: Where was it in Orlando? *The DEMM Perspective,* 19 (3): 9–11.

Gagne, R. M., L. J. Briggs, and W. W. Wager (1992). *Principles of Instructional Design,* 4th ed. Orlando, FL: Harcourt Brace Jovanovich.

Hansell, K. (1989). *The Teleconferencing Manager's Guide.* White Plains, NY: Knowledge Industry.

Hudson, L. (1985). Audio teleconference and freeze-frame technologies combined for distance learners. *Proceedings of First Annual Society for Applied Learning Technologies Conference for Health Sciences, 1.*

Hudson, L. (Winter 1987). Audio teleconferencing at the University of Central Florida. *Journal of Educational Media and Library Science,* 25(2): 177–185.

Hudson, L., and D. Bunting (August 1982). Telenetwork system: A viable alternative for distance instruction. Educational Technology, 17-19.

Hudson, L., and T. Casey (1985). Freeze-frame compressed video in the classroom: A cooperative study with the University of Central Florida and Racal-Milgo. In C. Olgren (ed.), *Teleconferencing and Electronic Communications, V.* University of Wisconsin, Center for Interactive Programs.

Hudson, L., P. Kinser, and J. Cragan (1985). Interactive audio telecommunications: A cooperative community venture. *Electronic Communication, IV.* In L. Parker and C. Olgren (eds.), University of Wisconsin, Center for Interactive Programs, p.1–7.

Hudson, L., R. Paugh and P. Olmstead (1990). Extending the RJ11 connection for audio and computer conferencing. In A. Miller (ed.), *National Conference on Applications of Computer Conferencing to Teacher Applications and Human Resource Development.* Columbus, OH: College of Education.

Hudson, L., S. Sorg, and B. Keene (1984). Teleconferencing instruction: A pilot approach. [monograph]. *Ideas in Education.* University of Central Florida, College of Education, pp. 30–37.

Johansen, R., R. Adler, J. Charles, B. McNeal, R. Plumber, E. Baker, M. Boone, C. Bullen and E. Gold (1984). *Teleconferencing and Beyond: Communications in the Office of the Future.* New York: McGraw-Hill.

Jordahl, G. (1991). Breaking down classroom walls: Distance learning comes of age. *Technology and Learning*, 11: 73–78.

Kelleher, K. and T. Cross (1985). *Teleconferencing*. Englewood Cliffs, NJ: Prentice-Hall.

Kemp, J. E. (1985). *The Instructional Design Process*. New York: Harper & Row.

Kemp, J. E., and D. C. Smellie (1989). *Planning, Producing, and Using Instructional Media*. New York: Harper & Row.

Kinnaman, D. (1990). Staff development: How to build your winning team. *Technology and Learning*, 11: 24–30.

Lewis, S. (1984). *Plugging in: The microcomputerist's guide to telecommunications*. Radnor, PA: Chilton Book Company.

Mager, R. F. (1984). *Preparing Instructional Objectives*, revised 2nd ed. Belmont, CA: David S. Lake Publishers.

Marsh, P. O. (1983). *Messages That Work*. Englewood Cliffs, NJ: Educational Technology Publications.

Mayer, I. (1985). *The Electronic Mailbox*. Hasbrouck Heights, NJ: Hayden.

Norton, R., and R. Stammen (May 1990). LONG – distance learning. *Vocational Education Journal*, 26–27, 41.

Olgren, C. and L. Parker (1983). *Teleconferencing Technology and Applications*. Dedham, MA: Artech.

Orwig, G., and L. Hudson (1985). Telecommunications and the school media program. *School and Library Media Annual, III*. S. Aaron and P. Scales (eds.). Englewood, CO: Littleton Libraries Unlimited, pp. 387–396.

Prosser, C. and T. Quigley (1949). *Vocational Education in a Democracy*. Chicago, IL: American Technical Society.

Trudell, L., J. Bruman, and D. Oliver (1984). *Options for Electronic Mail*. White Plains, NY: Knowledge Industry.

18

Uses of Future Technology: What's Next?

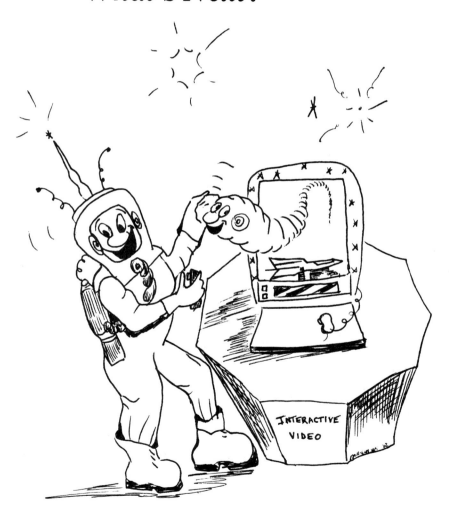

☞ APPLYING INTERACTIVE VIDEO

Interactive videodisc (IVD) programs offer an exciting and effective means for providing instruction in many areas of vocational health occupations programs (VHO). Studies have reported a number of advantages for IVD over other methods of instruction. One characteristic of a well-designed IVD program is that it is consistent; lesson content, method of presentation, and instructional features are predetermined. Studies have also demonstrated increased student retention, reduced learning time, and increased motivation for IVD. Because of the realism required for many of the procedures and scenarios in health care education, IVD is often the medium of choice. In fact, the health sciences support one of the largest and fastest-growing markets for videodisc programs. The tremendous potential of this technology makes learning about IVD a necessity for all educators in health fields. This section includes an overview of videodisc technology, illustrations of hardware configurations, discussions of health care applications, and lists of IVD resources.

Videodisc Formats

A videodisc is a durable medium for storing video and audio information. The video recorded on a disk is produced by shooting and editing a master videotape. One limitation is that only 30 or 60 minutes of motion video will fit on each side of a 12-inch disk (depending on the format). In addition, once the video has been recorded onto the videodisc, it cannot be changed or erased. Videodiscs are recorded by encoding microscopic pits on a platter and covering them with a protective plastic coating. Videodiscs are a form of optical media—that is, they are read with a tiny light beam. The combination of the durable coating and contact-free reading process produces a medium that is resistant to wear and maintains a consistent quality.

There are two different formats used to record a videodisc. These formats are referred to as constant angular velocity (CAV) and constant linear velocity (CLV). Both formats offer certain advantages and disadvantages.

Motion video consists of a series of individual frames that display at a rate of 30 frames per second to create the illusion of motion. When video is recorded in the CAV format, it is configured in concentric circles on the disk, with each circle representing one frame of video. This configuration allows the video to freeze-frame. In other words, the laser beam can play one of the frames (circles) over and over again, creating the same effect as pausing a videotape. A videotape can become damaged if it is paused for more than 20 seconds; however, in the case of a disk, a picture can remain in the still mode for hours. Each side of a CAV disk can store a maximum of 30 minutes of motion video.

The ability to freeze-frame, however, also allows a user to access individual frames on the disk. With 30 minutes of motion on each side of the disk, and 30 frames per second, one can access any of 54,000 still frames (30 frames per second × 60 seconds per minute × 30 minutes per side = 54,000 frames per side). It is easy to access a desired frame with a remote control unit or computer because a number (from 1 to 54,000) is automatically encoded on every frame of a CAV disk during the recording process.

The CAV format also provides features such as step-frames (going forward or backward one frame at a time), scanning (jumping rapidly through the disk content), and multiple speeds (playing at two or three times the normal speed, forward or in reverse). These features, and the fact that the laser beam can quickly (in less than 3 seconds) jump to any frame, make the CAV format the most popular format for creating educational videodisc programs.

The CLV format utilizes a different configuration to record the disk. The CLV format is much more linear (hence the expression constant linear velocity), and the video frames are encoded in a spiral pattern. On a CLV disk, the inner circle contains one frame, whereas the outer circle may contain many frames. This format allows twice as much video to be stored on each side (60 minutes). However, many of the features, such as freeze-frame, step frame, and multiple speeds are not available. CLV discs are often used to store movies and documentaries that are designed to be linear, rather than interactive. CLV disks do not contain frame numbers. Instead, they have time code embedded on the disk, which is listed in hours, minutes, and seconds. For example, 0:06.31 would refer to the section that is 6 minutes and 31 seconds into the video material. It is important to note that although you can use a remote control to search for a particular time code on a CLV disk, you will not get a still picture. Instead, you can search and then start to play from that particular location. Figure 18-1 summarizes some features of CAV and CLV videodisks.

Features of CAV and CLV formats: Both formats of videodiscs (CAV and CLV) provide two separate audio tracks. These tracks can be played together or independently. In many cases, each track will contain a different language. For example, many videodisc programs for schools now contain one audio track in English and an identical track in Spanish. The audio is heard only if the videodisc is playing at the standard rate of 30 frames per second.

Levels of Interactive Videodisc

Interactivity is a communication process between the user and the videodisc delivery system. Interactive systems allow students to make decisions, receive

FEATURE	CAV	CLV
Minutes per Side	30	60
Normal Play	Yes	Yes
Still Frame	Yes	No
Step Frame	Yes	No
Multispeed	Yes	No
Scan	Yes	Yes
Frame Search	Yes	No
Time Search	Yes	Yes
Chapter Search	Yes	Yes

FIGURE 18-1: *Features of CAV and CLV formats. (CAV = constant angular velocity; CLV = constant linear velocity)*

feedback, and choose their own sequence. There are three different levels (I, II, and III) of interactivity that are commonly used to refer to the delivery of videodisc programs. These levels differ in the amount of control available and hardware configuration required.

Level I systems consist of a videodisc player, a television monitor, and a manual control device. The manual control device is usually either a remote control unit or a barcode reader. The advantage of level I delivery is that it allows the user to exercise some control over the program without the expense and trouble of connecting a computer. Many level I videodiscs are designed with chapter stops and/or picture stops. These features allow you to use a remote control unit to search for and access a particular chapter. For example, if a disk had five chapters, you could press "search chapter 3" on the remote control unit to jump to chapter 3. At the end of chapter 3, the disc would automatically stop (on a picture stop) until you made your next choice.

Both CAV and CLV videodiscs may have chapter and picture stops on the disk. The exact number of chapters varies depending on the purpose of the disk and its intended use. Barcode readers are also popular input devices for

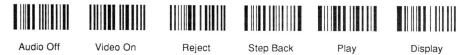

FIGURE 18-2: *Sample barcodes.*

level I videodiscs. Generic barcodes are usually provided with the disk player (Figure 18-2). In addition, many programs now provide books with barcodes to access a particular still frame or chapter on the disk.

The hardware for level II interactivity is the same as for level I. However, the videodisc player must contain a built-in microprocessor to read a special computer code that is embedded onto the videodisc. This allows the user more flexibility through the remote control unit. For example, a multiple-choice question may be placed on a still frame of the disk. The user presses the number for the answer on the remote unit, and the videodisc branches automatically to the next segment or to remediation. The advantage of level II interactivity is increased control of the disk without connecting a computer. The disadvantages are that only certain videodisc players have the components required, and the controlling software cannot be changed because it is embedded on the videodisc.

Level III interactivity combines the control and interactivity of a computer with the audio and visual realism of the videodisc. This level is usually referred to as IVD. The advantage is the increased flexibility that the computer can provide. In addition, management records can be stored on the computer

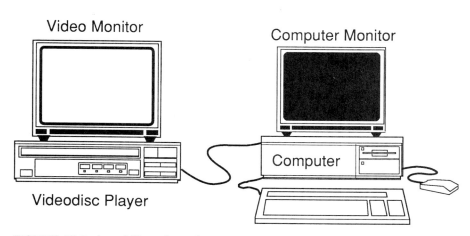

FIGURE 18-3: *Level III configuration.*

to track students' progress with the programs. The hardware required for level III is shown in Figure 18-3. It has the same configuration as level I, with the addition of a computer, monitor, and interface cable. An alternative configuration is to use a multisync monitor, such as InfoWindows. Multisync monitors allow both the video and the computer outputs to be displayed on the same monitor; however, they are more expensive.

Level III can configure with two monitors. When purchasing a system for level III delivery, it is extremely important to note the required hardware. Although a videodisc player can be connected to any computer (IBM, Macintosh, or Apple II), the software is not interchangeable. Therefore, if the program is designed for an IBM computer, a Macintosh will not work. In addition, if the program is designed for an InfoWindow system, an IBM PS/2 monitor will not be able to provide the proper display. Many programs in the health field are designed for touch screens (which are quite expensive). However, in most cases, a mouse may be substituted for the touch screen.

Applications

There are a wide variety of IVD programs available for VHO education. Many of the programs are designed to teach in the tutorial format; others use a simulation or role-playing approach. A comprehensive index of contact points for videodisc resources referred to in this section (and others) is provided in the appendix. Linear movies and documentary videotapes have been a valuable asset to health science education for many years. Many of the existing videotapes (and some new ones) are now being recorded on videodisc format, providing a durable medium for inexpensive delivery. Additional advantages for videodiscs (as opposed to videotapes) are that they do not degenerate with use, and they are easy to store.

The Incredible Human Machine, by National Geographic, is an excellent videodisc (in CLV format) for about $30. It offers an inside look at the human body, its systems, and their functions. Similar disks, focusing on the human brain and the nervous system, are available from Encyclopaedia Britannica.

Many interactive health programs are designed as tutorials that present students with new information and then reinforce the information with questions. Students can often branch off to different segments of the lesson based on their interests or needs. Interactive tutorials provide an excellent method for delivering visual and procedural information. In addition, most programs have a built-in management system to generate reports and records for students and instructors.

Volumetric Devices, by Synergistic Educational Technology Systems, is a level III tutorial program that operates on most major MS-DOS configurations. It provides the student with a demonstrate/practice approach to commonly used infusers, clinical uses of intravenous infusion pumps, and administration of intravenous medications. Questions with remediation and enhancement material are embedded in the instructional content. Student tracking is also included for reports.

Therapeutic Communication, by Fuld Institute for Technology in Nursing Education, examines the art of effective communication with patients. It provides basic communication theory and skills and progresses to specific techniques for nurse-patient relationships. The lessons are enhanced by exercises, practice scenarios, and embedded questions to reinforce the information. The program is designed for the IBM InfoWindow system.

MultiMedia libraries are offered by some of the IVD programs. These give users the opportunity to explore a wide array of interrelated information in video clips, still frames, sound, maps, text, and graphics. Users can interact in any number of ways and with a multitude of approaches to investigate their interests. These programs make excellent presentation tools for teachers and research tools for students. *Understanding Ourselves*, by Optical Data Corporation (produced by ABC News Interactive), consists of three videodisc programs — AIDS, Drugs and Substance Abuse, and Teenage Sexuality — which are designed to provide young adults with factual information on these important but controversial topics. For example, the AIDS program shows interviews and discussions with Ryan White and other young adults who talk frankly and openly about the disease. The programs consist of a double-sided videodisc, a guidebook with barcodes, and a control program written in HyperCard for the Macintosh.

Many disks are designed as a series of still frames or pictures called visual databases. They can be equated to a slide carousel with up to 54,000 slides (that will never be in upside-down or backwards). These still frames can be accessed in a matter of seconds with either the remote control unit, the barcode reader, or a computer. Most of the disks provide a written log with the frame numbers for easy access. As example, *The Slice of Life III*, from the University of Utah, contains over 26,000 still images contributed by medical schools across the country. The disk is level I and is updated every year. A corresponding index of all of the frame numbers is available to facilitate access to the video. *The Living Textbook: Life Science*, by Optical Data Corporation, focuses on all the basic concepts in high school and college life sciences and biology studies. The program contains thousands of slides, an image directory, and a lesson guide. These programs are designed for either Macintosh or Apple IIe delivery with two monitors.

Simulations re-create real-life situations that may be dangerous or expensive for students to experience in person. Students can explore various alternatives and make life-and-death decisions without harm to themselves or others. Examples: *Emergency*, by DataStar, provides simulations of real emergency situations and is designed for emergency personnel. Scenarios are enacted that allow students to see outcomes of their decisions regarding emergency situations. If the student does the right procedures, the patient stabilizes. If the student makes a fatal mistake, you can guess the result. *Emergency* is designed for delivery on most of the major MS-DOS platforms with touch screen. *The American Heart Association Cardiopulmonary Resuscitation Program*, by Actronics, Inc., includes electronic adult and infant mannequins to provide realistic CPR practice and testing. The mannequins are connected to the computer, which can then read and respond to correct and incorrect procedures. The hardware (IBM) for the system may be purchased as a complete package or in individual components.

Some videodisc programs are designed to teach soft skills or interpersonal techniques by use of role-playing. Programs generally set up a series of scenarios with actors, and the student can make decisions and see enacted the result of the decision. *Communication Challenges in Nursing: Establishing Rapport and Trust* focuses on developing feelings of trust between health care professionals and patients. The system allows the learner to build various interchanges with a patient and to witness the consequences of the communications used. This program is produced by Intelligent Images, Inc., and is delivered on IBM InfoWindow systems or compatibles. *When Your Parent Drinks Too Much*, by Coronet/MTI, allows the viewer to witness how children can deal with family drinking problems. Designed for young adults, this program includes a teacher's guide with additional information. This videodisc is level I.

An exciting feature of some videodisc programs is the ability to repurpose video segments and create documentaries or reports. This allows teachers to customize a presentation and enables students to create video reports for class. *The ABC News Interactive Programs* (AIDS, Drugs and Substance Abuse, and Teenage Sexuality) include a video report maker feature that provides access to all video stills and motion segments. The user can rearrange the sequence of the video and change the length of the segments. The selected segments are added to a Video Listing for presentation. Documentary maker can save up to fifteen segments in one listing and provides a word processing feature to add scripts or notes for the video. In addition, the AIDS program includes options for recording sound (using a MacRecorder) and for generating video overlays for titles and captions.

Implementation

The following are suggestions for the implementation of videodisc technology into your curriculum.

1. Educate yourself and your staff first. Inservice classes are available in many districts, and many colleges and universities offer classes and degree programs in technology.
2. Choose a champion supporter and a small group to begin with. The enthusiasm will spread, and soon you will be implementing IVD with more and more classes.
3. Ask for a demonstration before purchasing a system or a program. In many cases, the vendor will demo the product or provide a demonstration program for review. If possible, request input from students, instructors, and administrators.
4. One of the most difficult problems encountered in the selection of materials is incompatibility. Be sure that you have or can afford the correct hardware for the program. Most of the programs are not interchangeable between hardware platforms.
5. Check storage requirements. Some IVD programs require many megabytes of hard-drive space.
6. Choose the software that best supports the school's curriculum. Instructors are usually more likely to utilize a program that enhances their content area and provides support materials.
7. Order catalogs, attend conferences, read product reviews, and ask others in your field for their recommendations. Some conferences focus strictly on the use of interactive video in health care.
8. Investigate grants and other funding sources to purchase software and hardware. Some subject areas, such as AIDS, have a high level of public interest and are therefore a potential area for grant activity.
9. Contact medical schools at nearby universities. Medical schools are leaders in the production of videodiscs; however, many of them never advertise their efforts.

With videodisc technology, vocational health care professionals can enjoy the combination of audio and visual realism with the interactivity of a computer. A single videodisc can incorporate many forms of instructional media — text, charts, graphs, audio, and video motion. In addition, a videodisc player provides easy access to information stored on the disk. The user can randomly search for any frame or chapter, vary the direction of play (forward or reverse), and vary the speed (normal, fast, slow, or still frame). When capacities of a videodisc and player are combined with the power of a computer, the system becomes a tool for delivering individualized interactive instruction, illustrating lecture material, or providing a multimedia research library. The integration of this technology can help make educators more efficient and students more productive.

Videodisc Terminology

Baud rate: The speed at which binary data are transmitted. Common baud rates are 1,200, 2,400, 4,800 and 9,600.

Chapter: One linear segment of a videodisc. Chapter searches can be achieved through the remote control unit or the barcode reader.

Chapter stop: A frame on the disk that can be accessed by performing a chapter search with the remote control.

Constant Angular Velocity (CAV): A videodisc format that can address each frame separately and can store a maximum of 30 minutes of motion on each side.

Constant linear velocity (CLV): A videodisc format that can store 60 minutes of motion on each side but cannot address or display an individual frame.

Frame: A single, complete picture in a video recording.

HyperCard: A Macintosh-based software program that allows access to a variety of information, including text, audio, and videodisc.

InfoWindows: A computer monitor produced by the IBM Corporation that is multisnyc and has a touch screen.

Interactive Videodisc (IVD): Generally refers to level III interactivity in which a computer is used to control the videodisc player.

Level I interactivity: Control of the videodisc player is achieved through the player, a remote control, or a barcode reader. The player is not connected to a computer.

Level II interactivity: The videodisc contains a control program as well as the video material. The player is not connected to a computer.

Level III interactivity: A computer is used to control the videodisc player.

Monitor: A visual display device capable of accepting video and audio signals.

Receiver: A visual display device capable of receiving and displaying a broadcast signal.

Scan: A mode of play in which the player skips over several frames at a time. Scanning can be done in forward or reverse.

Step frame: A videodisc player function that moves from one frame to the next (can be forward or reverse).

Still frame: A single video frame presented as a static image.

Call or write to the following companies for catalogs and information on videodiscs.

Actronics
810 River Avenue
Pittsburgh, PA 15212
412-231-6200

AIMS Media
6901 Woodley Avenue
Van Nuys, CA 91406-4878
800-367-2467

American College of Radiology
1891 Preston White Drive
Reston, VA 22091
703-648-8989

American Journal of Nursing
Educational Services Division/E47
6555 West 57th Street
New York, NY 10019

Applied Learning International
1751 West Diehl Avenue
Naperville, IL 60540
312-369-3000

Cognitive Design Technologies
1501 Westview Drive
Coralville, IA 52241
319-337-8109

Coronet/MTI Film & Video
108 Wilmot Road
Deerfield, IL 60015
800-621-2131

Darox Interactive
1103 West Isabel Street
Burbank, CA 91506
800-733-1010

DataStar Education Systems
4220 98th Street, Suite 110
Edmonton, AB T6E 6A1
Canada
403-463-3327

Encyclopedia Britannica
Educational Corporation
310 South Michigan Avenue
Chicago, IL 60604
800-554-9862

FITNE
28 Station Street
Athens, OH 45701
614-592-2511

Health EduTech
7801 East Bush Lake Road, Suite 350
Minneapolis, MN 55435
612-831-0445

Health Sciences Consortium
201 Silver Cedar Court
Chapel Hill, NC 27514
919-942-8731

IBM Corporation
InfoWindow Educational Videodisc Catalog
3301 Windy Ridge Parkway
Marietta, GA 30067

Image Premastering Services
1781 Prior Avenue North
St. Paul, MN 55113
612-644-7802

Intelligent Images Inc.
1103 West Isabel Street
Burbank, CA 91506
818-563-1100

Interactive Health Network
400 Colony Square, Suite 152
51201 Peachtree Street, NE
Atlanta, GA 30361

Learning Arts
P.O. Box 179
Wichita, KS 67201
316-682-3066

Medical Interactive
3708 Mount Diablo Boulevard,
Suite 120
Lafayette, CA 94549
415-283-7995

Minnesota Educational
Computing Corp.
3490 Lexington Avenue North
St. Paul, MN 55126-8097
800-685-6322

National Geographic Society
Educational Services
Washington, DC 20036
800-368-2728

Optical Data Corporation
30 Technology Drive
Warren, NJ 07059
800-524-2481

Society for Visual Education Inc.
Department BM
1345 Diversey Parkway
Chicago, IL 60614-1299
800-829-1900

Stewart Publishing, Inc.
6471 Merritt Court
Alexandria, VA 22312
703-354-8155

Synergistic Educ. Tech. Systems
15717 Crabbs Branch Way
Rockville, MD 20855
800-422-SETS

Teaching Technologies
P.O. Box 3808
San Luis Obispo, CA 93403-3808
805-541-3100

Videodiscovery
1700 West Lake Avenue, North,
Suite 600
Seattle, WA 98109-3012
800-54V-DISC

Voyager Company
1351 Pacific Coast Highway
Santa Monica, CA 90401
800-446-2001

Ztek Company
P.O. Box 1055
Louisville, KY 40201
800-247-1603

☞ PROMISING VIRTUAL REALITY

As a VHO teacher, you are about to enter into a new era of curriculum design and computer technology. Virtual reality (VR) is a term that represents the cutting-edge collection of hardware and software. Your students will be able to create and enter a world of 3-D computer-generated sound and graphics that is custom fitted to their curriculum needs. Once inside, they can move about freely, interact with the environment, and physically reshape what surrounds them.

The equipment required includes EyePhones, DataGloves, a DataSuit, a Convolvotron, and Polhemus™ tracking devices. These will be described in more detail below. Your imagination sets the limits on how this new technology can be utilized in classroom and training instruction. If you can imagine any scenario, multimedia design, or learning environment, you can create and use it in a virtual world. Your students will be able to experience this and more while sitting in class or in a special computer laboratory.

Setting the Stage

You are no doubt familiar with the contribution that existing technology has made to education, medicine, engineering, and other sciences. As health care professionals, you are about to experience another remarkable advancement called VR. The potential impact it will have on the health education profession will become apparent as you read further.

Through the pioneering efforts of companies such as VPL Research, Inc., and agencies such as NASA, an integrated collection of computer software and hardware has become available that allows you to enter a simulated computer-based environment, complete with 3-D images, sound, interactivity, freedom of movement, and eventually, tactile feedback. The components are as follows. EyePhones™: This piece of hardware, developed by researchers at NASA Ames Research Center (Caruso, 1990), resembles an oversized scuba-diving mask. Mounted in front of each eye is a small liquid crystal display (LCD), much like the ones used in color Sony Watchman™ TVs. The clarity of the newest model rivals that of color TVs. If you are familiar with the concept behind 3-D pictures, you will remember that each eye sees a slightly different perspective of the same image. The physical separation of each eye's perspective allows the brain to integrate the two into a composite image with depth, or 3-D.

The Eyephones™ and similar head-mounted displays (HMDs) receive their images from a computer (or two computers) that generates the required perspectives and ports them to the correct LCD (Staff, 1989). The end result is 3-D, just like the ViewMaster™ disk slides you saw as a child. At the Human Interface Technology Laboratory at the University of Washington in Seattle, researchers are developing a display device that will directly scan 3-D images onto the retina, thus obviating the need for EyePhones™ or similar head-mounted displays (Meyer, 1991).

DataGloves™ and DataSuit™: Architects and engineers use computer-aided design (CAD) software packages to design buildings and mechanical devices. Each point in the wireframe drawing has a unique X-Y-Z coordinate. The points are connected by lines, and the result is a representation of the intended building or mechanical part. The key concept in CAD is that every object has an associated set of 3-D coordinates.

Your body also has an associated set of 3-D coordinates but happens to be outside the computer. By wearing the DataGloves™ and DataSuit™, your real-world 3-D coordinates can be determined as you move within a low-level magnetic field generated by Polhemus Isotrak hardware (Fisher, 1990).

We can represent your body in the computer display in any way you desire, as long as your simulated body movements are duplicated by your own physical movements (Kelly, 1989). Within the computer, your real-world 3-D coordinates can be integrated with the 3-D coordinates of the computer-generated CAD images.

What you see in the Eyephones™ is a perspective view as if you were inside the CAD image. When you turn your head to the side to look around, it is as if you have shifted your view to the side in the 3-D computer-generated world. You can walk around inside the building, turn, and view the scene (world) from any angle. Your physical body is still outside, but you imagine you are inside. You suspend disbelief. The potential of VR to bring you as a participant into any situation or simulation should begin to be obvious.

Convolvotron™: Because stereo audio equipment cannot duplicate real 3-D sound, you cannot tell the difference between equivalent sounds coming from directly in front or behind you. With the Convolvotron™, however, computer-enhanced sounds can be perceived from any direction (Wright, 1990). You are left with the impression of being surrounded by sounds just as you would be in the real world. All you need to wear is a set of sophisticated earphones.

Current Limitations

At present there are several major drawbacks to using this technology. For one, the costs are prohibitive for individuals, but time will eventually reduce them. Another involves the reality of the images you see in the EyePhones™ or other HMDs. It takes a considerable amount of computing power to generate images that look photographic in quality. Coupled with the need to move about inside any virtual world in real time (with no distortion or blurriness of the images due to your speed of movement), a trade-off is necessary. The less realistic the images you see, the faster the computer can generate them, and the closer you come to real-time movement. At this time, real-time movement with low resolution is preferable to slow-motion photographic imagery. What you see is not exactly what you would expect in the real world. The cartoonlike character of these worlds, however, is still quite remarkable.

Tactile Feedback

In the near future, there should be products available on the market that allow you to feel what you see inside a virtual world. When you reach out and touch an object, some kind of tactile feedback mechanism built into the DataGloves™ and DataSuit™ will respond. Eventually, you will be able to feel textures and distinguish hot from cold surfaces (Zimmerman, 1987).

The Institute for Simulation and Training's Visual Systems Lab in Orlando, Florida, under the direction of Dr. Mike Moshell, is doing basic research in all these areas with the help of students and faculty at the nearby University of Central Florida, area businesses, and the military.

Ongoing Research in Applications of VR

A considerable effort is currently under way at several research institutions and companies to apply VR to the everyday world of work and leisure. Here are a few examples that may directly affect you as a health care education professional. As you read, keep in mind the potential to integrate what is being done (or some variation) into your curriculum needs. What you eventually bring into your classroom will depend quite a bit on how far you are willing to carry your ideas. You must be able to explain and demonstrate the equipment to your students as these technologies become more widely used in the health care education system.

Once your teaching facility sees the potential that VR will have on curriculum, teaching, and training, you will probably be given the tools required to generate your own virtual worlds and directly affect the lives and careers of your students. Work is being done in the computer industry to make computers as userfriendly as possible. VR research along these lines is also progressing to the point where soon, it will also be user friendly and accessible to the average person. You will not be required to be a programmer in order to use VR in the classroom.

Current Applications of VR

At Stanford University, researchers are designing virtual cadavers. Three-dimensional images are generated by nuclear magnetic resonance imaging, computerized axial tomography, and other scanning techniques (Kelly, 1989). After assembling a complete set of body coordinates, the computer generates a 3-D cadaver with all the body parts in their proper places. Software programming will eventually allow for simulated blood flow. Further enhancements will mimic normal body chemistry functions. The ultimate use of VR will occur when doctors can perform virtual medical procedures on these 3-D images produced from the patient's own scans — before actually entering the operating room. Because cadavers are often difficult to obtain, reusable VR cadavers will revolutionize instruction of new doctors. Instructors will have available a host of teaching scenarios and capabilities inside the classroom, risk free.

Because the computer allows for changes in scale as well as perspective, one's viewpoint can become as small as possible. Through the EyePhones™, you will be able to travel through the arterial network or into any organ and see what is inside. The level of detail depends considerably on what the scanning techniques can divulge. For teaching scenarios, cellular-level detail unavailable through conventional scanning can come from independent photographic evidence gathered elsewhere. These data can be mapped into the virtual cadaver in their proper locations.

In the area of physical therapy (Ditlea, 1988), the DataSuit™ could be directly applied. Because the wearer's body coordinates are available to the computer, a physically impaired patient can proceed through full range-of-motion exercises. Knowing the extremes, the doctor can develop a rehabilitation program tailored to the individual. It is even possible for patients to see their own range of motion increasing through the EyePhones™ during exercise, with built-in audio inducements to push the patient just a little further toward reaching the incremental goals set by the doctor (Pausch, 1991).

At the University of North Carolina at Chapel Hill, researchers are developing a mechanical, force-feedback system, which allows chemists to manipulate computer-generated molecules (Pollack, 1989). By exploring the physical constraints within a molecule, scientists are able to move 3-D molecules into the cavities of other molecules. If a molecule will not fit, the force-feedback arm will prevent docking. This technology, when combined with other VR technology, will help scientists discover substrate-enzyme connections and other molecular-level interactions vital to cancer and medical research.

Sentient Systems Technology of Pittsburgh, has developed an eye-tracker, which allows one to enter information into a computer by simply focusing on a certain point on the keyboard (Tello, 1988). A natural use in the health care system involves operation of prosthetic devices and wheelchairs by patients with limited mobility. In the classroom, a teacher should be able to focus on a screen to bring any number of curricular multimedia aids or scenarios into operation in the virtual environment for use by students.

Researchers at Kurzweil Applied Intelligence in Waltham, Massachusetts, have developed a voice recognition system used by doctors and health care professionals to input standardized text by single-word voice commands (Tello, 1988). Specific numbers and data necessary to fill in the appropriate blanks are also required. Through voice recognition, the health care instructor can activate and control curriculum-based scenarios to fit any variation of instructional inquiry from the students in a timely manner.

Because VR technology can be combined with robotics, a host of applications will be available to the health care profession. The user will wear the DataGloves™, DataSuit™, and EyePhones™ to remotely control a surgical robot. In the harsh environments of radiation, deep space, combat, and toxic contamination, procedures carried out by the doctor can be mimicked by a remotely controlled robot.

Applications in Health Care Education

As indicated before, applications are limited only by the imagination of the health care professional. With proper training in the use of VR technology, you will be able to integrate this new field into your health care curriculum. Because you are a future teacher, you must be able to develop effective and efficient learning experiences. Part of that process includes designing instructional materials.

To expand on an earlier example, suppose you plan to become a teacher in corrective therapy, and the lesson you are developing involves teaching proper exercises to wheelchair patients. After the patient is fitted with the DataGloves™ and DataSuit™ (or an appropriate version), you can take him or her through a preliminary round of range-of-movement exercises. Programmed into your lesson will be the daily goals to be reached. Because proper body movements have associated limits in 3-D space, patients can be taught to use the equipment and be signaled when their movements are outside of these limits. Eventually, patients are able to monitor their own movements with little assistance. As inducements to reaching proper goals, they can be entertained with simulated trips inside virtual worlds of their choosing, be it through the rings of Saturn, through a field of grass, through the inside of an engine block, or to different vacation sites. Their progress can be tied directly to whatever incentives they desire.

As an instructor of future emergency medical technicians and paramedics, your lesson may involve the proper use of emergency vehicles during transport. A complete mock-up of the vehicle is provided in the virtual world. With the DataSuit™, DataGloves™, and EyePhones™, a simulated emergency trip to the hospital is programmed. The instructor can control the amount of traffic encountered, pedestrian congestion, unexpected hazards, and the like. The student must be able to drive the vehicle and maintain proper procedures in order to be successful. Meanwhile, inside the van, other students are performing medical procedures on virtual patients while wearing the same equipment. Using the correct medication and intervention practices, they can monitor their virtual patients enroute.

With a few innovative tools provided by VR companies, teachers of dental hygienists will also have a host of possibilities. Imagine a physical mock-up of the head and teeth that can be moved in every possible direction. The teeth can be twisted and turned to duplicate almost any possible patient. With the EyePhones™ on, plaque, gum disease, and nerve centers, can be programmed to reflect an individual patient. A simulated face, mouth, and throat would match the mock-up you are working on. If you clean the teeth properly, the plaque will disappear. If you hit the wrong nerve endings, the patient may scream or bite, all in a risk-free simulation. With real dental hygiene equipment equipped with the Polhemus™ devices, your real movements will be duplicated precisely at the correct location.

As an instructor of future LPNs or RNs, your lesson may involve examining a virtual patient for signs of illness or disease progression. The lesson may involve specifics or combinations of problems the student is required to distinguish. Virtual medications can be administered to the patient, and virtual monitoring equipment can be used. The range of possibilities is endless and can be determined in part by the kind of patient the student will likely encounter. Scenarios can also be programmed to simulate emergency situations.

If you are a teacher of animal medicine technicians, your students will likely perform a variety of laboratory chemical tests on specimens. Inside the virtual lesson, they can handle chemicals, formulate proper mixes, and apply the proper wet tests. If they make mistakes in mixing or measuring, warning lights can be triggered. If they use improper sanitation procedures, other warnings can appear when appropriate. There is less risk to the student in such situations, and a host of possible scenarios is available. Technicians in the virtual world will have a lab manual to follow until they are competent enough to perform the procedures unaided. An added variety and extension to the lesson may involve seeing a host of rare animals that require specialized lab tests. If microscopes are necessary, simulated slides can show up through the virtual eyepieces for examination. Real slides can be electronically scanned and included for realism. If the student performs the tests properly, a succession of expected slides will follow indicating good technique.

The radiologic personnel instructor can develop lessons for students as well. In a full virtual mock-up of the medical facilities, your future radiology, X-ray, dosimetry, and sonography technicians can perform their procedures on the virtual patients. Any chemical processing of the images can be completed afterward. With a virtual patient to work with, improper focusing or location of equipment can result in poor quality images. Techniques can improve with little cost and effort. The student can take one image after another until the procedure is correct. In the more advanced lessons, students will have to pay attention to the amount of radiation used and the dangers it presents to patients and themselves.

A Call to Action

As you can see, the list of possibilities could go on forever. As teachers of future health care professionals, your area of interest dictates what can be incorporated into your curriculum. Because the technology described above will no doubt affect you after you have taken up your position as a teachers, you need to be aware of what lies ahead. The above descriptions are the procedures possible at this moment, and is some planning and front-end thinking on your part are needed to incorporate them into your curricular needs.

VR in the schools will become more widespread as people like you dream up scenarios and describe in detail exactly what your needs are to implement them. Popular demand will spur further development, but popular demand will be stifled unless you act. It is a curious situation in that you must both demand it and be involved in the development of it at the same time. The hardware and software are available, but industry needs your focus and input to apply them to specific situations.

Pick up a textbook or any other appropriate curriculum aid you are using. Think about the existing technology. It is really as simple as this: If you see it done or know it can be done in real life, it can be built into a virtual world. You simply need to think about the learning situation for your students, how the lack of educational funding affects their training, and all the possibilities that could be realized if students had the time to be trained on any available equipment or under any situation. That is where the impetus to creating virtual worlds originates.

You now have a better understanding of how these remarkable advancements in technology and computers will aid you in your lesson designs. When you use EyePhonesä, DataGlovesä, DataSuitä, Convolvotronä, Polhemusä tracking devices, and other specialized hardware and software, your students will be able to enter a computer-generated world. They will be surrounded by 3-D sound and graphics. They will be free to move about inside the virtual world, see any perspective, move any object, and interact with other users as they would in the real world. In the comfort of the classroom or laboratory, they can experience the latest training and use the most expensive equipment available in their fields.

Training can occur at any simulated location and under most conditions. The major considerations to remember when incorporating this technology into your curriculum are the flexibility it gives you as an instructor and the vast possibilities it creates for your students. There is every reason to expect mobile versions of virtual environments that can be moved from location to location. Education will be able to go to students in isolation.

In order for VR in education to become widespread in use, you as thinkers and innovators must design virtual scenarios, discuss them with colleagues, and gather support. It is a curious situation in that you must design the worlds and promote the technology simultaneously. Only when the word has spread about the seemingly limitless possibilities VR has to offer education, will more people devote the time necessary to make it happen and become a reality.

References

Battiloro, J. and R. Bowe (Spring 1991). "Digital: The Future of Technology Today." *Video Times*, 61–64.

Beam, G., and P. Wright (1988). "Interactive Laser Video Disc. Health Occupations Education." ERIC Document ED297164.

Bolwell, D. (1990). *Nursing Education: A Promising Market for Interactive Video*. Alexandria, VA: Stewart Publishing.

Caruso, D. (August 1990). "Virtual Reality, Get Real." *Media Letter, 1*(3), 1–2.

Chaffin, E. (1989). "How to Say No: Substance Abuse Education." Electronic Learning, 8(4), 20.

Christie, K. (April 1989). "Interactive Media Primer." *Audio Visual Communications*, 23(4), 28–31.

Christie, K. (May 1989). "Media Primer: Part Two. *Audio Visual Communications*, 23(5), 21–35.

Ditlea, S. (September 1988). "Artificial Intelligence: DataSuit." *Omni*, p. 22.

Fisher, S. S. (1990). "Virtual Interface Environments." In B. Laurel (ed.), *The Art of Human-Computer Interface Design* (pp. 423–38). New York: Addison-Wesley

Helsel, S. (1990). Interactive Optical Technologies in Education and Training Markets. Presented at the Society for Applied Learning Technology, Orlando, Florida, February 1990.

Hertzberg, L. (1991). "Teaching About AIDS: Two Videodiscs to Help Teach a Difficult Subject." *Electronic Learning*, 10, 38.

Kelly, K. (Fall 1989). "Virtual Reality: An Interview with Jaron Lanier." *Whole Earth Review*, pp. 108–19.

Mageau, T. (1990). "Software's New Frontier: Laser-Disc Technology." *Electronic Learning*, 9 (6), 22–28.

Meyer, K. (May 1991). "The First Industry Symposium from the Perspective of a Small Company." *Virtual Reality Report*, 1(4), pp. 3–4.

O'Neill, P. N. (1990). "Developing Videodisc Instructions for Health Sciences: A Consortium Approach." *Academic Medicine*, 65(10), 624–27.

Pausch, R. (March 1991). "Virtual Reality on Five Dollars a Day." *ACM*, pp. 265–70.

Piemme, T. (1988). "Computer-Assisted Learning and Evaluation in Medicine." *Journal of the American Medical Association*, 260(3), 367(6).

Pollack, A. (April 10 1989). "What Is Artificial Reality? Wear a Computer and See." *New York Times*, pp. C1, C7.

Ross, R. (1988). "Technology Tackles the Training Dilemma." *High Technology Business*, September, 1988.

Rubeck, R. F. (1990). "The Interactive Videodisc in Health Care." *Academic Medicine*, 65(10), 624.

Salpeter, J. (February 1991). "Beyond Videodiscs: CompactDiscs in the Multimedia Classroom." *Technology and Learning*, 11(5), 32–40, 66–67.

Staff. (June 27 1989). "Appendix B: Specifying Stereo Views." *EyePhone Operation Manual: VPL Research, Inc.*, pp. B1–B8.

Stewart, S. A. (1990). *Interactive Video Primer: Medical Education*. Alexandria, VA: Stewart Publishing.

Stewart, S. A. (1990). *Videodiscs in Healthcare: A Guide to the Industry*. Alexandria VA: Stewart Publishing.

Tello, E. R. (September 1988). "Between Man and Machine: New Advances in User-Interface Technology Could Change the Way We Interact with Our Computers." *BYTE*, pp. 288–292.

Ullmer, E. J. (1990). "Videodisc Technology." ERIC Document ED311887.

Van Horn, R. (1991). *Advanced Technology in Education*. Pacific Grove, NY: Brooks/Cole Publishing.

Videodisc Compendium (1990). St. Paul, MN: Emerging Technology Consultants.

Videodisc Directory (1991). Alexandria, VA: Stewart Publishing.

Weaver, D. (1989). "Software for Teaching About AIDS and Sex: A Critical Review of Products." ERIC Document ED305524.

Wiist, W. H. (1988). "Update on Computer-Assisted Video Instruction in the Health Sciences." Health Education, 18(6), 8–12.

Wright, K. (December 1990). "An Earful of 3-D Music." *Discover*, pp. 34–35.

Zimmerman, T. G., J. Lanier, C. Blanchard, et al. (June 1987). "A Hand Gesture Interface Device." *CHI + GI*, pp. 189–92.

19

Making a Difference as a VHO Teacher: What It's All About

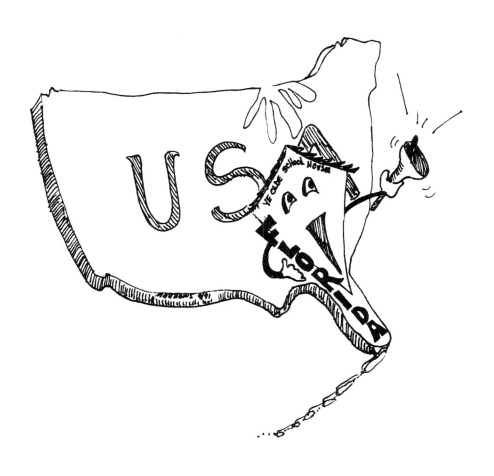

☞ WELCOME TO A NEW BEGINNING

A beginning that has no end, really. For, as Henry Brooks Adams, a Boston educator in the 1600s, said, "Teachers affect eternity; you never know where their influence leaves off." People in need of health care will feel your influence somewhere, sometime, forever.

Teachers in every discipline have been an inspiration to all of us, including those of us who have become teachers. I think of Dr. Burke at Suncoast High School in Florida. Son of a migrant sugarcane worker, he attended a one-room schoolhouse overseen by one teacher, Mr. King. Mr. King drilled into those migrant children: "Get an education. Get an education." Over and over again he told them. He told them the heights to be achieved through education, through persistence, through courage. Dr. Burke earned a doctorate and now teaches high school mathematics. His eyes well up when he mentions Mr. King. Mr. King made a profound difference in his life.

When I taught TV production in Miami's vocational education system, I had an especially wonderful, enthusiastic student named Cynthia Morgan. Twenty-three years later, I saw a newspaper article with her name in it. She had become an assistant principal at Morgan Vocational School in South Miami. I called to congratulate her. She replied, "I owe it all to you." I asked how that could be, and she answered, "Because you told me I could do anything, and I believed you." Just one of those spontaneous moments in which words were spoken, honest words, words that made a difference in her life.

A couple of years ago, when I was making a presentation at the annual American Vocational Association Health Occupations Education group meeting, I asked for volunteers to tell me about their master teacher, the one who most influenced their life. A teacher from Tampa offered the story of how she became a health care practitioner. She had told her father she was leaving Alabama to go to nursing school. Her father thought that was "low rent." She left with her father's words ringing in her ears: "If you don't make it, don't come back." She told us all how terribly shy she was at that time. She was afraid to speak out in class. The teacher noticed, cared, and counseled her. Her master teacher involved her in clubs and associations in which, in time, she would have to open up. The teacher told her how vital confidence in communication is for a nurse. "If that teacher hadn't taken me aside and helped me, I hate to think where I'd be today. She made a big difference in my life."

One of the greatest psychologists of our time, Abraham Maslow, whose influence has been felt in business, psychology, counseling, and health care, was inspired by teachers. Listen to his own words as quoted by Hoffman (1988): "My investigations on self-actualization were not planned to be research and did not start out as research but as the effort of a young intellectual to try to understand two of his teachers whom he loved, adored, and admired, and who were very, very wonderful people. I could not be content simply to adore, but sought to understand why these two people were so different from the run-of-the-mill people in the world." Millions and millions of people are leading a more fulfilled life because of Maslow's studies. He, as a teacher, has made a difference in so many of us. And all because of . . . two teachers.

The book you are holding in your hands was written because people cared. These respected educator contributors are dedicated to helping you make the transition from clinician to teacher comfortably and are unquestionably people of sincere commitment to the service they have been called to. It is on the record. They have all made a difference in the field of VHO education.

Our country is crying out for teachers who care, who care to make a difference. Our nation is going through a time of great uncertainty. The pessimists see us as all washed up. But for the of optimists, this is a decade of great awakening! With your leadership—teachership—you can awaken a sense of urgent dedication in every student you touch. And whereas some will be consumed in seeking plaudits and headlines for themselves, remember that it is people like you who will carry on the everyday miracle of making a difference in the life of people you touch—by your knowledge, by your experience, by your caring. Please, don't waver.

We need your strength, your courage.

We need you to . . . make a difference!

Reference

Hoffman, E. (1988). *The Right to Be Human.* Los Angeles, CA: Jeremy P. Tarcher, p. 50.

APPENDIX A
Recommended References

American Vocational Association (1990). *The AVA Guide to the Carl D. Perkins Vocational and Applied Technology Education Act of 1990*. Virginia: American Vocational Association.

Annas, G. J., L. H. Glantz, and B. F. Katz (1981). *The Rights of Doctors, Nurses, and Allied Health Professionals*. New York: Avon Books.

Barlow, M. L., and L. A. Burkett (1988). *The Legacy of M. D. Mobley and Vocational Education*. Virginia: The American Vocational Association.

Bass, M. R. (1983). *Fifty Hints for Teachers of Vocational Subjects*. Chicago: American Technical Society.

Bjorkquist, D. C. (1982). *Supervision in Vocational Education: Management of Human Resources*. Boston: Allyn and Bacon.

Bott, P. A. (1987). *Teaching Your Occupation to Others*. New York: National Publishers.

Brawer, M. P., and W. D. Hunter (1983). *Developing Vocational Education Programs from V-TECS Catalogs*. Florida: Department of State.

Carpenito, L. J., and T. A. Duespohl (1985). *A Guide for Effective Clinical Instruction* (2nd ed.). Maryland: Aspen Systems Corporation.

Center for Instructional Development and Services (1988). *Microcomputer Programs for Health Occupations Education: A Bibliography*. Florida: Florida Department of Education.

Christian, N. K. (1982). *Education in the 80s: Vocational Education*. Washington: National Education Association.

Clinical Instruction (module series) (1988). Macomb, IL: Western Illinois University, p. 800.

Copa, G. H., and J. Moss Jr. (1983). *Planning and Vocational Education*. New York: McGraw-Hill.

Cross, A. A. (1980). *Vocational Instruction*. Virginia: American Vocational Association.

Dare B. F., and E. J. Wolfe (1966). *You and Your Occupation*. Chicago: Educational Opportunities Project.

Directory of Health Occupations Education Programs in Florida Public Schools (1991). Tallahassee, FL: Florida Department of Education.

Ducanis, A. J., and A. K. Golin (1979). *The Interdisciplinary Health Care Team*. Maryland: Aspen Systems Corporation.

Evans, R. N., and E. L. Herr (1978). *Foundations of Vocational Education* (2nd ed.). Columbus: Charles E. Merrill.

Finch, C. R., and J. R. Crunkilton (1984). *Curriculum Development in Vocational and Technical Education: Planning, Content, and Implementation* (2nd ed.). Boston: Allyn and Bacon.

Flexner, A. (1910). *The Flexner Report on Medical Education in the United States and Canada.* Washington: Carnegie Foundation for the Advancement of Teaching.

Ford, C. W. (1978). *Clinical Education for the Allied Health Professions.* St. Louis: Mosby.

Ford, C. W., and M. Morgan (1976). *Teaching in the Health Professions.* St. Louis: Mosby.

Fryklund, V. C. (1942). *Occupational Analysis.* New York: Bruce Publishing.

Goetsch, D. (1983). *Learning How to Teach.* Virginia: American Vocational Association.

Goetsch, D. (1982). *The Vocational Instructor's Survival Guide.* Florida: Florida Department of Education.

Goetsch, D., and P. Szuch (1985). *The Vocational Administrator's Survival Guide.* Virginia: American Vocational Association.

Hall, C. W. (1973). *Black Vocational Technical and Industrial Arts Education: Development and History.* Chicago: American Technical Society.

Hamburg, J. (1974, 1976, 1979, 1981, and 1985). *Review of Allied Health Education: 1–5.* Kentucky: University Press of Kentucky.

Henderson, J. T. (1970). *Program Planning with Surveys in Occupational Education.* Washington: American Association of Junior Colleges.

HOSA People Development Video Services (1990). *Helping Members Become the Best They Can Be!* Texas: Health Occupations Students of America.

Hudson, L. R. (1986). *HOSA: A Handbook for School Leaders.* University of Central Florida.

Journal of Vocational Education Research. American Vocational Education Research Association.

Law, G. F. (1971). *Contemporary Concepts in Vocational Education.* Washington: American Vocational Association.

Miller, M. D. (1985). *Principles and a Philosophy for Vocational Education.* Ohio: National Center for Research in Vocational Education.

Moore, B. A. *Health Occuations Teacher Education: Model Curriculum.* Louisiana: Louisiana State University.

Morgan, M. K., and D. M. Irby (1978). *Evaluating Clinical Competence in the Health Professions.* St. Louis: Mosby.

Myers, G. E. (1941). *Principles and Techniques of Vocational Guidance.* New York: McGraw-Hill.

National Center on Education and the Economy (1990). *America's Choice: High Skills or Low Wages!* Rochester, NY.

National Center for Research in Vocational Education (Winter 1984–Spring 1986). Facts and Findings. Ohio: Ohio State University.

National Center for Research in Vocational Education (1988). *On Becoming a Teacher: Vocational Education and the Induction Process.* California: University of California, Berkeley.

National Center for Research in Vocational Education (1991). *Products Catalog.* California: University of California, Berkeley.

National Center for Research in Vocational Education (1991). *Subject Matter of Vocational Education: In Pursuit of Foundations.* California: University of California, Berkeley.

National Center for Research in Vocational Education (1991). *Vocational Preparation and General Education.* California: University of California, Berkeley.

National Commission on Allied Health Education (1980). *The Future of Allied Health Education.* San Francisco: Jossey-Bass.

1980 Yearbook of the American Vocational Association (1979). *Vocational Instruction.* Virginia: American Vocational Association.

1983 Yearbook of the American Vocational Association (1982). *The Politics of Vocational Education.* Virginia: American Vocational Association.

1984 Yearbook of the American Vocational Association (1983). *Collaboration: Vocational Education and the Private Sector.* Virginia: American Vocational Association.

1985 Yearbook of the American Vocational Association (1984). *Adults and the Changing Workplace.* Virginia: American Vocational Association.

Newcomb, L. H. (1977). *The Heart of Instruction Series.* Ohio: Ohio Department of Education.

Nystrom, D. C., G. K. Bayne, and L. D. McClellan (1977). *Instructional Methods in Occupational Education.* Indianapolis: Bobbs-Merrill.

Pautler, A. J. (1971). *Teaching Shop and Laboratory Subjects.* Ohio: Charles E. Merrill.

Rose, H. C. (1961). *The Instructor and His Job.* Chicago: American Technical Society.

Shea, M. L. (1985). *Health Occupations Clinical Teacher Education Series for Secondary and Secondary Educators.* Illinois: Department of Vocational and Technical Education.

Sievers, R. A. (1982). *The Politics of Vocational Education.* Virginia: American Vocational Association.

Snell, M. (1991). *Bioethical Dilemmas in Health Occupations.* Illinois: Macmillan/McGraw-Hill.

Snyder, H. M. (1982). *Kentucky Allied Health Project Final Report.* Kentucky: Commonwealth of Kentucky.

Stadt, R. W., and B. G. Gooch (1977). *Cooperative Education: Vocational, Occupational, Career.* Indianapolis: Bobbs-Merrill.

Stakenas, R. G., D. B. Mock, and K. M. Eaddy (1985). *Educating Hand and Mind: A History of Vocational Education in Florida.* Maryland: University Press of America.

Stanfield, P. S. (1990). *Introduction to the Health Professions.* Boston: Jones and Bartlett.

State of Florida Department of Education (1984). *Summaries of Florida Research in Vocational Education.* Florida: Department of State.

Swanson, G. I. (1981). *The Future of Vocational Education.* Virginia: American Vocational Association.

Third Biennial National Health Occupations Education Curriculum Conference (1990). *Theme: Health Occupations Education—1990 to 2000 and Beyond.* Sacramento.

Third National Research Conference (1989). *The Need for Research in Education of Human Service Workers.* Washington: U. S. Department of Education.

Twining, J., S. Nisbet, and J. Megarry (1987). *Vocational Education.* New York: Kogan Page.

Vocational Instructional Services (1977). *Handbook for Vocational Industrial Education Shop Teachers.* Texas: author.

Vocational-Technical Education Act of 1983 (1984). Washington: U.S. Government Printing Office.

Walter, N. (ed.). *Journal of Health Occupations Education* (1986–present). Pennsylvania State University.

Walters, R. G. (1939). *Methods of Teaching Commercial Subjects.* Cincinnati: South-Western Publishing.

Wentling, T. L., and T. E. Lawson (1975). *Evaluating Occupational Education and Training Programs.* Boston: Allyn and Bacon.

Wolansky, W. D. (1985). *Evaluating Student Performance in Vocational Education.* Iowa: Iowa State University Press.

APPENDIX B
LIST OF FINAL AUTHORS

(w=work phone; h=home phone)

Karen G. Allen, M.Ed., CDA
Co-chairperson
Dental Science Department
Indian River Community College
3209 Virginia Avenue
Ft. Pierce, FL 34981
    407-468-4726 (w)
    407-337-3406 (h)

Shirley Baker-Loges, PH.D.
1711 Avenue J
Nederland, TX 77627
    409-727-0853 (h)

Chandra Bandhu
Manager
Employment and Staff Development
Davis Medical Center
University of California — Davis
Medical Center
Sacramento, CA 95817
    916-734-5000 (w)

Anne Barron, Ed.D.
Assistant Professor
Instructional Computing
College of Education
University of South Florida
Tampa, FL 33620-5650
    813-974-3470 (w)
    407-352-0309 (h)

Brenda Benda, RN, B.S.N., MEd
Instructor
Francis Tuttle Vocational
Technical Center
12777 North Rockwell
Oklahoma City, OK 73142-2710
    405-722-7799 ext 200 (w)
    405-720-3790 (fax)
    405-263-4587 (h)

Holly L. Bennett, B.H.A., RN
Nursing/Medical Education
Department Chair
Mt. Diablo Adult Education Center
1266 San Carlos Avenue
Concord, CA 94518
    510-685-7340 (w)
    510-687-8217 (fax)
    510-672-8179 (h)

Beverly Campbell
Program Manager
Health Careers Education
California Department of Education
721 Capital Mall, 9th Floor
Sacramento, CA 95814-4785
    916-657-2541 (w)
    916-677-1700 (h)

Carol Darling, Ph.D.
Co-director
Sex Equity Project
Vocational Education
College of Education
University of Central Florida
Orlando, FL 32816
    407-823-5060 (w)
    813-355-9613 (h)

Richard Cornell
Associate Professor
Department of Educational Services
College of Education
University of Central Florida
Orlando, FL 32816

Richard A. Dietzel, M.A.
Curriculum and Instruction
Educational Foundations
Department
College of Education
University of Central Florida
Olando, FL 32816
    407-823-2057 (w)
    407-330-3740 (h)

Roberta Driscol, Ed.D., MFT
Associate Professor
Counselor Education
University of Central Florida,
1200 Volusia Avenue Box 2811
Daytona Beach, FL 32115-2811
    904-823-2013 (w)
    904-696-4073 (h)

O.J. Drumheller, M.S., RRT
Cardiopulmonary Sciences
Program Director
College of Health and Public Service
University of Central Florida
Orlando, FL 32816
    407-823-2214 (w)
    407-823-5821 (fax)
    407-327-2249 (h)

Lois Drumheller, RRT
    407-327-2249 (h)

Lou Ebrite, Ph.D., RN
Department Chair
Administration, Vocational, Adult
and Higher Education Department
College of Education
University of Central Oklahoma
100 North University Drive
Edmond, OK 73034-0120
    405-341-2980 ext 5801 (w)
    405-341-4964 (fax)
    405-478-7826 (h)

Tom Edwards, Ed.D., Rt (R)
Associate Professor and Director
Radiological Sciences Program
College of Health and Public
Service University of Central
Florida
Orlando, FL 32816
    407-823-2747 (w)
    407-823-5821 (fax)
    407-699-8010 (h)

John T. Gentry, CDT
Instructor, Dental Lab
Moore-Norman Area Vo-Tech Center
4701 12th Avenue, NW
Norman, OK 73069
    405-364-5763 (w)
    405-222-2292 (h)

Judi Hansen
Regional Recruitment Director
Kaiser Permanente Medical Care
Program
393 Walnut Center, 6th Floor
Pasadena, CA 91188
    800-331-3976 (w)
    818-405-2611 (h)

Larry Holt, Ed.D.
Assistant Professor
Department of Educational
Foundations
College of Education
University of Central Florida
Orlando, FL 32816
    407-823-2004 (w)
    407-823-5990-X 32004# (VM)
    407-823-5135 (fax)
    407-365-7607 (h)

Larry R. Hudson, Ph.D., RRT
Associate Professor
Health Occupations/Vocational
Education, Instructional Programs
Department
College of Education

University of Central Florida
Orlando, FL 32816
    407-823-2007 (w)
    407-823-5135 (fax)
    407-678-0807 (h)

Maxine Hudson, B.S., RN, CIC
Quality Assessment Director
Winter Park Memorial Hospital
200 North Lakemont Avenue
Winter Park, FL 32792
    407-646-7003 (w)
    407-678-0807 (h)

Elizabeth Kerr (deceased)
Former Director
Programs in Health Occupations Education
University of Iowa
Iowa City, IA 52242

Jacquelyn King, Ph.D., RN
Lecturer
Vocational Education Studies
Southern Illinois University
Carbondale, IL 62901
    618-453-3321 (w)
    618-453-1646 (fax)
    618-549-5703 (h)

Lisa Long, B.L.S., CDA, RDH
Instructor
Dental Hygiene Department
Indian River Community College
3209 Virginia Avenue
Ft. Pierce, FL 34981
    407-468-4700 (w)
    407-337-3406 (h)

Judy Mabrey, RN
Inservice Coordinators
Cookeville Health Coordinator
815 Bunker Hill Road
Cookeville, TN 38501
    615-528-5516 (w)
    615-268-0625 (h)

Carla J. Maloy, B.S.N., RN
Chisolm Trail Area Vocational Center
Route 1, Box 60
Omega, OK 73764
    405-729-8324 (w)
    405-375-5291 (h)

Shannon Manuel, CMA
Instructor
Medical and Dental Assisting Programs
O. T. Autry Area Vo-Tech Center
1201 West Willow
Enid, OK 73703
    405-242-2750 (w)
    405-234-8830 (h)

Barbara Matthews, LPN, CMA
Lead Instructor
Medical Assisting Program
Winter Park Adult Vocational Center
901 Webster Avenue
Winter Park, FL 32789
    407-647-6366 (w)
    407-260-0312 (h)

Michael McCumber, M.Ed., RRT
Clinical Coordinator
Respiratory Therapy Program
Daytona Beach Community College
P.O. Box 1111
Daytona Beach, FL 32015
    904-255-8131 (w)

Richard Merriam, A.A.
Electrical Instructor
Industrial Electricity
Mid Florida Technical Institute
2900 West Oak Ridge Road
Orlando, FL 32809
    407-855-5880 (w)
    407-657-2609 (h)

Elaine L. Mohn, Ed.D., RN
Second Level Coordinator
Associate Degree Nursing Program
Chemeketa Community College
4000 Lancaster Drive
Salem, OR 97309
   503-399-5256 (w)
   503-636-1498 (h)

Joan Mucciarone, M.A., RN
Instructor
Medical Assistant Program
Atlantic County Vocational School
2000 Atlantic Avenue
Mays Landing, NJ 08330
   609-641-6562 (w)
   609-822-3645 (h)

Phyllis Olmstead, M.Ed.
Curriculum and Instruction
College of Education
University of Central Florida
620 Sherwood Oaks Circle (h)
Ocoee, FL 34761
   407-299-6159 (h)

Rebecca Osterhout, B.A., RN
Instructor
Practical Nursing Program
Withlachoochee Vocational
Technical Center
1201 West Main
Inverness, FL 32650
   904-726-2430 (w)
   904-726-4532 (h)

Ruth Ellen Ostler, Ph.D.
Retired Chief
Bureau of Health Occupations
Education
New York State Education
Department
4117 Center Pointe Drive (h)
Sarasota, FL 34233
   813-378-3371 (h)

Jacquelyn T. Page, M.Ed.
Chair
Student Services, Testing, and SAIL
Orlando Vocational Technical Center
301 West Amelia Street
Orlando, FL 32801
   407-425-2756 (X4813) (w)
   407-849-3372 (fax)
   407-423-7377 (h)

Jack A. Powers, A.A.S., RRT
Director
Respiratory Care Technical Program
Great Plains Area Vocational
Technical School
4500 West Lee Boulevard
Lawton, OK 73505
   405-355-6371 (w)
   405-357-6658 (fax)
   405-355-2523 (h)

Nancy Raynor, M.Ed., RN
Chief Consultant
Health Occupations Education
State Department of Public
Instruction
DVTES 116 West Edonton Street,
Room 558
Raleigh, NC 27603-1712
   919-733-2518 (w)
   919-733-0648 (fax)
   919-848-3295 (h)

Beverly Richards, Ph.D., RN
Associate Professor
College of Education and
Psychology
North Carolina State University
Raleigh, NC 27695-7801
   919-737-2231 (w)

Rita Richardson, RN
Instructor
Nursing Assistant Program
Indian River Adult Evening School

1426 19th Street
Vero Beach, FL 32960
   407-770-5555 (w)
   407-562-3158 (h)

Jane Rocque, B.A., CDA
Chair and Instructor
Dental Assisting Program
Gateway Technical College
3520-30th Avenue
Kenosha, WI 53144-1690
   414-656-6947 (w)
   414-656-7209 (fax)
   414-633-7085 (h)

Janice R. Sandiford, Ph.D., RN, ARNP
Associate Professor
Health Occupations/Vocational Education and Associate Dean
College of Education
Florida International University, North Miami Campus
North Miami, FL 33181
   305-940-5820 (w) 475-4179
   305-424-6919 (fax) 424-6919
   305-940-2606 (h)

Judy Sheehan, M.Ed., RN, CMA
Curriculum Resource Teacher
Winter Park Adult Vocational Center
901 Webster Avenue
Winter Park, FL 32789
   407-647-6366 (w)

Karen Shores
Coordinator
Careers Academy
Encina High School
   916-971-7570 (w)
   916-663-4449 (h)

Steven Sorg, Ph.D.
Associate Professor
Vocational Education
College of Education
University of Central Florida
Orlando, FL 32816
   407-823-5060 (w)
   407-695-2726 (h)

Sharon Thomas
Lead Health Careers Teacher
c/o San Mateo County ROP
101 Twin Delphin Drive
Redwood City, CA 94065-1064
   415-802-5409 (w)

Arnie Warren, B.A.
President
Arnie Warren Corporation
Consultant, Motivational Speaker on "Master Teachers"
7027 West Broward Blvd, Suite 272
Fort Lauderdale, FL 33317
   305-475-9895 (w)

Cynthia Woodley, Ed.D.
Research Associate
Center for Education Research and Development
College of Education
University of Central Florida
Technology Point II, Suite 210
3051 Technology Parkway
Orlando, FL 32826
   407-658-5551 (w)
   407-658-5557 (fax)
   407-644-5957 (h)

Delmar Contacts

Marion Waldman
Administrative Editor, Health Services

Lisa Santy
Delmar Electronic Publishing

Delmar Publishers Inc.
3 Columbia Circle, Box 15-015
Albany, NY 12212
   800-347-7707

INDEX

ABC News Interactive Programs, 308
Accident procedure, 121
Accreditation, 230–31, 257–58
  compliance, 123–26
Advertising, 97, 98
Affiliation agreement, 114–16
  developing, 58–61
Affirmative action/equal employment opportunities, 112
AIDS, 36–37, 172
Allied Health Fields: Problems and Opportunities, 101n.2
American Association for Vocational Instructional Materials (AAVIM), 199
  See also Health Occupations Students of America (HOSA)
American Federation of Labor (AFL), 215, 216
American Heart Association Cardiopulmonary Resuscitation Program, 308
American Industrial Arts Student Assoc. (AIASA), 206
American Medical Association
  Committee for Allied Health Education Accreditation (CAHEA), 257
  definition of accreditation, 123
American Vocational Association (AVA), 324
  the AVA-HOE division, 234–35
  choosing the appropriate organization, 232–33
  funding for programs, 237
  involvement in, 236–37
  purpose and structure of, 234–35
  specific benefits of, 235–36
  and the teacher, 232
Aspergillosis, 34
Assessment. *See* Learning assessment
Attendance and promptness, 162
Attire
  for job interviews, 63
  professional, 122
  setting guidelines for, 5
Audiovisual materials and equipment, 272–84
  advantages and disadvantages of, 282–83
  instructional systems design (ISD), 272, 273–74
  focused topic video production, 283–84
  medium as teacher, 274–75
  problems, and how to handle them, 278–82
  projected materials, mute
    filmstrips, 276
    overhead transparencies, 276–77, 280
    slides, 277, 280–81
  projected materials, with sound and motion, 277–82
  teacher as medium, 274
  unprojected material, 275–76
Audit mechanisms
  for formative evaluations of the program, 123–26
AVA-HOE Division Newsletter, 235

Barlow, M., 215
Bauer, V. Devine, 202
Behavior
  modification, 84
  professional, 122
Bennett, William J., 206
Benson, P., 66
Birchenall, Joan M., 202, 203
Board of Curators of the U. of Missouri v. Horowitz, 169
Boyer, Ernest, 206
Bureau of Adult, Vocational and Technical Education, 226

Career
  advancement
  mobility, 228, 229
  opportunities for, 228
Carl Perkins Vocational and Applied Technology Education Acts 71, 72, 219, 257
Carnegie Council, 66
Centers for Disease Control (CDC)
  "Guidelines for Isolation Precautions in Hospitals," 36
  "Recommendations for the Prevention of HIV Transmission in Health Care Settings," 36
  Study on the Efficacy of Nosocomial Infection Control, 32–33
Checklists, 39, 44, 139, 140
Civil Rights Legislation, 92–93
Clarity
  for effective teaching, 16–18
Classroom
  arrangement, for self-paced instruction, 161
  environment
    creating a safe and comfortable, 18
    for the adult student, 77
  management, 5, 161–62
  protocol, 5
  setup, 5
Clinical instruction, 52–63
  answering and handling student criticisms, 55–57, 59–60
  developing affiliation agreements, 58–61
  evaluating student performance, 55, 57–58
  faculty, recruiting and orienting, 61–63
  making clinical practice relevant, 54–55
  planning clinical experiences, 52–53
  reality vs the ideal, 56–57
  supervision of students, 53–54
Clinical rotation, 108
Clinician
  responsibilities as, 3
Commitment, to place of employment, 63–64
Committees, advisory
  use of, 99–101
Communication
  effective skills, 122
  learning the language of education, 7–11
Communication Challenges in Nursing: Establishing Rapport and Trust, 308

Community contact
  maintaining, 96–97
Competence, 63, 64
Competency-based education, 146–65
  benefits of, 162–63
  classroom management, 161–62
  converting to, from traditional program, 163
  curriculum development for, 150–54
    occupational analysis of, 150–51
    and sequence core competencies, 151
    competency-based test item bank, 152
    course sequences and outlines, 151–52
    program and course specifications, 152–53
    program/course blueprints, 153
    supplemental resources, 153–54
    units of instruction per course, 153
  curriculum maintenance, 154–55
  defined, 146
  evaluating student progress, 162
  for teachers, 227
  implementation in a VHO program, 155–59
    organization, 157–58
    planning and preparation, 156–57
    responsibility for, 150
    testing and evaluation, 160
    writing instructional materials for, 158–60
  the instructor and, 160–61
  scheduling, 162
  what it can do, 146–48
  what it cannot do, 148–49
  the Wheel, 163–65
Computer-assisted instruction mode (CAI), 286–87
Computer disks, 192
Computerized axial tomography, 315
Computers, 285–88. *See also* Virtual reality (VR)
  applications, 285–86
  integrating with the telephone, 290–97
    computer conferencing, 296–97
    educational resources, 295–96
    electronic bulletin board system (BBS), 291–94
    how to call, 292–93
    electronic mail, 290–91
    health care resources, 294–95
  recordkeeping with, 286
  software, method for reviewing, 287
  for teaching, 286–87
  test construction by, 287–88
  usefulness of, 22
Conferencing and advisement
  approaches to, 84
  determining readiness and appropriateness, 80–83
  the instructor as conferencing agent, 83–85
Confidentiality, 122
  oath of, 120
Connelly v. University of Vermont, 169
Continuing education programs, 228
Convolvotron™, 312, 314

337

Cost control, 48–49
Counseling, 84, 96, 250
Credentialing, 231
Cremin, L. A., 213, 214, 215
Curriculum
  definitions of, 128–29
  development
    accommodation and articulation, 229
    competency-based education, 150–54
  identifying, 128–34
    conduct a needs assessment, 130
    identifying create curriculum design/model, 131–33
    organize advisory committee, 130–31
  materials, bias-free, 89
  performance-based, 112
  sources for curriculum-related information, 133

DataGloves™, 312–19
DataSuits™, 312–19
Della Vos, Victor, 213, 214
Dependability, 63, 64, 82
Developmental counseling, 84
Dismissal, of students. *See* Legal issues
Dixon v. Alabama State Board of Education, 168
Drinks Too Much, 308

Educational materials, 109. *See also* Audiovisual materials and equipment; Interactive videodisc (IVD) programs
Electronic bulletin board system (BBS), 291–94
Elias, Karen, 204, 205
Ely, Don, 274
Emergency, 308
Employee recruitment, 112
Equipment and tools
  acquiring, 47–49, 109
Evaluation. *See* Learning assessment
Experience
  prior clinical, as requirement for teaching, 2
EyePhones™, 312–19

Facsimile, 289–90
Faculty
  assistant instructor, duties of, 62–63
  principal instructor, duties of, 62–63
  recruiting and orienting, 61–63
Federal laws
  addressing special needs students, 71, 72, 73
Feedback
  from students, 19–22
    criteria for useful, 21–22
    defined, 19–20
    effect of, 21
    giving and receiving, 21–22
    rating instruments for, 20
    reliability of, 20–21
  to students, 59
Feirer, J. L., 213, 214
Field trips, 88–89
Filmstrips, 192, 276
Financial appropriations, 226
Financial assistance
  for the adult student, 76
  information about, 81, 109
  for special needs students, 73
Finn, Jim, 274
Flexibility, 74
Foley catheterization, 34
Formative evaluation, 23
Froebel, 214, 216
FTE (full-time equivalent), 174

Gagne, R. M., 274
Gaspary v. Bruton, 169.
Gillespie, Wilma B., 202
Glaser, Robert, 136
Grading, methods of, 140
Graham, Lois, 204
Greenhill v. Bailey, 169
Grievance committees, 176, 179

Hatfield, Jack, 201
Head-mounted displays (HMDs), 313–19
Health Amendments Act (1956), 217, 225–26
Health care site
  policy of, 123
Health clearance, 118, 120, 121
Health Occupations Education (HOE), 224–37
  accreditation of specialized fields of study, 230–31
  as a division of AVA, 232–37
  administrative responsibility for, 230
  basic principles for, 229–30
  categories of health care workers, 225
  citizen-consumer participation in, 230
  need for health care, 224–25
  programs, 225–26
  teachers, 226–31
  USDOE-HOE program specialist, 268–69
Health Occupations Educators Association, 248
Health Occupations Students of America (HOSA), 184–94, 257
  becoming a chapter advisor, 184
  the beginning, 203–4
  competitive events, 190–91, 207–8
    list of, 208
  development of, 200–8
  establishing a chapter, 186–87
  handbook, using, 184–86
  HOSA creed, 206
  integrating HOSA into the classroom, 188–92
  local officers' perspectives, 192–93
  national HOSA
    board of directors, 206–8
    management/headquarters, 204–5
    motto/emblem/uniform policy, 205
  officers, 189–90
  organizing
    the chapter, 187–88
    the students, 187
  pre-HOSA history, 201–3
  recognition by U.S. Dept. of Education, 206
  resources, 192
  secondary school students' perspectives, 193–94
  terms of importance, 194
Hepatitis, 36, 37
Hitchens, Howard, 274
HIV disease, 36–37
Hoffman, E., 324
Holstein, Mary, 202
Homework, 5
Howser, M. A., 21
Hubbard v. John Tyler Community College, 169
Human Interface Technology Laboratory, 313
Hunkins, F. D., 213

Identification badge, 120
Incredible Human Machine, The, 306
Individualized Education Plan (IEP), 72, 75
Individuals with Disabilities Act, 71
Infection control, 32–37
  barrier precautions, 35–37
  community acquired infections, 32
  defined, 32
  and hepatitis, 36, 37
  and HIV disease, 36–37
  implications for the VHO teacher, 37
  importance of, 32–33
  nosocomial infections, 32–33
  prevention, 33, 35
  transmission of infection, 33–35
    infectious agent, 33–34
    movement of organisms, 34
    person at risk, 35
    place of entry, 34–35
    portal of exit, 34
    reservoir, 33–34
Instructional systems design (ISD), 272, 273–74
Instructors. *See also* Teachers; VHO Instructors
  clinical, use of, 53–54
Intellectual development
  of middle school students, 69
Interactive videodisc (IVD) programs, 302–11
  applications of, 306–8
  catalogs and information about, 311–12
  formats, 302–3
    features of CAV and CLV, 304
  implementation of, 308–9
  levels of, 303–6
  sample barcodes, 305
  terminology, 310
Interviews
  preparing student for, 63

James, Barbara, 204
Job opportunities
  placement, 63–64, 246
  summer/off track, 111
Job Training Partnership Act (JTPA), 72, 73
Johnson, A., 66
Joint Commission on Accreditation of Healthcare Organizations and infection control requirements, 32
Junge, Catherine, 201

Kaufman, J. J., 215
Kemp, J. E., 274

Kenora Enterprises, 204, 205
Kerr, Elizabeth E., 224
Knowledge
  for effective teaching, 16
Koeninger, Jim, 204, 205
Kurzweil Applied Intelligence, 316

Laboratory work
  assessing student performance, 39-46
  equipment and supplies
    ordering and acquiring, 46-49
    requests for, 38
  planning laboratory simulations, 37-39
  preparing students for, 30
  safety
    plan for, 38
    procedures, 30-31
Ladder and lattice concepts, 229
Language
  of education, 7-11
  stereotyping in, avoiding, 90-91
Learning
  affective, 23
  cognitive, 23
  modalities of, 4-5
  psychomotor, 23
Learning activity packets (LAPS), 73-74
Learning assessment, 22-25
  of affective learning, 23
  of cognitive learning, 23
  evaluating student performance, 55, 57-58
  performance instruments, 39-44
  of psychomotor learning, 23
  relationship between curriculum and, 22
  reliability of, 24-25
  validity of, 24
Legal issues, 168-81
  and AIDS, 172
  due process, application to VHO, 168-71
  failing an unsatisfactory student and, 173-78
    developing a plan for dismissal, 176-77
    emotional issues, 173-74
    importance of effective communication, 175-76
    process of dismissal, guidelines for, 174-75
  grievances, handling student, 178-81
  malpractice, 172
  reducing tort liability, 171-72
Legal requirements
  for health care site use, 114-21
Legionellosis, 34
Legislation, federal vocational education, 215-19
  precursor events, 215-16
  Smith-Hughes Act, 216-17
Legislation and Teachers
  civil rights and, 92-93
Lessner, M. W., 171-72
Liability coverage, 117
Lindbeck, J. R., 213, 214
Living Textbook:Life Science, 307
Loyalty
  oath of, 121
Lyons v. Salve Regina College, 169

McClure, A. F., 212, 215, 216
McEwin, K., 66, 68
McGee, Lynne, 203
Mager, R. F., 274
Majorowicz, K., 175, 180
Malpractice, 172
Management Action Plan (MAP), 235
Manpower Development Training Act (1962), 218
Marketing the program, 98-99
Mars, Jerry, 274
Maslow, Abraham, 324-25
Mentors, 109-10
Mitstifer, D. I., 140, 143
Mobile units (rotating occupational labs), 110
Morill Land-Grant Act, 215

National Association of Health Occupations Teachers (NAHOT), 10, 11, 235
National Association of Manufacturers (NAM), 215, 216
National Association of State Administrators of Health Occupations Educators (NASAHOE), 10
National Defense Education Act (1958), 217
National Society for the Promotion of Industrial Education (NSPIE), 215
Navera, James L., 201
Networking, 110, 112
Niedringhaus, L., 169
Nosocomial infections, 32-33
Nuclear magnetic resonance imaging, 315

O'Driscoll, D. L., 169
Office of Adult and Vocational Education, 266-68
Omnibus AIDS Act, 37
Organization
  for effective teaching, 16
Organizations, professional, 10. *See also* names of individual organizations
Ornstein, A. C., 213
Ostler, Ruth-Ellen, 204

Packets
  student informational, 6-7
Parental consent forms, 117, 118
Partnerships, with the healthcare industry, 101-23
  describing the partnership proposal, 113-14
  establishing, 103-8
    form advisory committee, 106, 108
    forum to discuss training needs, 104, 106
    identify local education agencies, 103
    identify local health care sites, 103-4
    obtain initial site contact, 104, 105
    provide ongoing information, 106, 108
    survey identified partners, 104, 106, 107
  identifying resources and services
    offered by education partners, 111-13
    offered by healthcare partners, 108-11
  legal requirements, for healthcare site use, 114-21
  recommended membership, 102
Pell Grant Program, 81
Performance instruments, 39-41, 39-46
  checklists, 39
    performance, 40
    product, 44
  rating scales
    performance, 41-44
    product, 45
  rules for developing, 45-46
Performance objectives, 136-44
  condition, 137
  criteria, 138
  performance, 137
  samples of, 138
  testing
    achievement, 140, 142
    checklists, 139, 140
    criterion-referenced measurement, 136-37, 143-44
    methods of grading, 140
    norm-referenced, 142-43
    simulation/work sample, 138, 139
    types of, 138-44
Personality
  for effective teaching, 18-19
  as your best asset, 60
Pestalozzi, Johann H., 213, 214, 216
Petersen, Dale J., 201
Physical development, of middle school students, 66-67
Piaget, J., 69, 242
Polhemus™ tracking devices, 312, 313, 318, 319
"Position Paper on Student Organizations in the Field of Health Occupations Education," 202
Powers, Helen K., 201
Powers, Jack A., 26
Practical nurse training, 226
Professional image, 122-23
Professionalism, 236
Prosser, Charles A., 216
Publicity, 110
Public relations, 112
Pulliam, J. D., 212
Punctuality, 5

Qualities, of health care workers, 63, 64

Radiation monitoring, 121
Randall, Mary, 204
Rating scales, 41-45, 140, 141, 142
Recruiting students, 96-97, 110
Rehabilitation Act of 1974, 71
Reliability, 63, 64
Relicensure, 228
Respect
  earning the students', 70-71
Responsibilities
  as a clinician, 3
  of the health care professional, 82
  as teacher, 3-4
Robotics
  and VR technology, 316
Runkle, John D., 214

Safety
  plan for, 38
  procedures, 30–31
Schaefer, C. J., 215
Science of Education and Psychology of the Child, The, 69
Scope of practice, rules and regulations
  understanding, 118
Security clearance, 120
Self-discipline, 64
Self-evaluation, 16
Semmelweis, Ignaz, 35
Sentient Systems Technology, 316
Sex-role stereotypes, 89–91
Shareware programs, 293–94
Site tours, 109
Slice of Life, The, 307
Smith, Ken & Nora, 204
Smith-Hughes Act, 216–17
Social development
  of middle school students, 67–69
Speakers, 110–11
Special needs students, 71–75
  categories of handicapping conditions, 71
  curriculum adjustments for, 73–74
  federal laws addressing, 71, 72, 73
  post/secondary adult programs for, 73
  secondary programs for, 72
  teaching techniques for, 74
Spink, L. M., 168
Stereotyping
  in language usage, 90–91
Stoddard, Joan B., 201
Strahan, D., 66, 67, 68, 69
Students. *See also* Special needs students; Work force: nontraditional students
  adult, 75–77
    classroom environment for, 77
    differences, 75
    responsibilities of, 76–77
  feedback from, 19–22
  high school, 69–71
  middle school, 66–69
  procedure demonstrations by, 30
  participation, setting standards for, 5
  recruitment of, 96–97, 110
  as volunteers, 112–13, 113
Summative evaluation, 23
Supplies
  acquiring, 109
  ordering, 46–47
Swartout, Sherm, 274
Symanski, M. E., 173, 174
Systems operator (SYSOP), 293

Teachers. *See also* VHO instructors
  and clinical supervision of students, 53–54
  as medium, 274
  medium as, 274, 274–75
  professional support for, 111
  responsibilities as, 3–4
  as role model, 6
  transition from clinician to, 2–4
  as volunteers, 113
Teaching. *See also* Clinical instruction
  characteristics of effective, 20
  classroom
    management, 5
    protocol, 5
    setup, 5
  defining the role of, 4–6
  first day, preparing for, 6–7
  lesson plans, 5
  MICRO TEACH exercise, 17–18
  modalities of learning, 4–5
  motivating students, 14–15
  setting standards for, 5–6
  special needs students, 74
  techniques
    selecting, 16–19
    for special needs students, 74
Teamwork, 7
Teleconferencing
  audio, 288–89
  facsimile, 289–90
  freeze-frame video, 290
Telephone
  integrating with computers, 290–97
  teleconferencing, 288–89
Television
  use of, in VHO education, 297
Tests and testing, 5
  achievement, 140, 142
  construction of, 25–26
    by computers, 287–88
  criterion-referenced measurement, 136–37, 143–44
  methods of grading, 140
  norm-referenced, 142–43
  rating scales, 140, 141, 142
Therapeutic Communication, 307
Thomason, J., 66, 68
Training
  no-cost or low-cost, 112
  plans, 117, 119
  sites, 111
Two-plus-two programs, 227
Tyler, R. W., 123–24

Understanding Ourselves, 307
U. S. Dept. of Education (USDOE)
  Office of Adult and Vocational Education, 266–68
  personnel, 265–69
  USDOE-HOE program specialist, 268–69

VanHoose, J., 66, 67, 68, 69
Vaughn, Paul R., C. Rosco, and D. Lanette, 199
Video camera
  using, for self-evaluation, 16
Video resources, for HOSA, 192
Virtual reality (VR), 312–19
  applications of, 315–16
  in health care education, 317–18
  research in, 315
  limitations of, 314
  introduction to components, 312–3
  tactile feedback, 314–15
Vocational education, history of, 212–14
  apprenticeship, 212
  in colonial America, 212–13
  early American, 213–14
Vocational Education Act of 1963, 218, 226
Vocational Education Journal, 235
Vocational Health Occupations (VHO) Instructors
  at adult vocational center, 245–47
  in community colleges
    counseling, 250
    providing handbooks, 249–50
    responsibilities toward students, 249
    serving on committees, 250
  curriculum
    guides, sources for, 256
    revision, 256
  department chairpersons, roles of, 251–53
  in the high school, 243–44
  in community colleges, 247–51
    budget preparation, 248
  influence of, making a difference, 324–25
  in the middle school, 240–43
    exploratory programs, 242
    orientation program, 241
    orientation resources, 242–43
  pay scales for, 2
  requirements for, 2
  school district supervisor, 253–59
    consultant
      background and preparation, 254
      duties and responsibilities, 255–57
      course offerings, 258
      evaluation of textbooks, 257
      interpretation of state standards, 258–59
      professional improvement, 258
      program review, audit and accreditation preparation, 257–58
  state department personnel, 259–64
    expectations, 261
    HOE program administrator, 261–62
    resolving teacher problems, 263–64
    mission, purpose, structure, 260–61
  teacher certification, 255
  teacher educator, 264–65
  U. S. Dept. of Education (USDOE) personnel, 265–69
Vocational Student Organizations (VSOs)
  advisor's creed, 199
  general understanding of, 198–200
  those recognized by U.S. Dept. of Education, 198
Vocational-technical education, 226–27
Volumetric Devices, 306–7
Volunteer/community service, 111

Watson, Linda, 203
Wedberg, Des, 274
Wheel, The, 163–65, 243
Williams, D., 66
Williams, Robin, 14, 15
Woodward, Calvin, 214
Word processors
  usefulness of, 22
Worker's Compensation Authority
  sample letter, 117
Work force
  adapting to the changing, 85–93
  nontraditional students
    classroom instruction for, 88–91
    clinical instruction for, 91
    recruitment of, 86–87
    retaining, 87–88
Workforce 2000 Committee
  Competing in a Seller's Market, 101n.1
  reports of the, 85–86
Wotruba, T R., 20
Wright, P. L., 20
Written assignments, 5

Zimmerman, T. G., 314